AF672615

Health Informatics

This series is directed to healthcare professionals leading the transformation of healthcare by using information and knowledge. For over 20 years, Health Informatics has offered a broad range of titles: some address specific professions such as nursing, medicine, and health administration; others cover special areas of practice such as trauma and radiology; still other books in the series focus on interdisciplinary issues, such as the computer based patient record, electronic health records, and networked healthcare systems. Editors and authors, eminent experts in their fields, offer their accounts of innovations in health informatics. Increasingly, these accounts go beyond hardware and software to address the role of information in influencing the transformation of healthcare delivery systems around the world. The series also increasingly focuses on the users of the information and systems: the organizational, behavioral, and societal changes that accompany the diffusion of information technology in health services environments.

Developments in healthcare delivery are constant; in recent years, bioinformatics has emerged as a new field in health informatics to support emerging and ongoing developments in molecular biology. At the same time, further evolution of the field of health informatics is reflected in the introduction of concepts at the macro or health systems delivery level with major national initiatives related to electronic health records (EHR), data standards, and public health informatics.

These changes will continue to shape health services in the twenty-first century. By making full and creative use of the technology to tame data and to transform information, Health Informatics will foster the development and use of new knowledge in healthcare.

Christina Eldredge
Sue S. Feldman
Mohammad A. Faysel • Arif M. Rana
Editors

Introductory Textbook in Health Informatics

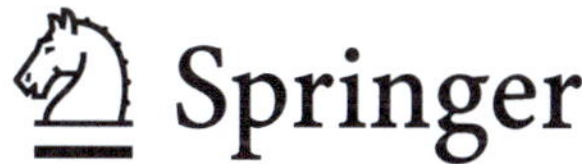

Editors
Christina Eldredge
School of Information
University of South Florida
Tampa, FL, USA

Sue S. Feldman
Graduate Programs in Health Informatics
University of Alabama at Birmingham
Birmingham, AL, USA

Mohammad A. Faysel
Health Informatics Program
SUNY Downstate Health Sciences
University
Brooklyn, NY, USA

Arif M. Rana (deceased)
College of Health Sciences
SUNY Polytechnic Institute
Utica, NY, USA

ISSN 1431-1917 ISSN 2197-3741 (electronic)
Health Informatics
ISBN 978-3-032-16656-2 ISBN 978-3-032-16657-9 (eBook)
https://doi.org/10.1007/978-3-032-16657-9

This Springer imprint is published by the registered company Springer Nature Switzerland AG
The registered company address is: Gewerbestrasse 11, 6330 Cham, Switzerland

Contents

1 Health Informatics Education: Textbook Overview, Book Structure, and Foundational Domains

Christina Eldredge, Sue S. Feldman, and Mohammad A. Faysel

1.1 Introduction

Welcome to the field of health informatics! We are excited to introduce our readers to this maturing and changing field. This textbook was developed to fulfill the need for an introductory-level resource tailored to students and professionals who are new to the field of health informatics (HI), as well as to those who are needing to fill some knowledge gaps. It originated as an idea from a community of health informatics professionals dedicated to education at the baccalaureate level and grew into a textbook that stretches across knowledge and skill levels. The American Medical Informatics Association's (AMIA) ten foundational domains of health informatics education at the baccalaureate level were used as the guiding principles in writing this book (Khariat 2023). These will be discussed in more depth below.

This text is meant to provide a survey or overview of the major concepts in the field of health informatics. Each chapter introduces concepts that lend themselves to deeper exploration as students advance in a program, or as an early professional explores gains breath in HI. If you are just beginning to learn about this important field, you may notice the interdisciplinary nature of HI. Students from different backgrounds, career stages, and/or majors may take a course in HI to support their career path in fields such as premedicine, health sciences, nursing, information science, data analytics, computer science, or biomedical engineering.

1.2 Background

AMIA developed a framework for the competencies required for comprehensive education in health informatics and to effectively prepare the health informatics workforce of the future. This framework was developed at a time when the

C. Eldredge (✉)
School of Information, University of South Florida, Tampa, FL, USA
e-mail: celdredge2@usf.edu

S. S. Feldman
Graduate Programs in Health Informatics, University of Alabama at Birmingham, Birmingham, AL, USA
e-mail: sfeldman@uab.edu

M. A. Faysel
Health Informatics Program, SUNY Downstate Health Sciences University, Brooklyn, NY, USA

C. Eldredge et al. (eds.), *Introductory Textbook in Health Informatics*, Health Informatics,
https://doi.org/10.1007/978-3-032-16657-9_1

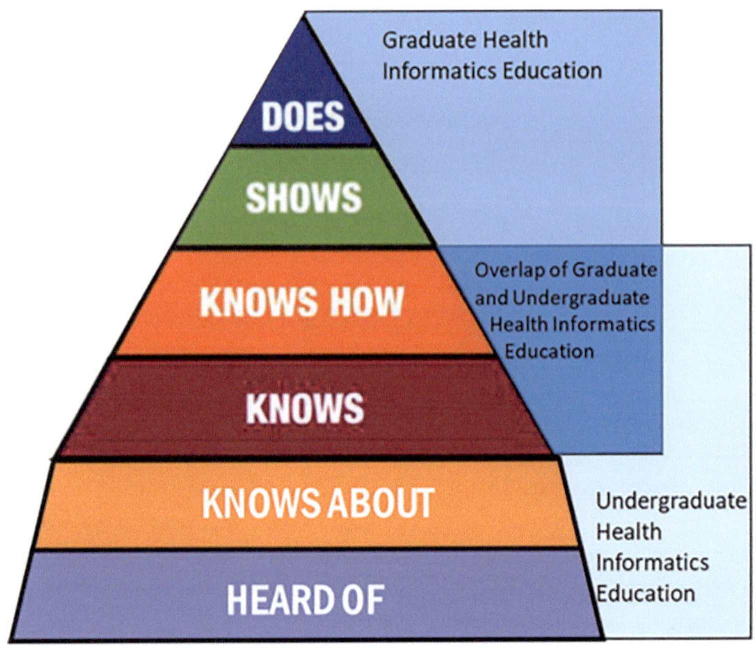

Fig. 1.1 Extended Miller's Pyramid for undergraduate HI education

field was moving away from content-based education and toward competency-based education [3]. In other words, health informatics educators wanted to prepare the next generation of professionals in the field by equipping them with the knowledge, skills, and attitudes required to be successful in the health informatics field. First, AMIA developed the ten foundational domains for master's level education in HI [3], which then followed with the development of the ten baccalaureate-level foundational domains [2] (Fig. 1.1).

The foundational domains in HI are based on three knowledge-based or "parent" domains (Health, Information Science and Technology, and Social and Behavioral Science) and three professional domains (Professionalism, Interprofessional Collaborative Practice, and Leadership). The overlap of these domains creates new domain intersections with corresponding knowledge, skills, and attitudes (KSA), or competencies. In other words, the interdisciplinary nature of the health informatics field inherently results in the application of one or more of these domains in the context of the others and creates new domain KSAs. AMIA presents this in a Venn diagram format where the overlap of the three parent domains is set upon the three professional domains, please see Fig. 1.2. For another way of looking at this concept, please see the mind map below, Fig. 1.3, for an illustration of this description.

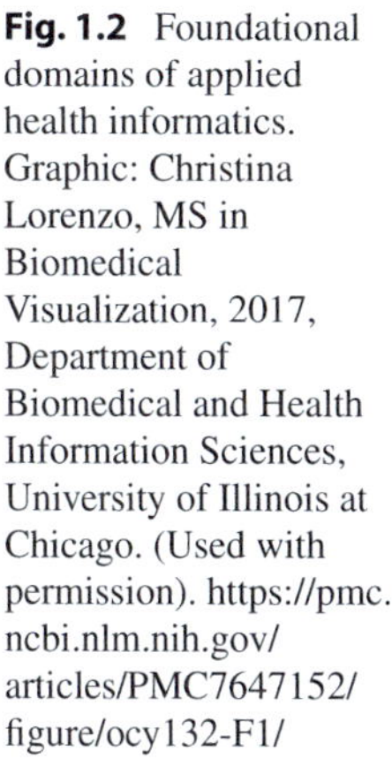

Fig. 1.2 Foundational domains of applied health informatics. Graphic: Christina Lorenzo, MS in Biomedical Visualization, 2017, Department of Biomedical and Health Information Sciences, University of Illinois at Chicago. (Used with permission). https://pmc.ncbi.nlm.nih.gov/articles/PMC7647152/figure/ocy132-F1/

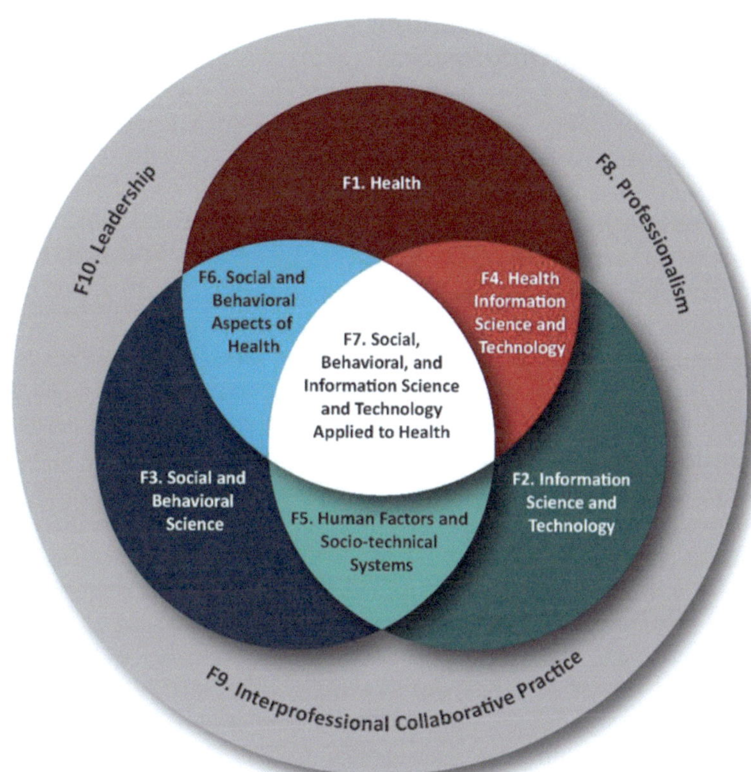

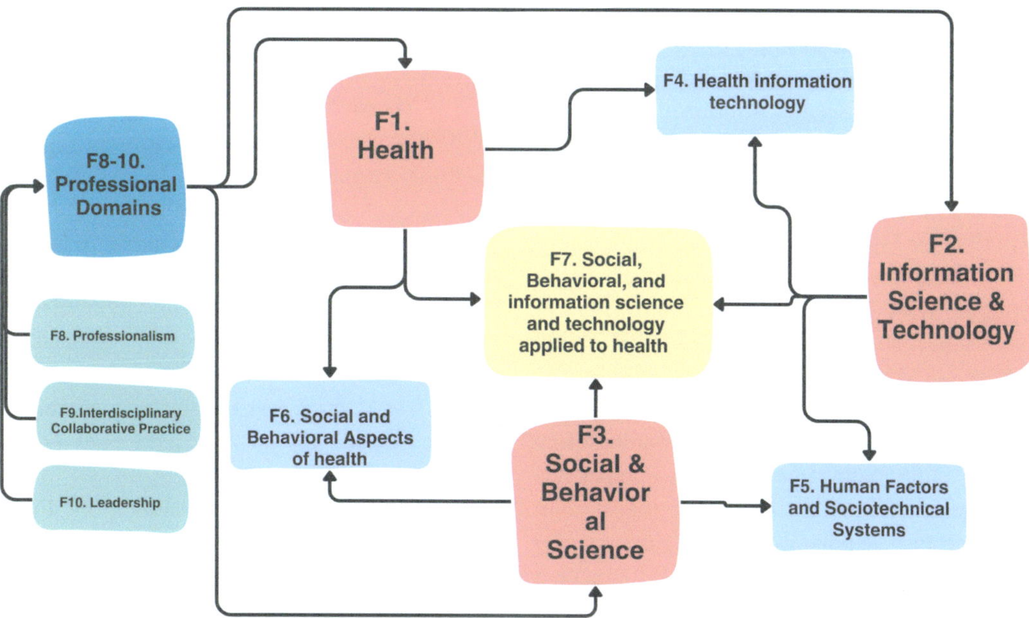

Fig. 1.3 Mind map of health informatics foundational domains [2, 3]

1.3 Domains, Accreditation, and Health Informatics Programs

The Commission on Accreditation for Health Informatics and Information Management Education (CAHIIM) is the accrediting body for HI education in the United States. As such, they have worked collaboratively with AMIA's Accreditation Committee to develop accreditation standards specifically tailored to accrediting HI programs. While those standards have been in place for graduate education for quite some time [1, 3], they were newly developed for undergraduate education [2]. The graduate accreditation standards adopted Miller's Pyramid Levels of competency demonstration and these proved very successful; hence they were adopted and modified for the undergraduate accreditation standards as well. While the AMIA Foundational Domains are detailed elsewhere in this text, the Miller's Pyramid levels of competency are not. The chapter cited here [1] provides an excellent and detailed background of how the Millers Pyramid was adapted for HI education, there are modifications specific to the undergraduate environment that are critical to acknowledge.

While most of these are laid out in the chapter on Undergraduate Health Informatics Education [2], it is important to note two levels have been added to the Miller's Pyramid as adapted for Health Informatics: HEARD OF and KNOWS ABOUT, see Fig. 1.1. These two new layers provide foundational learning at appropriate undergraduate KSA levels, while also allowing for competence at the KNOWS, KNOWS HOW, SHOWS, AND SHOWS HOW levels of graduate-level competence. HEARD OF and KNOWS ABOUT provide a level of domain awareness that often lays the foundation for further competence development, frequently involving demonstration of competence, in other words *how* to use the new knowledge, and therefore, is a critical foundation of competence in undergraduate education.

Consistent with the competencies established by AMIA, Foundational domains 1–3 are at the knowledge level while foundational domains 4–10 include the demonstration level. This structure provides great flexibility to the accreditation of programs and the content delivered, and further accommodates learning needs and competence anywhere along the Miller's Pyramid as adapted for HI.

1.4 Foundational Domains and Textbook Structure

Each chapter in this textbook includes a list of the domains covered within the chapter. This is meant to guide students and instructors as they are learning the foundational domains and levels of competence of the field. Students will enter the field with varying degrees of knowledge and competence across these ten domains and therefore, each student may need to personalize their study based on their gaps in their knowledge. From the faculty perspective, the textbook can be tailored toward a course(s) by noting which domain(s) are covered in each chapter. The book serves to introduce the concepts for further student exploration which can be facilitated using the additional resources and references found within each chapter.

1.5 Book Chapter Organization

The book chapters are organized to first introduce the history of the field, potential careers, professional organizations, and certifications in Chaps. 1, 2 and 3. These are followed by Chaps. 4, 5, 6 and 7, covering the basics of information science, computer science data science, and and decision analysis. Chapter 8 provides an overview of human factors (and systems thinking approach) and the relationship of this field with health informatics.

In the next quarter of the textbook, the focus shifts to application areas of health informatics. Chapters 9, 10, 11, 12, 13 and 14 focus on clinical applications of health informatics including electronic health records, telehealth, imaging informatics, and clinical decision support. However, in Chaps. 15 and 16, the focus moves to a population-level application of health informatics with topics on public and population health. Lastly Chaps. 17, 18, and 19, will explore into the fields of genomics, precision medicine, and translational science.

In the third quarter of the textbook, the reader will explore how health informatics relates to healthcare quality in chapters on patient safety (Chap. 20) and quality improvement (Chap. 21). Topics on health informatics standards development, standards organizations (Chap. 23), and controlled vocabularies and terminologies (Chap. 24) will also be covered. These fields will be interwoven with important health informatics topics of interoperability (Chap. 22) and privacy and security (Chaps. 25 and 26).

In the last quarter of the textbook, important concepts on project management and data governance will be covered. Finally, the last chapter of the book will provide a basic overview of artificial intelligence and how it relates to the HI field.

Each chapter includes a brief abstract, a list of foundational domains covered in that chapter, learning objectives, and a list of references and resources. Most chapters include knowledge check questions and a case study to help students apply context to the topic. Chapter 4 (The Basics of Data Science), Chap. 27 (Project Management), and Chap. 29 (Data Management) all use the case study approach throughout the chapter to help contextualize the information and its application to the health informatics field in an easy-to-understand format. Specific to Chap. 29 is an overarching connection with many concepts from the other chapters in the textbook and this chapter can serve as a review of the importance and application of data management principles in HI. The book concludes with artificial intelligence and the look toward the future.

Acknowledgments We would like to acknowledge the support of the AMIA Academic Forum, especially the members of the Baccalaureate Educators Community.

Dedication "In cherished memory of our esteemed co-editor, Dr. Arif M. Rana, Ph.D., Ed.S., M.S., M.P.H., M.A., who passed away unexpectedly during the editing of this book and contributed greatly to the early stages of this project."

References

1. Feldman SS, Boren SA, Tesch LH, Valenta AL. Accreditation of health informatics programs. In: Berner ES, editor. Informatics education in healthcare. Health informatics. Cham: Springer; 2020. https://doi.org/10.1007/978-3-030-53813-2_17.
2. Khairat S, Feldman SS, Rana A, Faysel M, Purkayastha S, Scotch M, Eldredge C. Foundational domains and competencies for baccalaureate health informatics education. JAMIA. 2023;30(10):1599–607. https://doi.org/10.1093/jamia/ocad147.
3. Valenta AL, Berner ES, Boren SA, Deckard GJ, Eldredge C, Fridsma DB, Gadd C, Gong Y, Johnson T, Jones J, Manos EL, Phillips KT, Roderer NK, Rosendale D, Turner AM, Tusch G, Williamson JJ, Johnson SB. AMIA Board White Paper: AMIA 2017 core competencies for applied health informatics education at the master's degree level. JAMIA. 2018;25(12):1657–68. https://doi.org/10.1093/jamia/ocy132.

The History of Health Informatics 2

David Gibbs and Mohammad A. Faysel

Foundational Domains
This chapter addresses the following AMIA Foundational Domains: F4—Health Information Science and Technology, F10—Leadership.

Learning Objectives
At the end of reading this chapter, the reader should be able to:

1. Explain the origins, periods, and important milestones achieved during the evolution of health informatics.
2. Describe the challenges faced by the field and how they were overcome as the field progressed.
3. Identify key standards which have enabled advancement in the field.
4. Describe current challenges which still need to be addressed as the field moves into the future.

Definitions
None

D. Gibbs (✉)
Department of Health Informatics & Information Management, Texas State University, Round Rock, TX, USA
e-mail: dgibbs@txstate.edu

M. A. Faysel
Health Informatics Program, SUNY Downstate Health Sciences University, Brooklyn, NY, USA

2.1 Introduction

The relatively short history of health informatics has been well documented by several pioneers in the field and other authors striving to acknowledge the accomplishments of those early innovators. Details about the earliest uses of computers and digital data in medicine, nursing, and health professions are rightfully explained in several books, journal articles, websites, and other sources. This chapter provides a few brief highlights drawn from previous works intended to establish a context for the remainder of the textbook. Readers seeking additional details are encouraged to explore the references provided and other sources.

Some of the major milestones in health informatics are organized in this chapter by decades to summarize the sequence and pace of development.

The first uses of computers in healthcare were associated with administrative functions rather than clinical applications. Following effective administrative applications, some clinicians recognized the potential of using computers and digital data to improve the delivery of clinical care to patients. According to Collen [1], there were several names associated with the use of computers and digital data in medicine including medical computing, computer medicine, medical computer science, and many more. It was after these clinical applications were already in use

C. Eldredge et al. (eds.), *Introductory Textbook in Health Informatics*, Health Informatics,
https://doi.org/10.1007/978-3-032-16657-9_2

that pioneers realized a new discipline had been created and a name for the discipline was needed.

Part of the naming challenge was that the new discipline incorporated elements from multiple existing distinct fields of science, engineering, and technology. Based on earlier publications from England, France, Poland, and Russia where forms of the term *informatics* had been associated with medicine and health, the terms *medical informatics* and *health informatics* began to be more widely adopted. In recent years, genomics research generated the term *bioinformatics*. Academic programs providing broad coverage of content adopted the combined term *biomedical informatics* [2]. While sometimes used interchangeably, health informatics is often interpreted more broadly than medical informatics and is largely synonymous with biomedical informatics to include the range of applications of science, engineering, and technology applied across the spectrum of human health and wellness.

"Computers are especially suited to help the physician collect and process clinical information and remind him of diagnoses which he may have overlooked" [3].

These foretelling words published in 1959 have increased in accuracy during the ensuing decades. The following sections highlight only a few representative milestones that have contributed to health informatics.

2.2 1950–1959 Origins

Before health informatics and today's digital health could develop, computers and digital emerged to address challenges at the time.

The first commercially available computer capable of handling both numeric and alphabetic text, the Universal Automatic Computer (UNIVAC I), was deployed into production in 1951. A primary feature was the ability to support applications requiring large volumes of data. While initially developed and implemented for the US Bureau of the Census, the benefits of the computer rapidly expanded to other fields. For example, within the first 8 months, the UNIVAC was being used to generate premium notices for a life insurance company [4].

Early computers were very large and very expensive, which limited availability to the government and other large organizations. The US military health organizations recognized the early potential for computers in healthcare. In 1956 and 1957, a series of conferences sponsored by the US Air Force's Air Research and Development Command were held to explore the application of computers in medicine and biology. One early innovation was an automatic electroencephalogram analyzer that reduced the time required to evaluate wave patterns. The conference participants envisioned similar applications to analyze additional bioelectrical phenomena such as electrocardiogram and galvanic skin responses could be performed by specialized devices [5].

Later in the decade, Ledley & Lusted wrote about how computers could be used to aid physicians in making medical diagnoses. The article explained how mathematical principles of probability and symbolic logic relate to the foundations of reasoning for medical diagnosis. The authors were clear that computers could not replace physicians but could enable physicians to focus on more complicated tasks and develop new knowledge [3]. These are some of the earliest writings about what would evolve into augmented intelligence.

2.3 1960–1969 Early Innovations

Specialized intensive care unit (ICU) information systems were developed early in this decade at several medical centers across the United States. For example, the Texas Institute for Research and Rehabilitation (TIRR) created a bedside computer to monitor physiological indicators in patients after surgery. The TIRR ICU system continued to evolve and expand capabilities throughout the 1960s. Computer-based solutions were also developed at other medical centers including Los Angeles County General Hospital monitoring for circulatory shock and Hollywood Presbyterial Hospital developed a severity index for ICU patients and applied algorithms to predict survivability. George Washington University advanced work in electrocardiography analysis [2, 6].

The Massachusetts General Hospital Utility Multi-Programming System (MUMPS) was developed at Massachusetts General Hospital (MGH) in 1965 as a language for clinical data management. Features of MUMPS included rapid application development and modifications along with manipulation of hierarchically organized textual data [7]. MUMPS was used to develop Computer Stored Ambulatory Record (COSTAR), an early computerized patient record system at MGH. MUMPS enabled many of today's commercial electronic health record systems [8].

Around 1967, a technical committee on medical informatics was established by Dr. François Grémy of France in the International Federation for Information Processing. The first meeting occurred in Paris in 1968 and over time the committee became the International Medical Informatics Association (IMIA) [9]. Since its origin, the IMIA has facilitated global collaboration to advance the field [10].

2.4 1970–1979 Electronic Medical Records and Clinical Decision Support

The Regenstrief Medical Record System (RMRS) was deployed in 1974 at Wishard Memorial Hospital as one of the earliest EMRs. Use of the system expanded from the initial diabetic clinical to general medicine. Clinical decision support was recognized as the most interesting benefit of the system and would require standardized, structured data [11].

MYCIN was developed as a prototype at Stanford University as an early clinical decision support system incorporating artificial intelligence (AI). The purpose of the project was to develop an interactive computer-based tool to provide advice and explanations to physicians regarding antimicrobial therapy. The system used a series of questions and responses based on a collection of rules developed by clinical experts. MYCIN inspired further research and development of AI in clinical decision support.

The Health Evaluation through Logical Processing (HELP) system was initiated at LDS Hospital in Utah. HELP continued to evolve into a comprehensive clinical information system including a patient medical record and clinical decision support [12, 13].

2.5 1980–1989 Microcomputers

In 1983, the US Veteran's Administration began using the internally developed electronic health record system which later became the Veterans Health Information Systems and Technology Architecture (VistA). The system is based on MUMPS and provides electronic medical documentation, ordering, and decision support [14].

The American Medical Informatics Association (AMIA) was first proposed in 1980 to advance medical informatics in the United States. The First Congress of the American Medical Informatics Association was held in 1982. Through the merger of three previous organizations that had evolved separately with overlapping membership, the AMIA was incorporated in 1988 and the first president was elected in 1989 [15].

2.6 1990–1999 The HIPAA Era

In 1996, the Health Insurance Portability and Accountability Act (HIPAA) was passed. This federal legislation established laws to protect the privacy of healthcare data while also enabling patients access to their own medical records and to move between jobs without compromising access to healthcare [16].

The landmark publication *To Err is Human: Building a Safer Health System* was released on December 1, 1999 by the Institute of Medicine (IOM), now known as the National Academy of Medicine [17]. This first report from the Committee on the Quality of Health Care in America brought widespread attention to the high rate of medical errors. The report had a lasting effect and inspired more IOM publications in subsequent years that continued to emphasize patient safety and encourage the use of electronic health records to improve the quality of care and outcomes [18, 19].

The first issue of the Journal of the American Medical Informatics Association (JAMIA) was published in January 1994 [2].

2.7 2000–2009 A Focus on Patient Safety and Quality

The second report from the IOM was released in 2001 entitled *Crossing the Quality Chasm: A New Health System for the twenty-first Century*. This report draws further attention to the relationship between technology such as electronic health record systems and patient safety. Among the recommendations included in the report was a nationwide infrastructure for health information exchange [20].

The Office of the National Coordinator (ONC) for Health Information Technology was initially established in 2004 by an executive order creating the position of National Coordinator and in 2009 mandated by Congress as part of the Health Information Technology for Economic and Clinical Health (HITECH) Act. The charge of the ONC was to ensure patients have access to their health information and to improve healthcare through interoperability and sharing data [21].

In 2005, AMIA initiated a multi-year effort that led to the Clinical Informatics Subspecialty for physicians who apply knowledge of informatics and patient care.

Congress passed the American Recovery and Reinvestment Act (ARRA) in 2009 which provided significant funding of $20 billion to the healthcare industry including specific support for health information technology. Within ARRA was the Health Information Technology for Economic and Clinical Health Act (HITECH) which directed federal funds to incentivize eligible healthcare professionals and healthcare organizations to implement and demonstrate "meaningful use" of electronic health record (EHR) systems [2, 22].

2.8 2010–2019 The Meaningful Use Era

Prior to HITECH Act 2009, the adoption of EHRs was very low among hospitals, less than 10% [23]. The lack of wide adoption of EHR had been a serious impediment toward advancing healthcare, especially for making health information sharable for improved care coordination and efficient of care delivery. The HITECH Act 2009 created a concept called "Meaningful Use"(MU) initiative that aimed to encourage the use of EHRs in a "meaningful" way to ensure improvement in the quality, patient safety, and overall efficiency in healthcare delivery through a financial incentive [24]. This initiative was called the Medicare and Medicaid Electronic Health Record (EHR) Incentive Programs introduced in 2011 by Centers for Medicare and Medicaid Services (CMS) for eligible hospitals, critical access hospitals (CAS), and other providers "to adopt, implement, upgrade, and demonstrate meaningful use of certified electronic health record technology (CEHRT)" [24, 25]. In 2010, the Department of Health and Human Services published the standards for the first stage of "meaningful use" incentives. Stage 1 provided incentives for capturing patient data electronically using prescribed medical coding standards. This stage also included e-prescribing and alerts for drug interactions [22]. These financial incentives directly influenced the rapid expansion of EHR systems in the United States.

To be eligible for the financial incentives, providers were required to demonstrate effective use of EHRs through three incremental stages: Stage 1 (expected in 2011–2012), Stage 2 (expected in 2012–2013), and Stage 3 (expected in 2015), and each stage required a specific set of requirements for eligible hospitals and providers [26]. Stage 1 required the adoption of a certified EHR and laid the foundation for capturing clinical data in electronic format and sharing of information, while Stage 2 required the expansion of the baseline clinical data capture and encouraged the capture of clinical quality measures and more structured data for health information exchange and continuous quality improvement that were aligned with the objectives of the National Quality Strategies to advance clinical processes [26].

In October 2015, the Center for Medicare and Medicaid (CMS) consolidated Stage 1 and Stage 2 into a more simplified Modified Stage 2 program to simplify some of the complexities of measures that existed in the two original stages [27]. Stage 3 requirements focused on interoperability and improved patient outcomes through various objectives and measures addressing protection of protected health information (PHI), use of clinical decision support (CDS), electronic prescribing (eRx), computerized provider order entry (CPOE), patient access, coordination of care through patient engagement, health information exchange (HIE), and public health and clinical data registry reporting [28].

Although the meaningful use initiative was the driving force behind wide adoption of EHRs among hospitals and eligible providers (59% in 2016), there were challenges with hospitals meeting the criteria, especially due to substantial costs associated with EHR implementation [29]. Recognizing the importance of interoperability for efficient healthcare delivery, in April 2018, CMS changed the EHR Incentive Programs to continue to promote health information exchange, interoperability, and patient access, and renamed it to the Medicare and Medicaid Promoting Interoperability Programs. Although the Medicaid Promoting Interoperability Program ended in 2022, a version of Medicare Promoting Interoperability Programs is currently in existence for only eligible hospitals and CAS [25].

2.8.1 HIEs/Interoperability Challenges

There was a significant improvement in the use of EHRs in a meaningful way and a higher EHR adoption rate among hospitals (96% and 80% for hospitals and office-based practice, respectively), CAS, and other providers resulted from the Medicare and Medicaid Electronic Health Record (EHR) Incentive Programs that promoted the use of CEHRT [30]. Despite these achievements, there were significant challenges in health information exchange (HIE) among healthcare entities and interoperability in the existing EHRs that were resulted primarily from technological, financial, cultural (stakeholders work in silos), and regulatory barriers [30]. A December 2015 Report to US Congress included lack of adoption of standards-based EHRs, complex regulations that were overburdening for vendors and providers, providers' burnout resulting from documentation burden using EHR in daily workflow, issues with preserving patient information privacy and data security related to health information exchange, lack of collaboration from stakeholders, and unclear EHR incentives as the major categories of barriers toward achieving interoperability [31].

2.8.2 EHR and Burnout

Early design of EHRs (known as legacy systems) did not consider interoperability and user-centered design. Moreover, Stages 1 and 2 of the MU incentive programs focused more on certified EHR adoption, data capture and clinical documentation without providing a clear guideline for interoperability and many of the certified EHRs were not designed to be interoperable while providers faced staggering costs associated with creating interfaces to communicate with other EHRs to make them interoperable (only 6% providers achieved interoperability with disparate EHRs in 2015) [29]. Perceived benefits of "meaningful use" of EHR supposed to increase efficiency and improve quality of care, but substantially added documentation burden using EHR and manual data entry, poorly designed interfaces and lack of usability, and other administrative duties that required over use of EHR resulted in providers' burnout [32].

2.8.3 Privacy and Security/Data Breaches

During this decade, there was an influx of incidents related to healthcare data privacy and security, especially due to storing sensitive electronic health records in vulnerable network environments and devices that were not strongly secured. Oftentimes, these sensitive data were unintentionally exposed on the "Business Associate (BA)", usually vendors who deal with patient data on behalf of the CAs, side that posed a direct threat to patient privacy and security of health records. In 2010, covered entities were required to implement the changes to the HIPAA Security Rule that were required by the HITECH Act 2009 to ensure that the BAs were compliant with the HIPAA Security Rule [33]. To deter increased number of privacy breaches occurred among BAs of healthcare providers in the United States, HIPAA Omnibus Rule was enacted and implemented in 2013 that ensured a more stringent compliant requirements for the BAs [34]. Major types of healthcare privacy and security incidents that took place during this decade were related to hacking or cyberattacks, unauthorized accessing of protected data (malicious intentions), theft or loss of laptops and/or portable storage devices that stored sensitive patient PHI, and disposing PHI and health data without properly destroying them [35]. Because of high financial gain associated with sensitive health records on the dark web, it made healthcare data breach lucrative to hackers which resulted in an increase in financially motivated data breaches toward the end of this decade [35]. There was also an increase in malware and ransomware attacks on hospital systems toward the end of this decade costing billions of dollars that were previously not widely known to the healthcare community [35]. The HITECH Act 2009 also included a Breach Notification Rule to HIPAA that resulted in the creation of 45 CFR 164.408—Notification to the Secretary in 2010 which required health entities to report any breach of unsecured protected health information to the Secretary of Health and Human Services (HHS) within a specific time period [36]. The Office of the Civil Rights (OCR) of HHS maintains a publicly available database of healthcare data breaches with detailed information including the organization where the data breach originates [38]. The database can be accessed from the OCR website (https://ocrportal.hhs.gov/ocr/breach/breach_report.jsf).

During the decade of 2010, there was a rapid improvement in internet connectivity and advancement in Internet of Things (IoT) that led to the emergence of Internet of Medical Things (IoMT) [37]. IoMT enabled integration of a range of technologies in healthcare that served as a catalyst toward the development and wide use of mobile health (mHealth) applications (such as smartphone-based daily health activity monitoring, etc.), remote monitoring, wearable sensors and devices, telehealth, and other patient-centered technologies that with improved patient engagement and remote monitoring and management of patient's health conditions [38]. The emergence of these technologies led to the advancement of health informatics field, especially toward the later part of this decade, advancing in developing systems and methods to deal with large volume of complex health-related data from EHR and various monitoring and wearable devices and analyzing them using more advanced AI and machine learning powered algorithms and "big data" tools [39].

This decade also witnessed the rapid emergence of personalized or precision medicine, an approach that aims to consider individual's characteristics such as genetic markup, lifestyle, environmental exposure and other unique factors and offers individualized or tailored patient care and improves patient outcome [40, 41].

In 2011, the American Board of Preventive Medicine (ABPM) Committee on Certification (COCERT) approved the proposal for the Clinical Informatics Subspecialty which was recognized as a subspecialty of medicine by the American Board of Medical Specialties [42].

2.9 2020-Present Dawn of Augmented Intelligence

ChatGPT became available to everyone with a web browser on November 30, 2022. This widespread availability and easy-to-use AI tool sparked a new era for artificial intelligence. Using generative pretrained transformer (GPT) models developed by OpenAI, users may have online chat sessions by submitting prompts that generate natural language responses. Subsequent prompts may continue the conversation within the continuing context. Competing GPT solutions soon emerged from many major vendors such as Microsoft's Copilot, Google's Gemini, Meta's Llama, and Anthropic's Claude. The American Medical Association prefers the term augmented intelligence to emphasize that technology should enhance rather than replace human intelligence [43]. More recently in 2025, another Open Source generative AI platform named DeepSeek, that was originated from China, has drawn attention to health informatics community, especially because of its low computing resource requirements and other attractive features compared to other proprietary generative AI platforms [44]. It is too early to evaluate its suitability in clinical setting due to privacy and security concerns. Although there are potential benefits of using of AI-driven applications in healthcare given the availability of a large volume of complex health data and improved connectivity, existing healthcare data privacy and security concerns need to be addressed. Among other methods, blockchain is becoming popular to secure healthcare data in a limited scale but its full potential to secure sensitive health data is yet to be realized [45]. Current era has been witnessing an ever-increasing cyberattacks including ransomware on US healthcare systems. To address that, HHS, through OCR, updated the HIPAA Security Rule in December 2024 to strengthen cybersecurity protections to safeguard PHI [46].

The COVID-19 pandemic had a profound impact on how care has been delivered, especially how rapidly hospitals and other healthcare providers embraced telehealth technologies to continue to provide care during this pandemic. The pandemic also revealed the need for a more modernized national public health data infrastructure, interoperable health systems, and the urgency for the availability of timely and accurate data for decision making at the population level. The American Rescue Plan Act of 2021 was enacted that included funding for modernizing public health related systems and health IT infrastructure in the United States [47].

In May 2020, the HHS enacted Twenty-first Century Cures Act: Interoperability, Information Blocking, and the ONC Health IT Certification Program Final Rule and the ONC created ONC's Cures Act Final Rule to support "seamless and secure access, exchange, and use of electronic health information" and to support patient's access to their health information in electronic format to implement the requirements of the twenty-first Century Cures Act [48, 49]. In 2024, the ONC name changed to Assistant Secretary for Technology Policy and Office of the National Coordinator for Health Information Technology (ASTP/ONC) [50].

The current decade has already witnessed a significant evolving of the field of health informatics. There exist rising concerns of "Digital Divide" and health equity which address the inequalities in access to technology and health informatics oriented patient care and their utilization by vulnerable populations [51].

2.10 Conclusion

The relatively new field of health informatics has been growing and evolving for over 75 years. Energized by innovations in computing, healthcare, and data science, health informatics has become a mainstream global profession and academic discipline with program accreditation at undergraduate and graduate levels. Organizations of health informatics professionals exist in countries around the globe to meet local workforce, research, and academic needs. The history of the health informatics field is as intriguing as its bright future.

Knowledge Check Questions (3–5) These Should Be Multiple Choice for the Test Bank

1. How did reports from the Institute of Medicine impact the field?
   (a) IOM reports inspired the creation of AMIA
   (b) IOM reports encouraged the use of EHR systems
   (c) IOM reports highlighted the low rate of mistakes in healthcare
   (d) IOM reports inspired the HIPAA legislation

2. What was the impact of the HITECH Act on the pace of EHR implementation?
   (a) The HITECH Act incentivized the meaningful use of EHR systems
   (b) The HITECH Act inspired the HIPAA legislation
   (c) The HITECH Act inspired the creation of AMIA
   (d) The HITECH Act established legislation to prohibit medical error

3. How did the COVID-19 pandemic drive awareness of public health and dashboards?
   (a) The pandemic demonstrated that EHR systems are no longer needed
   (b) The pandemic highlighted that telehealth services are rarely effective and that funding should be redirected to other purposes
   (c) The pandemic demonstrated the need for information blocking to help restrict dissemination
   (d) The pandemic inspired the American Rescue Plan Act of 2021 to fund modernization of public health infrastructure

Answers

1. (b)
2. (a)
3. (d)

References

1. Collen MF. Origins of medical informatics. West J Med. 1986;145(6):778.
2. Collen MF, Ball MJ, editors. The history of medical informatics in the United States. Springer; 2015. Available from: https://link.springer.com/content/pdf/10.1007/978-1-4471-6732-7.pdf
3. Ledley RS, Lusted LB. Reasoning foundations of medical diagnosis: symbolic logic, probability, and value theory aid our understanding of how physicians reason. Science. 1959;130(3366):9–21. https://doi.org/10.1126/science.130.3366.9.
4. Eckert JP Jr, Weiner JR, Welsh HF, Mitchell HF. The UNIVAC system [includes discussion]. International workshop on managing requirements knowledge; 1951 Philadelphia. 6-16. IEEE.
5. Weinrauch H, Patishall E. The air force and applications of computers to medicine and biology. Mil Med. 1958;122(3):178–80. https://doi.org/10.1093/milmed/122.3.178.
6. Clemmer TP. Computers in the ICU: where we started and where we are now. J Crit Care. 2004;19(4):201–7. https://doi.org/10.1016/j.jcrc.2004.08.005.
7. Zimmerman J, Rothmeier J. History and future of MUMPS in medical computing. Med Inform (Lond). 1979;4(1):5–11. https://doi.org/10.3109/14639237909044355.
8. Patel SY, Palma JP, Hoffman JM, Lehmann CU. Neonatal informatics: past, present and future. J Perinatol. 2024;44:773–6. https://doi.org/10.1038/s41372-024-01924-4.
9. Lorenzi NM. 40 years of IMIA: shaping medical informatics worldwide. Yearb Med Inform. 2007:163–4.
10. Haux R. Medical informatics: past, present, future. Int J Med Inform. 2010 Sep;79(9):599–610. https://doi.org/10.1016/j.ijmedinf.2010.06.003.
11. Biondich P, Dixon BE, Duke J, Mamlin B, Grannis S, Takesue B, et al. Regenstrief medical informatics: experiences with clinical decision support systems. In: Clinical decision support. 2nd ed. Elsevier; 2014. p. 165–87. https://doi.org/10.1016/B978-0-12-398476-0.00005-1.
12. Warner HR. Knowledge sectors for logical processing of patient data in the HELP system. In: The second annual symposium on computer application in medical care; 1978. p. 401–4. Available from: https://research.ebsco.com/linkprocessor/plink?id=ad618d48-576f-3bd9-8534-4c7c101523c1.
13. Gardner RM, Lundsgaarde HP. Evaluation of user acceptance of a clinical expert system. J Am Med Inform Assoc. 1994;1(6):428–38. https://doi.org/10.1136/jamia.1994.95153432.
14. Brown SH, Lincoln MJ, Groen PJ, Kolodner RM. VistA—US Department of veterans affairs national-scale HIS. Int J Med Inform. 2003;69(2–3):135–56. https://doi.org/10.1016/S1386-5056(02)00131-4.

15. American Medical Informatics Association (AMIA). AMIA's role in CIS and history. Retrieved February 25, 2025, from https://amia.org/careers-certifications/clinical-informatics-subspecialty/amias-role-cis-and-history.
16. Rosenbloom ST, Smith JR, Bowen R, Burns J, Riplinger L, Payne TH. Updating HIPAA for the electronic medical record era. J Am Med Inform Assoc. 2019;26(10):1115–9. https://doi.org/10.1093/jamia/ocz090.
17. Kohn LT, Corrigan JM, Donaldson MS. Committee on quality of health care in america. To err is human: building a safer health system. Washington, dc: national academies press; 2000. https://doi.org/10.17226/9728.
18. Havens DH, Boroughs L. "To err is human": a report from the institute of medicine. J Pediatr Health Care. 2000;14(2):77–80. https://doi.org/10.1067/mph.2000.105383.
19. Bates DW, Singh H. Two decades since to err is human: an assessment of progress and emerging priorities in patient safety. Health Aff (Millwood). 2018;37(11):1736–43. https://doi.org/10.1377/hlthaff.2018.0738.
20. Committee on Quality of Health Care in America. Crossing the quality chasm: a new health system for the 21st century. Washington, DC: National Academies Press; 2001. https://doi.org/10.17226/10027.
21. DeSalvo KB, Dinkler AN, Stevens L. The US Office of the National Coordinator for Health Information Technology: progress and promise for the future at the 10-year mark. Ann Emerg Med. 2015;66(5):507–10. https://doi.org/10.1016/j.annemergmed.2015.03.032.
22. Burde H. The HITECH act: an overview. AMA J Ethics. 2011;13(3):172–5.
23. https://www.hipaajournal.com/what-is-the-hitech-act/.
24. Classen D, Bates D. Finding the meaning in meaningful use. N Engl J Med. 2011;365(9):855–8. https://doi.org/10.1056/NEJMsb1103659.
25. Centers for Medicare & Medicaid Services [CMS]. Promoting interoperability programs. Centers for Medicare & Medicaid Services; 2024. Retrieved February 19, 2025, from https://www.cms.gov/medicare/regulations-guidance/promoting-interoperability-programs?redirect=/EHRIncentivePrograms/30_Meaningful_Use.asp
26. Anumula N, Sanelli PC. Meaningful use. AJNR Am J Neuroradiol. 2012;33(8):1455–7. https://doi.org/10.3174/ajnr.A3247. Epub 2012 Jul 12. PMID: 22790244; PMCID: PMC7966550.
27. American Medical Association [AMA]. Meaningful use: Electronic Health Record (EHR) incentive programs. American Medical Association; n.d.. Retrieved February 19, 2025, from https://www.ama-assn.org/practice-management/medicare-medicaid/meaningful-use-electronic-health-record-ehr-incentive.
28. American Medical Association. Meaningful Use (MU) stage 3 and 2015 certification rules. American Medical Association; n.d.. Retrieved February 19, 2025, from https://www.ama-assn.org/system/files/corp/media-browser/premium/washington/meaningful-use-stage-3-certification-final-rule_0.pdf.
29. Inverso G, Flath-Sporn S, Monoxelos L, Labow B, Padwa B, Resnick C. What is the cost of meaningful use? J Oral Maxillofac Surg. 2016;74(2):227–9. https://doi.org/10.1016/j.joms.2015.10.010.
30. Reisman M. EHRs: the challenge of making electronic data usable and interoperable. P T. 2017;42(9):572–5. PMID: 28890644; PMCID: PMC5565131.
31. Health Information Technology Policy Committee. Report to congress: challenges and barriers to interoperability. 2015. Retrieved February 20, 2025, from www.healthit.gov/facas/sites/faca/files/HITPC_Final_ITF_Report_2015-12-16%20v3.pdf.
32. Wu Y, Wu M, Wang C, Lin J, Liu J, Liu S. Evaluating the prevalence of burnout among health care professionals related to electronic health record use: systematic review and meta-analysis. JMIR Med Inform. 2024;12:e54811. https://doi.org/10.2196/54811. PMID: 38865188; PMCID: PMC11208837.
33. Modifications to the HIPAA privacy, security, enforcement, and breach notification rules under the health information technology for economic and clinical health act and the genetic information nondiscrimination act; other modifications to the HIPAA rules. Fed Regist. 2013;78(17):5565–702. PMID: 23476971.
34. Yaraghi N, Gopal RD. The role of HIPAA omnibus rules in reducing the frequency of medical data breaches: insights from an empirical study. Milbank Q. 2018;96(1):144–66. https://doi.org/10.1111/1468-0009.12314. PMID: 29504206; PMCID: PMC5835681.
35. Healthcare Data Breaches: Insights and Implications – PMC. 2020. https://pmc.ncbi.nlm.nih.gov/articles/PMC7349636/.
36. Breach Reporting – HHS.gov. 2023. Retrieved February 10, 2025, from https://www.hhs.gov/hipaa/for-professionals/breach-notification/breach-reporting/index.html.
37. Vishnu S, Ramson S, Jegan R. Internet of Medical Things (IoMT) – an overview. In: 2020 5th International Conference on Devices, Circuits and Systems (ICDCS); 2020. p. 101–4. https://doi.org/10.1109/ICDCS48716.2020.243558.
38. Habibzadeh H, Dinesh K, Rajabi Shishvan O, Boggio-Dandry A, Sharma G, Soyata T. A survey of Healthcare Internet of Things (HIoT): a clinical perspective. IEEE Internet Things J. 2020;7(1):53–71. https://doi.org/10.1109/JIOT.2019.2946359.
39. Ristevski B, Chen M. Big data analytics in medicine and healthcare. J Integr Bioinform. 2018;15(3):20170030. https://doi.org/10.1515/jib-2017-0030. PMID: 29746254; PMCID: PMC6340124.
40. Marcon AR, Bieber M, Caulfield T. Representing a "revolution": how the popular press has portrayed

personalized medicine. Genet Med. 2018;20:950–6. https://doi.org/10.1038/gim.2017.217.
41. Goetz LH, Schork NJ. Personalized medicine: motivation, challenges, and progress. Fertil Steril. 2018;109(6):952–63. https://doi.org/10.1016/j.fertnstert.2018.05.006. PMID: 29935653; PMCID: PMC6366451.
42. Lehmann CU, Shorte V, Gundlapalli AV. Clinical informatics sub-specialty board certification. Pediatr Rev. 2013;34(11):525–30. https://doi.org/10.1542/pir.34-11-525. PMID: 24187144.
43. American Medical Association (AMA). Augmented intelligence in medicine [Internet]. Retrieved February 12, 2025, from https://www.ama-assn.org/practice-management/digital/augmented-intelligence-medicine.
44. Peng Y, Malin BA, Rousseau JF, Wang Y, Xu Z, Xu X, Weng C, Bian J. From GPT to DeepSeek: significant gaps remain in realizing AI in healthcare. J Biomed Inform. 2025;10:104791. https://doi.org/10.1016/j.jbi.2025.104791. Epub ahead of print. PMID: 39938624.
45. Fonsêca ALA, Barbalho IMP, Fernandes F, Arrais Júnior E, Nagem DAP, Cardoso PH, Veras NVR, Farias FLO, Lindquist AR, Dos Santos JPQ, Morais AHF, Henriques J, Lucena M, Valentim RAM. Blockchain in health information systems: a systematic review. Int J Environ Res Public Health. 2024;21(11):1512. https://doi.org/10.3390/ijerph21111512. PMID: 39595779; PMCID: PMC11593537.
46. For 2020 on ward reference to HIPAA security rule change in 2024 to address cyber security: https://www.hhs.gov/hipaa/for-professionals/security/hipaa-security-rule-nprm/index.html.
47. Congress.gov. HR 1319—American Rescue Plan Act of 2021. Accessed 10 Feb 2025. https://www.congress.gov/bill/117th-congress/house-bill/1319.
48. Department of Health and Human Services. 21st century cures act: interoperability, information blocking, and the ONC health IT certification program [Internet]. Fed Regist. 2020; Available from: https://www.federalregister.gov/documents/2020/05/01/2020-07419/21st-century-cures-act-interoperability-information-blocking-and-the-onc-health-it-certification.
49. ONC'S cures act final rule | HealthIT.gov [Internet]. wwwhealthitgov. 2022. Available from: https://www.healthit.gov/topic/oncs-cures-act-final-rule.
50. Tripathi M. ONC'S next chapter [Internet]. HealthITbuzz. 2024; [cited 2025 Feb 26]. Available from: https://www.healthit.gov/buzz-blog/health-it/oncs-next-chapter.
51. Litchfield I, Shukla D, Greenfield S. Impact of COVID-19 on the digital divide: a rapid review. BMJ Open. 2021;11 https://doi.org/10.1136/bmjopen-2021-053440.

Careers, Professional Organizations, and Certifications

3

Shushawna DeOliveira and Adiebonye Jumbo

Foundational Domains

This chapter addresses the following AMIA Foundational Domains: F8—Professionalism, F9—Interprofessional Collaborative Practice, F10—Leadership.

Learning Objectives

After reading this chapter, you should be able to:

1. Identify the diverse careers in health informatics and health information systems.
2. Explain the significance of professional organizations in advancing health informatics career pathways.
3. Compare the categories and requirements of health informatics certifications.
4. Describe the roles and responsibilities of health informatics professionals.

3.1 Introduction

The twenty-first century has ushered in an unparalleled era of opportunity for informaticians. The field of health informatics (HI) has advanced swiftly, driven by continuous technological innovations, positioning the profession on the brink of vast new possibilities for informaticians [1]. The health informatics world has the potential to utilize new-age tools and technologies to help healthcare professionals improve the quality of care, improve patient outcomes, increase the efficiency, and accessibility of healthcare services [2]. These increased opportunities bring with them an increased need for specialists who can analyze health information systems, specialists who understand both health information and the health information systems that are integral to our healthcare systems [3]. Health informaticians are involved in the design, analytics, management, retrieval, and storage of data, information, and knowledge to optimize their use for improved communication and data-driven decision-making with a focus on improving patient care.

Currently, HI encompasses a wide range of specializations. These include clinical informatics, bioinformatics, and public health informatics, each of which reflects the diverse kinds of data utilized in the many facets of modern healthcare. Integrating artificial intelligence (AI), telemedicine, and big data analytics into the disciplines of health informatics presents today's health informatics professionals with unfathomable opportunities to implement these technologies in health service delivery [4].

Artificial Intelligence has the potential to transform healthcare and healthcare delivery. In this chapter, we will review the transformation, its implications, and how to navigate health infor-

S. DeOliveira (✉) · A. Jumbo
State University of New York Downstate Health Sciences University, Brooklyn, NY, USA
e-mail: sdeoliveira@downstate.edu; adiebonye.jumbo@downstate.edu

C. Eldredge et al. (eds.), *Introductory Textbook in Health Informatics*, Health Informatics,
https://doi.org/10.1007/978-3-032-16657-9_3

mation, including diverse career opportunities ranging from health data management to health information systems and HI [3, 5]. Central to this new landscape is the integration of HI and clinical operations [6]. Explored in this chapter are the organizations that began to appear and serve the needs of the informaticians.

As the field of HI evolved, so did professional organizations. Organizations such as the American Medical Informatics Association (AMIA), International Medical Informatics Association (IMIA), and Healthcare Information and Management Systems Society (HIMSS) are designed to serve as professional organizations for the informatics community to collaborate, network, and share resources. Such organizations help with motivation, support, and their value in the use of informatics methods and approaches across the healthcare ecosystem.

This chapter will wrap up with a discussion on the importance of certification as part of the informatician's career trajectory. Obtaining specialty certification showcases the knowledge and skills needed to perform tasks to the best of one's ability. It sets one apart from those who may think they can do the work, but do not have the proper training. A certified informatician demonstrates their expertise, competence, mastery, and understanding of HI [7]. Certification will also enhance one's career while validating the individual's expertise and showcasing to supervisors or potential employers that one is interested in growing and advancing in the field.

Health informatics occupies the intersection of technology and clinical operations. This chapter will trace the historical context of HI, explore its current circumstances, and discuss future opportunities for the profession. It will also cover some of the various facets of HI, including professional organizations and certifications. Knowing about career options, professional organizations, and various credentialing certification options is important for training the next generation of informaticians who will have an impact on the timely delivery of healthcare services.

3.2 Historical Background and Context

The advancement of the field of HI spread from a relatively small group of very talented informaticians to the establishment of professional organizations, and ultimately, the development of certifications [8].

3.2.1 Digital Shift

The origins of HI can be traced back to the 1960s with the integration of computer technology into clinical operations. While the initial focus was on automating administrative functions, as healthcare operations became more and more complex, the role of informaticians began to expand to include clinical applications. Since the 1970s and 1980s, people began to recognize how the use of computers can help with patient outcomes and patient care. In these decades, the term clinical informatics started to become well known as health professionals in collaboration with information technology (IT) specialists, implemented electronic health record (EHR) systems as well as clinical decision support systems (CDSS) [6]. That is, when it was first realized that clinical care could benefit from EHRs to achieve improved patient outcomes. The Health Information Technology for Economic and Clinical Health (HITECH) Act of 2009 pointedly enhanced the digital shift of healthcare. The HITECH Act sought to streamline clinical operations through what it termed "improved health information technology" and "enhanced patient care" [9]. The Act provided financial incentives to healthcare providers to adopt the EHRs, which paved the way toward the digital equivalent of the paper chart. The HITECH Act can be viewed as the footing for deploying digital health system infrastructures.

In alignment with the goals of the HITECH Act is the Office of the National Coordinator for Health Information Technology (ONC) which was established to provide leadership in seeing that the "adoption and meaningful use" of EHR systems occur under the tutelage of that office [10]. Furthermore, the ONC also serves as a chaperon for those healthcare organizations that have made the digital health transformation such as improved patient outcomes, streamlined coordination of care, and improved data sharing.

Clinical operations are now in an unprecedented digital era due to the joint power of the HITECH Act and the ONC, which has infused every element of the healthcare sector with HI. Not only is the use of electronic health records (EHRs) mandated for most healthcare providers, but these systems are also now intimately and intricately tied managing patient care, supporting clinical decisions, and enhancing the delivery of care [9]. This increased need for providing a skilled workforce of informaticians with diverse expertise ensures data integrity, system interoperability, and data harmonization, enabling health information exchange between organizations and widespread health systems.

3.2.2 HI Careers

The field of HI has matured over several decades to a place where it not only serves the needs of clinical operations but also serves the needs of individual patients in a personalized way. Today, the term "health informatics" carries with it an expectation that information technology solutions will be used in both direct patient care and in the meaningful analysis of services for the purpose of improving quality of life. The notable evolution of health informatics from the 1960s and 1970s to the present has not occurred without problems, however. Among the important issues that need to be addressed along the way are ethics, privacy, and security [11].

With the advancement of technology came the demand for healthcare professionals with specialized knowledge and skills in informatics. The "informatics revolution" took off after 2004, when the federal government called for the "decade of health information technology" [11]. This period has increasingly underscored the intelligent use of information and technology to improve patient care and has drawn rising attention (and funding) to the field. One of the stated goals during this time has been to push for a set of unified competencies in health informatics across all medical specialties.

3.2.3 HI Professional Organizations

Professional development of HI practitioners is deeply influenced by the formation of professional organizations. It was not until the late twentieth century that such organizations started appearing within the HI field to serve and support its growing community of professionals. One of the oldest and most well-known HI professional organizations is the Healthcare Information and Management Systems Society (HIMSS), which was founded in 1961 and has since become a major force behind the development and advancement of technology in the HI profession. Another influential HI professional organization is the American Medical Informatics Association (AMIA), which was founded in 1988 [12]. Initially called the American Association for Medical Systems and Informatics, AMIA has also played an important role in serving the growing HI community.

The value of professional organizations in HI cannot be overstated. By facilitating communication, collaboration, and knowledge-sharing among HI professionals, these organizations have contributed to the spreading of new knowledge, data acquisition, and skills commensurate with technological advances in clinical operations.

3.2.4 HI Certifications

The Healthcare Information and Management Systems Society has started the trend toward specialty certifications. As the industry emphasizes standardized skills and competencies in HI, certifications become more of a necessity. The Certification of Commission for Health Information Technology (CCHIT) was established in 2004 to certify EHR systems [13]. Moreover, certifications such as CPHIMS (Certified Professional in Healthcare Information and Management Systems) and CHISP (Certified Health Informatics Systems Professional) were implemented to ensure that professionals have expertise in the field [14].

The healthcare world continues to change, and skilled health informatics professionals are now in demand more than ever. These professionals leverage data and technology to improve patient outcomes. The history of health informatics careers, professional organizations, and certifications is rich and complex, and it mirrors the healthcare landscape's increasingly dynamic and crucial role in shaping its future.

3.3 HI Careers

AMIA offers various opportunities and resources for informaticians by creating communities and a platform that connects informaticians to serve in positions of leadership. The organization also supports networking, collaboration, and certifications, as well as hosting webinars and conferences that enable experts in the field to share the latest trends and innovations in the field. Forums such as this help to drive advancement in informatics. Health informatics is an interdisciplinary field that blends healthcare, information technology, and data management to optimize the delivery and quality of care. Figure 3.1 presents a framework encompassing a wide range of career paths and specialty areas, each contributing uniquely to the healthcare ecosystem. Below is an overview of key fields and specialties within health informatics, based on the framework provided:

Translational Bioinformatics Translational bioinformatics applies data management tools to turn biological and clinical data into healthcare insights. Professionals ensure accurate data collection and processing for clinical use. They manage health information systems like electronic health records, clinical decision support, health information exchange, telehealth, and ensure ethical, secure data governance across healthcare settings.

Clinical Informatics Clinical informatics enhances healthcare operations by using data to improve workflows and decision-making. Data analytics specialists provide insights for better patient care and efficiency. Clinical decision support (CDS) systems help clinicians make informed decisions at the point of care, while workflow informatics professionals integrate technologies to optimize healthcare processes.

Public Health Informatics (PHI) Public health informatics applies informatics tools to improve disease surveillance and health management. Population health surveillance systems monitor public health trends and outbreaks in real-time. Public health data management specialists organize and analyze data to support large-scale health initiatives and policy-making, enhancing overall population health and response to threats.

Research & Bioinformatics Bioinformatics integrates biology and data science to analyze genetic data, contributing to personalized medicine. Research informatics manages large clinical and genomic datasets to discover disease insights. Specialists analyze complex biological data, such as DNA sequences, while adhering to strict ethical standards to ensure patient data privacy and compliance in health informatics research.

Consumer Health Informatics (CHI) Consumer health informatics empowers patients to manage their health through tools for easy access to health data and services. Specialists ensure secure management of health records, while mobile health applications support health monitoring, appointment scheduling, and communication. Telehealth enables remote care, increasing accessibility, especially for underserved populations.

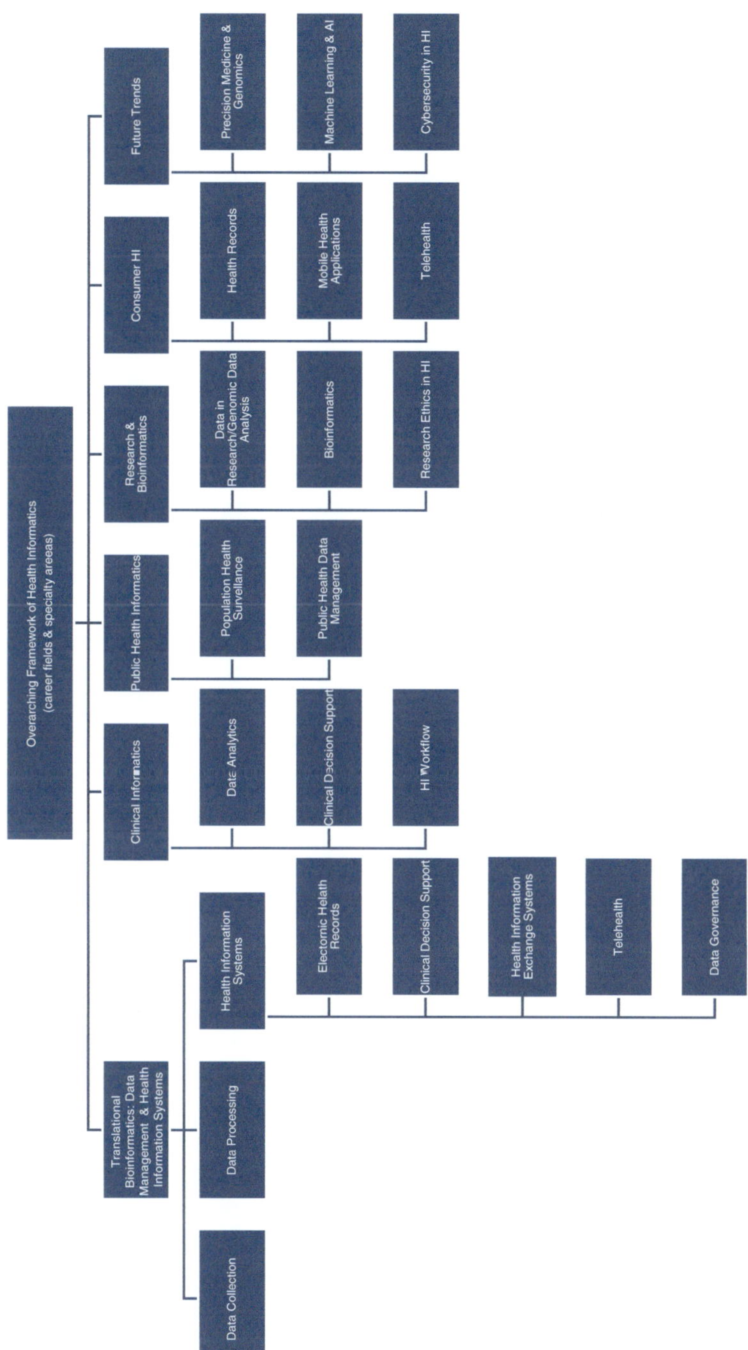

Fig. 3.1 Overarching framework for health informatics careers fields and specialty areas

3.3.1 Future Trends

As healthcare advances, health informatics will see growth in precision medicine, using genomic data to personalize treatments. Machine learning and AI will optimize patient outcomes and identify disease patterns. Cybersecurity experts will play a crucial role in safeguarding sensitive health information as digitalization increases, protecting it from potential cyber threats.

Public health informatics has become increasingly important, especially since the pandemic. Public health informaticians apply data-driven methods to prevent disease, promote health, and manage public health interventions at both the community and national levels. This area of concentration emphasizes the integration of health informatics with public health and community health approaches to tackle the major health challenges and achieve positive outcomes at the population and community levels.

Career opportunities within informatics have expanded because of the use of new Health Information Exchange (HIE) systems, telehealth, and data analytics. These new systems of health information have made it possible to manage individual patient care but have also made it possible to significantly enhance public health activities, such as surveillance, disaster response, and long-term population health management which are now areas that now employ a number of individuals in specialized roles such as clinical informaticists, clinical data analysts, HI researchers, health IT security specialists, and all the above positions previously mentioned.

As the result of this digital shift, healthcare clinical operations are now seeking skilled informaticians who specialize in specific areas like clinical informatics that use the EHRs data analytics based on the data the information had been collected about the patients [15], health IT project managers (individuals who set goals for information systems in an organization and ensure these goals are met), data analysts (individuals who analyze health data into graphs, tables, and trends) [6]. As would be expected with changes in technology and new advances in the environment, several different jobs have job titles and job descriptions that did not previously exist before the increased interest in informatics. Some of these job titles and descriptions are healthcare data analyst, healthcare data scientist, mobile health app developer, telehealth specialist, health information manager, healthcare quality improvement specialist, and clinical informatician [16].

More recently, the push for interoperability has shifted the healthcare environment to embrace data to make decisions. EHRs can generate profuse amounts of data, which can be connected to improve coordinated patient-centered care. The integration of artificial intelligence (AI) grew in the healthcare sector with roles such as healthcare AI specialist and machine language analysts (MLA) [17]. Additionally, there has been an increased focus on data security roles such as HI security officers and compliance analysts, leading to roles like HIPPA compliance officers.

Along with these technical advancements, the leadership of health informatics has become increasingly important. AMIA's foundational domain F.10 highlights leadership in health informatics which involves guiding the strategic vision for healthcare technology, fostering collaboration, and driving innovation; these are the fundamentals of health informatics leadership today [18]. Chief information officers (CIOs) and chief medical informatics officers (CMIOs) have pivotal roles in managing, governing, and exchanging health information. These leaders not only ensure the adoption and integration of technology but also oversee the compliance, protection, and full potential realization of digital health in their organizations.

Future trends in HI also include specializations (see Fig. 3.1) within informatics, such as becoming a population health manager who leverages informatics and data to address the healthcare needs of specific populations. Other specializations include clinical informaticists, clinical data analysts, health IT researchers, health IT security specialists, and the roles previously noted.

3.4 HI Professional Organizations

Professional organizations in HI have been crucial to the progress made in the field, setting standards and promoting professional development. The global leader among these organizations is the HIMSS, which was founded in 1961 as the Hospital Management Systems Society [19]. HIMSS is mainly focused on the key integration of healthcare systems and technology. Over the years, this organization has expanded its scope to effectively use the technology of computing in clinical operations and in the use of such things as electronic medical records.

Another key organization is the AMIA, founded in 1988 as the AAAMSI [12]. AMIA has taken a robust academic tactic to advancing HI with emphasis on workforce development, research, and the need to integrate informatics education into healthcare curricula. Through its focus on the academic foundation of HI, AMIA has contributed significantly to elevating the field's educational standards.

3.4.1 CAHIIM Accrediting HI Programs

As the field of HI continues to grow, it is more crucial to standardize education in the field. The Commission on Accreditation for Health Informatics and Information Management Education (CAHIIM) has played a pivotal role in this effort. Since its founding in 2007, CAHIIM has accredited health informatics programs to safeguard that they meet quality standards [20]. As a result, students and professionals have a clear pathway to achieving recognizable and valuable qualifications.

The growing complexity of the healthcare industry has highlighted the necessity of elevating and standardizing health informatics education. Since its founding in 2007, the CAHIIM has performed the invaluable service of accrediting health informatics programs, enabling prospective students to distinguish between programs of high educational quality and those of lower quality.

3.4.2 CAHIIM-AMIA Relationship for Accreditation Standards

The American Medical Informatics Association and CAHIIM work cooperatively to shape the educational framework for HI programs. Through this partnership, AMIA brings the voice of the profession and the needs of health informatics to the partnership, while CAHIIM represents the educational programs and students entering the profession in the near future. The partnership allows for the health informatics programs' "growing up" into a fully rigorous and relevant college-level curricular and accreditation model.

The partnership stresses the value of combining practical abilities with theoretical knowledge, thus providing graduates with the necessary competencies to confront and solve real-world problems. In addition, the collaboration serves as an excellent vehicle for establishing a continuous feedback loop between academia and industry. That loop allows both sectors to revise the standards of the partnership's programs in a timely fashion, responding to all sorts of trends and emerging technologies. This responsiveness is crucial in a rapidly developing field like health informatics. Because these graduates are trained in both sectors, they are not only knowledgeable but also adaptable.

Health informatics certifications, supported by organizations like HIMSS, AMIA, and CAHIIM, serve as vital tools for career advancement, upskilling, and enhancing professional credibility. Certifications offer a structured pathway for knowledge acquisition, boosting confidence and providing a competitive advantage in the job market. For professionals, these credentials not only validate their expertise but also demonstrate a commitment to ongoing professional development, ultimately increasing employability and opportunities for career advancement in an increasingly data-driven healthcare environment.

3.5 HI Certifications

Frequently, there is a disparity between the inherent worth of HI certifications and employer perceptions. This is due to most employers not fully grasping the nature of informatics certifications and the ways in which they can directly benefit their organizations. We should explore how to communicate the value of these certifications to employers more effectively. One way might be to draw parallels with other certifications, like those from Google, that are seen as rigorously earned and directly applicable to a job. Such certifications are valued by employers because they are supposed to lead to much-enhanced skills for the employees who earn them and to significantly enhanced performance by the organization as a whole.

In health informatics, the value of certification remains unclear due to limited employer awareness, creating challenges for professionals seeking validation of their expertise. Rob and Roy (2013) identify similar issues in IT certifications, where the perceived value varies by employer, leading to uncertainty about the return on investment. Health informatics faces the same problem, with inconsistent employer recognition reducing the impact of certifications. For these certifications to be meaningful, efforts must focus on aligning employer understanding with the value certifications provide, ensuring they are recognized as essential tools for skill enhancement and career growth.

Eventually, the path forward for HI certification lies in bridging the gap between certification and employer understanding. Just as Rob and Roy suggest more consistent recognition of IT certifications, similar efforts must be made in HI to ensure that these certifications are seen as valuable assets in the workforce, both for skill development and career advancement [21]. In the new area of HI, the significance of certification is still not clear. Why? Because many employers in the sector are not fully cognizant of the benefits that certification can provide. Consequently, HI professionals who wish to use certification as a means to "score" their level of "expertise" are somewhat stuck.

What is occurring now with HI certifications is similar to what has long been the case with IT certifications for some time. Both types of certifications, in the eyes of many employers, have pretty much the same image problem. They simply do not have a high "certification value" in the eyes of many employers. Employers' perception aside, if certification value is ever boosted to some more widely acknowledged level, then HI professionals will be able to reap the benefit of the appearance of having more certification value than they do now.

Although there are many certifications an informatician can obtain to validate their level of expertise and competence, the difficulty lies in determining which, if any, are the most appropriate. Health informaticians need to evaluate the specific health career goals they have for themselves and determine which certification would align with their current area of expertise and how would obtaining that certification be of benefit to the trajectory of their HI career [22].

Obtaining a certification in HI demonstrates competencies in the field, and it serves as a formal recognition of knowledge. When a health informatics degree is obtained, it shows that the individual has completed competency in the field. However, when certification is obtained, it exemplifies that the health informatician meets the knowledge and skill level to be marketable. In some positions, it is an employment or practice condition. Generally, certifications are available and are awarded by professional organizations and academic institutions whose primary goal is to provide a formal platform to enhance further and or supplement the knowledge base and advance the skill level of the health informatician. Specialty certification helps to separate and professionalize the health informatician from other professionals. In doing so, the certification helps to bring together experts and create distinction within the HI field, which helps with teamwork, professional development, and learning from the different experts across the domains using a mutual level of engagement [1].

The Commission on Accreditation for Health Informatics and Information Management Education accreditation of educational programs (see Table 3.1) can also facilitate access to certification programs as well as certificates in spe-

Table 3.1 Overview of common certifications [8, 11, 15, 18, 19]

Professional organizations	Certification	Who should pursue it	Requirements	Renewal	Benefit
Healthcare Information and Management Systems Society (HIMSS)	Certified Associate in Health Information and Management Systems (CAHIMS)	Pathway for careers in health IT	High school diploma; 45 h of continuing education related to health information	Every 3 years	Offers professional development, networking, and library resources
	Certified Professional in Healthcare Information and Management Systems (CPHIMS)	Experience in healthcare information and management systems professionals	Bachelor's degree and 5 years of experience in information management, including 3 years in healthcare	Every 3 years	
	Certified Professional in Digital Health Transformation Strategy (CPDHTS)	Interest in managing and securing health information	Bachelor's degree and 5 years experience in information and management systems with 3 years in a healthcare setting	Every 2 years	
American Medical Informatics Association (AMIA)	Advanced Health Informatics Certification (AHIC)	Interest in mastery of health informatics	Master's degree in health profession/ informatics	Every 4 years	Networking opportunities, publications, offers educational programs, conferences, and meetings on various professional health care topics
	Board Certified in Clinical Informatics (CIS)	Interest in the intersection of healthcare, information technology, and data science	Unrestricted, current valid license(s) to practice medicine; medical degree. See the website for additional requirements	Every 10 years	
American Nursing Informatics Association (ANIA) www.ania.org	Informatics Nursing Certification (NI-BC)	Current practicing nurses interested in informatics	Current, active RN license; bachelor's degree; 2 years full-time practice as an RN; 30 h of continuing ed. in nursing informatics within the last 3 years; see website for more eligibility requirements	Every 5 years	Provides networking, education, and information resources that help to strengthen the role of nurses in the field of informatics
American Society of Health Informatics Managers (ASHIM)	Certified Health Informatics Systems Professional (CHIP)	Interest in organizing and managing healthcare information	Complete the ASHIM health IT professional training program or have 3 years of IT experience or a degree in computer science. See the website for additional requirements	Annually	Provides online training

(continued)

Table 3.1 (continued)

Professional organizations	Certification	Who should pursue it	Requirements	Renewal	Benefit
Society for Imaging Informatics in Medicine (SIIM)	PACS certification	Interested in archiving and communicating medical records, especially imaging data	No minimum requirement: Recommend enrolling in a PACA program before taking the certification exam, which will give you the content needed to be proficient	Every 3 years, including 10 h of continuing ed. or retake the exam	

cific areas such as Health Data Analyst (CHDA) or for a special area of completion such as being Certified in Healthcare Privacy and Security (CHPS). Obtaining certifications such as the Certified Professional in Healthcare Information and Management Systems (CHHIMS) and AMIA Health Informatics Certification (AHIC) adds credibility to a health informatician's career portfolio, which can help to establish more career opportunities. Obtaining certifications also demonstrates to potential employers a commitment to continuous learning and professional growth [12].

3.6 Ongoing Advancements and Opportunities

The field of HI offers diverse career pathways. The demand for skilled professionals in HI continues to surge. The more technology intertwines with healthcare, the more HI opportunities will continue to unfold.

3.6.1 Diverse Career Pathways

Health Informatics Traditional Roles: Traditional career paths in HI include roles such as clinical informaticians, nurse informaticians, health informatics managers, health informatics directors, and clinical data analysts [2]. However, the health informatician is no longer confined to working in these traditional roles in the clinic or hospital setting. The health information world now spans across many growing areas of specialization, such as consumer health informatics, public health informatics, and emerging fields in AI. Within these emerging fields, there are roles that include telehealth specialists, mobile health application developers, and AI specialists [12].

Health Informatics Emerging Roles: The impact of technological advances has created new job opportunities for informaticians in artificial intelligence. In this subarea of HI, informaticians use AI to create solutions to aid clinicians in administrative tasks, data analytics, and decision support. Health informaticians may use machine learning algorithms to analyze large datasets more efficiently and to harness the findings to improve healthcare. Bioinformatics informatics is another emerging area that deals with the application of cellular and molecular biology [25], which paves the way for employing genomic data scientists to conduct genetic dataset analysis to inform clinicians and patients of courses of action.

The widespread adoption of EHRs is another one of the opportunities for informaticians to utilize their skills to streamline and optimize health processes and improve patient care. Informaticians can also leverage their skills to extract meaningful healthcare data to help facilitate evidence-based decision-making, giving opportunities for roles like clinical informaticists, HI analysts, data analysts, or informatics consultants [2]. They can also help to shape policies and improve performance in the healthcare industry using data-driven procedures.

Artificial Intelligence, machine learning, analytics from extensive data sets, and genomics are among a few of the latest formations in HI [9, 10]. While HI remains a unique field of study, it has come a long way from data management to a field that aligns with changing technology. The use of this technology with patient care streamlines interior healthcare and supports research. Health informatics will still have a long history in the health field, and there is no shortage of work to be done by professionals, possessions of professions by recent certifications, and participation in professional organizations.

3.7 Challenges

With the dynamic field of HI, technological advancements require health informaticians to remain proactive in continuous learning to keep up with emerging trends and remain at the forefront of their field. As such, the informatician must make a concerted effort to keep abreast with technological advances in healthcare implications and know how and when to pivot their skills to match these changes [2]. Informaticians will also need to leverage technologies to help improve healthcare delivery. Additionally, privacy and security issues, interoperability concerns, and health data exchange remain challenges for health informaticians.

As discussed later in this textbook in this chapter on interoperability, the complexity of the healthcare system can be an issue when it comes to the exchange of health information between healthcare providers. Therefore, health informaticians need to be able to come together and standardize information to promote the integration of health information regardless of the varying sources to maintain patient-centered care.

3.7.1 Overview

The future of the health informatics career is promising, driven by rapid advancements in medical technologies and increasing consumer demand for medical information [7]. As healthcare systems digitize their processes and more healthcare data becomes available, the role of HI professionals becomes crucial in transforming and integrating healthcare information technologies. This includes EHRs, telehealth, telemedicine, and utilizing artificial intelligence for predictive analysis of clinical data and implementing functional data privacy and security to ensure efficient patient care and safety [23].

As modern healthcare technologies and research continue to evolve, careers in health informatics will expand into emerging roles, such as opportunities in research, biotechnology, public health, and pharmaceuticals. Professional organizations like AMIA and HIMSS will also continue to offer specialized certifications, professional development, and networking opportunities in this field. The involvement of HI professionals, along with policies, interoperability standards, and platforms for collaboration, will ensure that the field is adequately positioned to meet the future needs of healthcare.

3.7.2 Navigating Success

The field of HI offers many rewarding career opportunities. However, it requires a combination of different knowledge in technical expertise, medical and information sciences, and strong leadership skills to succeed [24]. Professionals and individuals considering "up-skilling and re-skilling" to learn a new skill for a new career [25] and are interested in digitizing the healthcare systems should consider pursuing educational degree programs and obtaining specialized certificates to enhance their career prospects and earning potential. Another point is that succeeding in the world of HI requires active participation in HI professional organizations, engaging in networking activities, collaboration, and staying up to date on industry trends. It also requires dedication and practical application in healthcare settings.

3.8 Conclusion

In summary, delving into the realm of health informatics by exploring various career paths, professional organizations, and certifications can offer invaluable insights into this ever-evolving field. Table 3.2 provides a comprehensive list of free online resources that aspiring informaticians can use to further their knowledge. With the demand for specialized expertise growing rapidly, informaticians play a pivotal role in driving innovation and improving patient care delivery. Professional organizations offer a platform for networking and continued education, allowing informaticians to stay up-to-date with the latest industry best practices. Additionally, certifications serve as a tangible demonstration of one's competence and skill in the workplace, enhancing employment prospects. Given the constantly evolving nature of technology and healthcare, staying informed through ongoing education, professional development, and collaboration is critical to excel in the field of health informatics.

Table 3.2 Learning resources for students

Name	Description	Permalink
HealthIT.gov	Information on health IT: Case studies, data, quick stats, apps	https://www.healthit.gov/
Coursera.org	Online courses in health informatics including specializations and certification	https://www.coursera.org/search?query=informatics&
MIT OpenCourseWare	Free access to MIT course materials related to health informatics and data	https://ocw.mit.edu/search/?q=health%20informatics
Health Informatician	Online forum for students/professionals to take free courses and to discuss topics in health informatics	https://www.health-informatician.com/
Data.gov	Datasets related to healthcare and informatics	https://data.gov/
Open access journal	Access to a variety of journals/research articles/publications in the health informatics field.	https://www.openaccessjournals.com/journals.html

Case Study/Vignette for Discussion

Maryanne recently graduated with an undergraduate degree in health informatics and is undecided about which career path to pursue. She has several options regarding her career path; however, she is unsure (a) which certification to pursue and whether it will impact her job opportunities, (b) which professional organization to join and how to network effectively in the field.

Answer

(a) A certification will help Maryanne to grow professionally and improve her employability by specializing within the field of health informatics. When deciding on a certification, Maryanne should consider what her career interests are, including the demands within the job market, the cost and time commitment for pursuing such certification. Two certifications that Maryanne can choose from are:
   (i) Certified Associate in Healthcare Information and Management Systems (CAHIMS) is an entry-level certification that will help Maryanne to understand healthcare information systems and provide the foundations for a more advanced role related to her career in health informatics.
   (ii) Certified Professional in Healthcare Information and Management Systems (CPHIMS) will help Maryanne to develop leadership skills in health IT or healthcare systems management.

(b) As part of Maryanne's professional development, continuing education and networking opportunities, there are many professional organizations she could consider joining that would help her to keep abreast with trends in the industry, such as the American Medical Informatics Association and the Healthcare Information and Management Systems Society. Both organizations will offer Maryanne the opportunity to access resources, networking opportunity as well as the opportunity to attend webinars and conferences.

Please see Table 3.1 *for a list of certifications, professional organizations, and their benefits.*

References

1. Hersh W. A stimulus to define informatics and health information technology. BMC Med Inform Decis Mak. 2009;9(1):24.
2. McLane TM, Hoyt R, Hodge C, Weinfurter E, Reardon EE, Monsen KA. What industry wants: an empirical analysis of health informatics job postings. Appl Clin Inform. 2021;12(2):285–92.
3. Hersh W. Who are the informaticians? What we know and should know. J Am Med Inform Assoc. 2006;13(2):166–70.
4. Kuziemsky C, Maeder A, John O, Gogia S, Basu A, Meher S, Ito M. Role of artificial intelligence within the telehealth domain. IMIA Yearb Med Inform. 2019;28(1):35–40.
5. Kluge EW. Health information professionals in a global eHealth world: ethical and legal arguments for the international certification and accreditation of health information professionals. Int J Med Inform. 2017;97:261–5.
6. Detmer DE, Munger BS, Lehmann CU. Clinical informatics board certification: history, current status, and predicted impact on the clinical informatics workforce. Appl Clin Inform. 2010;1(1):11–8.
7. Fridsma DB. The scope of health informatics and the advanced health informatics certification. J Am Med Inform Assoc. 2016;23(4):855–6.
8. Cummins M, Gundlapalli AV, Murray P, Park HA, Lehmann CU. Nursing informatics certification worldwide: history, pathway, roles, and motivation. Yearb Med Inform. 2016;25(01):264–71.
9. The Health Information Technology for Economic and Clinical Health (HITECH) Act. 2009.
10. Office of the National Coordinator for Health Information Technology. Available from: https://www.healthit.gov/topic/about-astponc.
11. Paolo L, Nicola R, Luca G, Mariano C. Health care information systems: architectural models and governance. In: Christos K, editor. Innovative information systems modelling techniques. Rijeka: IntechOpen; 2012. Ch. 4.
12. American Medical Informatics Association. 2023. Available from: https://amia.org/.
13. Sapci AH, Sapci HA. Teaching hands-on informatics skills to future health Informaticians: a competency framework proposal and analysis of health care informatics curricula. JMIR Med Inform. 2020;8(1):e15748.

14. Certified Health Informatics Systems Professional (CHISP) 2010. Available from: https://ashim.com/health-it-certification/.
15. Mantas J. Accreditation and certification in health informatics: principles and procedures. In: Informatics empowers healthcare transformation; 2017. p. 272–5.
16. Available from: https://www.cdc.gov/drugoverdose/data/statedeaths.html.
17. Murdoch B. Privacy and artificial intelligence: challenges for protecting health information in a new era. BMC Med Ethics. 2021;22(1):122.
18. AMIA. What is Informatics and Areas of Practice. 2023. Available from: https://amia.org/about-amia/why-informatics/informatics-research-and-practice.
19. Healthcare Information and Management Systems Society 2023. Available from: https://www.himss.org/resources-certification/overview.
20. Commission on Accreditation for Health Informatics and Information Management Education (CAHIIM) 2007. Available from: https://www.cahiim.org/.
21. Rob MA, Roy A. The value of IT certification: perspectives from students and IT personnel. Issues Inf Syst. 2013;14(1):153–61.
22. Gadd CS, Williamson JJ, Steen EB, Fridsma DB. Creating advanced health informatics certification. J Am Med Inform Assoc. 2016;23(4):848–50.
23. Yogesh MJ, Karthikeyan J. Health informatics: engaging modern healthcare units: a brief overview. Front Public Health. 2022;10:854688.
24. HIMSS TIGER Interprofessional community. Global informatics definitions. In: Reform TIGE, editor. HIMSS20220.
25. Gratton L. New frontiers in re-skilling and upskilling. MIT Sloan Manag Rev. 2019; Available from: https://sloanreview.mit.edu/article/new-frontiers-in-re-skilling-and-upskilling/.

4 Information Science: The Basics

James E. Andrews

Foundational Domains

This chapter addresses the following AMIA Foundational Domain: F2—Information Science and Technology.

Learning Objectives

1. Explain the core features and foundational elements of information science as a discipline.
2. Describe the essential elements and functions of information retrieval.
3. Outline the major features and approaches to knowledge and information organization.
4. Explain the central role of human information behavior to information science research and practice.
5. Describe examples of how information science methods and tools can be applied to health settings.

4.1 Introduction

Information is central to virtually every aspect of our lives. Each day we must access information in myriad forms from disparate sources to help us to manage our personal lives, function in our careers, support our health, and any number of other everyday contexts. The rapid advances in information and communication technologies over the past several decades have accelerated our ability to create, access, and share information with others across the globe. It is within this intersection of information, technology, and people that the discipline of information science focuses its research and practice.

Information science is a broad, interdisciplinary field. The study and practice of information science is concerned with understanding information in and of itself, including its creation, curation, dissemination, communication, use, maintenance, and other related functions supporting users across contexts. The complexities inherent in the study of information in all these stages requires contributions from intersecting disciplines in the development and practice of information science, including computer science, library science, communication and information technology, education, philosophy, cognitive science, and others. It is through highly integrated interactions and sharing of knowledge, methods, and perspectives that this interdisciplinary domain has emerged; and it has been accelerated with concomitant advances in computing and related technological advances.

The foundations of information science might be seen as stemming from several broad areas: computing and data sciences, information and communication technologies, people and social sciences, and, of course, information objects

J. E. Andrews (✉)
University of South Florida, School of Information, Tampa, FL, USA
e-mail: jimandrews@usf.edu

C. Eldredge et al. (eds.), *Introductory Textbook in Health Informatics*, Health Informatics,
https://doi.org/10.1007/978-3-032-16657-9_4

themselves, as a form of recorded knowledge and meaning. These tend to be the dominant perspectives that an information scientist or professional might use to frame their work and inquiry. These are not discrete, of course, as interactions across these areas are common and necessary as we look to address complex, information-focused problems that span contexts and subject areas. *Health informatics (HI)* shares many common features with information science and so they can be seen as "sibling" disciplines, albeit regarding HI, the primary orientation is healthcare across the ecosystem, from research, to practice, to education and workforce development, and the information challenges therein are what drive research, development, and practice in informatics. Below we review some core areas of information science that also support the primary aims of health informatics once brought into the health context.

4.2 Information as the Focus of the Field

The common thread in information science domains is information or knowledge in a variety of recorded forms. However, a challenge in any subject of study is agreeing what information is and how to define it. Each of us might feel like the meaning of information is intuitive or common enough that we all know what we mean by this term. In the various information fields (information science, informatics, information management, etc.) deriving a universally accepted definition of information can be elusive and challenging. In part, this stems from the variety of contexts in which we experience or think about information,; or the different concepts associated with the term itself (i.e., polysemy).

Given the range of contexts in which information science might operate, it may be best to avoid some of the more restrictive definitions of information in favor of more flexible ones. To this end, Case [1] builds from Bateson's commonly cited definition of information by suggesting information to be "...whatever appears significant to a human being, whether originating from an external environment or the (psychologically) internal world." [p. 56]. Similarly, it is useful to consult with the Oxford English Dictionary, which suggests information can be either a process or a type of message: "(a) The action of informing. The action of telling or fact of being told of something, (b) That of which one is apprised or told; intelligence, news." [1]. Other definitions tend to facilitate a certain area of study or specific context, but the above are general enough to serve as a starting point.

Information is often used quasi-synonymously or interchangeably with other terms, such as data or knowledge. This can be misleading, so some common reference is helpful. Figure 4.1 is similar to many other hierarchical representations of data, information, knowledge, and wisdom [2].

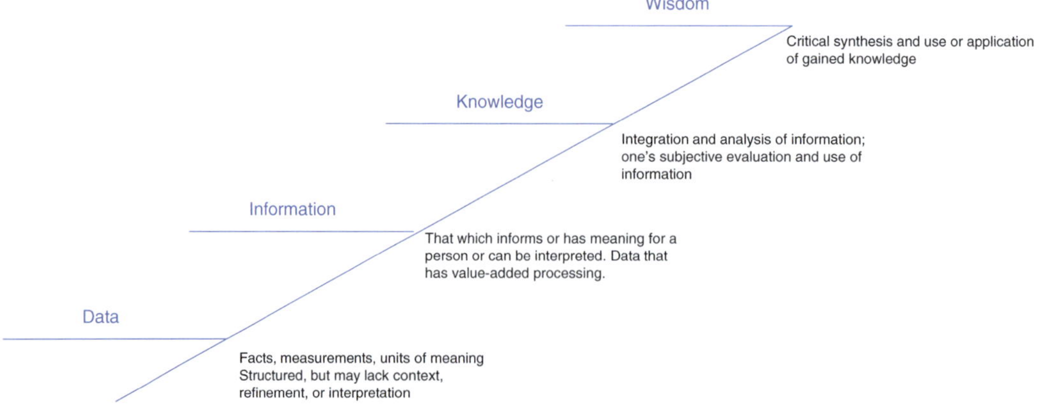

Fig. 4.1 Data, information, knowledge, wisdom hierarchy. (Adapted from Bawden and Robinson [2])

Though some may argue each of these terms has a more nuanced definition and relationships to one another that cannot be captured in a basic representation, such models have become a common starting point in many information-focused disciplines including information science and health informatics.

In the model, each layer builds upon the other and implies additional processing or value-added refinement as one moves up the hierarchy. Data would be at the bottom and has the most amount (volume) of content. We can consider data as facts or basic measured or observed elements that are the building blocks of information. That is, data are not information until they are processed or interpreted in some way so as to provide a level of meaning to them. Once value is added to data and it becomes information, then further, formal analysis and added value can lead to knowledge. Ultimately, how well one might draw from and apply certain knowledge can be seen as wisdom. Again, while this may be a rudimentary hierarchy it allows for a shared understanding of the distinctions in the concepts.

There are also various levels of communicating information, each with its own implied complexities [2]. The first level, *empiric*, is concerned with the physical transmission of information. Next is the *syntactic*, or the language or coding used to communicate a message. Third is the *semantic*, which refers to the meaning of the message; and fourth is the *pragmatic*, or the significance to the recipient, given a certain context [2, p.82]. These can each be envisioned in a common email: a message is to be sent using computing and communication protocols for sending email (empiric); it is encoded using some text formatting standard (such a Unicode) and translated into machine-readable format (syntactic); an attempt to communicate meaning comes from the phrasing of the message in some language, like English (semantic); and the effect or usefulness is determined by the recipient (pragmatic).

Information Theory is commonly evoked within formal discussions of information and communication. Information Theory was popularized by Claude Shannon in the 1940s, building on earlier work by Nyquist and Hartley, a few decades earlier [2]. The goal was to develop a mathematical approach to measuring transmission and successful communication of information in systems. As such, it is more relevant to the engineering and computing side of information (or, the empiric, as described earlier), and rather outside any detailed coverage in this chapter. This was originally for telegraph and telephone, and Shannon's statistical approach was meant to measure content of a message in terms of its symbols (i.e., not the "meaning" of a message) and how much of a message was accurately reproduced in transmission [2]. Thus, *entropy* is a core factor in information theory as it relates to the uncertainty, noise, or randomness that is introduced to a system that can impact amount and quality of information communicated.

4.3 Information Retrieval (IR)

Efficient and accurate retrieval of information objects from either formally or informally organized information sources has driven much work in information science and crosses many disciplinary boundaries. Most people in today's computationally sophisticated society are regular users of search engines (Google, Bing, etc.) and other tools that perform search and retrieval functions with amazing speed, and that present and link to the results and sources across the globe. While there are complex systems at work behind the scenes to enable these tools (not the least of which the miraculous advances in computing networks, standards, processing, and other features that have brought about our connected world), a brief discussion of the core features of IR can help guide future investigations.

Any discussion on IR implies information storage *and* retrieval. Although the storage of information can be relatively informal (such as a random collection of files or documents), we usually define *information storage* as "The transfer of information sources or some representation of knowledge to a durable material format, usually with the intention of being able to locate, retrieve, and logically manipulate documents or surrogates of documents for anticipated and unanticipated future needs." [3]. Other definitions show the IR portion of this; for instance: "The location and presentation to a user of information relevant to an information need expressed as a query" [4]. Reflected in each of these is that IR involves documents or information objects (widely defined), and their representation and organization to enable access and to meet some information need. This is all brought together with additional tools that enable processing, efficiency, and presentation.

In earlier days, before widespread access to personal computing devices that are able to access globally networked resources, retrieval would happen either physically (e.g., libraries, via card catalogs) or in a closed environment such as a local database or organization's information system. Today, the variety of information objects available in the digital realm, and places and means by which they are stored, is expansive to say the least. These can include tera- or petabytes of information in storage systems in the cloud, to other data repositories and warehouses of big data. A goal of IR is to efficiently retrieve the information from these and other sources. In other words, the *information problem* (per Baeza-Yates [3]) is how we can retrieve all documents related to a user's query while retrieving as few non-relevant ones as possible.

The below model (Fig. 4.2) represents the core elements of virtually any IR model or system. The simplicity of the model belies the complexity that underlies each of the components; however, it helps illustrate essential IR functions.

On the right, we might think of the various storehouses of information from which users have an interest in retrieving information. This can be the most complex of search engine databases generated by automated collection and indexing programs that scour the web, or a relatively straightforward student information system for a school, or even a personal database of one's pictures or other information. Moving toward the center, we recognize that these information objects must be logically represented to make them searchable in some way.

On the left side of the model is someone with an information need or needs. Like the information objects, the information need must be formalized into a query that is understandable and able to be processed by the IR system. The formalized queries (e.g., a formal or keyword search, say in PubMed or Google) would be processed by the IR system, compared to the information object surrogates (metadata), resulting in a set of matching items presented to the user. It is likely that there will be some non-relevant items retrieved, some partially relevant, and some relevant to what the user intended to find. A number of complex processes can be applied to the system to refine the retrieval set; also, users might refine their search criteria as they progress through the search process (e.g., as they learn more, the expressed need evolves). On the search side, there are many methods and standards to help guide in the classification and representation of information objects. Some of these are noted in the model above and briefly described below.

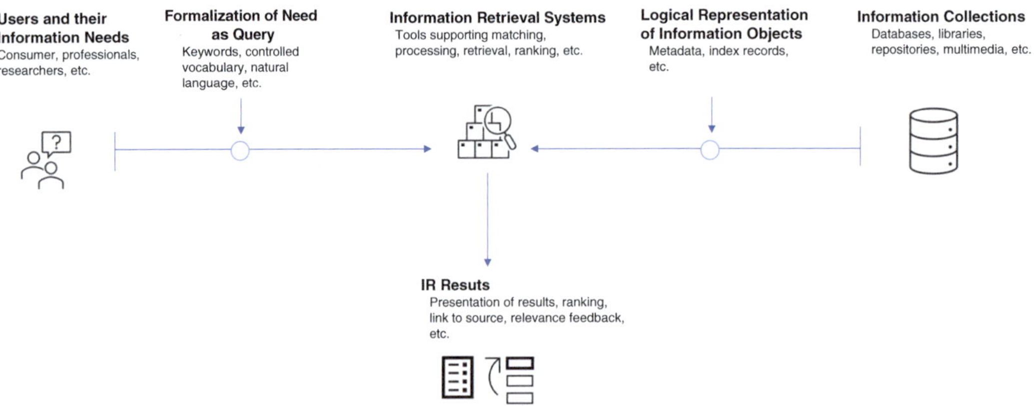

Fig. 4.2 Basic components of information retrieval. (Adapted in part from Baeza-Yates and Ribiero-Neto [3])

Of course, much of the information available to users today is in formats that are not easily represented by traditional standards and requires the use of advance computing methods.

In the early days of computing systems for IR, simple Boolean systems were used that could process search terms using Boolean operators (AND, OR, and NOT) in a logical sequence to help a user guide the IR system in refining a search. Eventually, systems advanced to include statistical approaches wherein term frequencies and distributions within a document and across a collection would be used to assign a term weight that can be used to discriminate relevant documents from non-relevant ones. The TF*IDF (Term frequency by Inverse document frequency) forumla is common to most modern IR systems that utilize term weighting or other text-based statistics. The highly technical systems of today (many of which are proprietary to search engine companies) are built on these earlier models with advanced technologies and approaches, such as probabilistic retrieval, inference-based models, AI of various kinds, and others.

4.3.1 Intersection of IR and Health Informatics

IR is one of the areas where information science and health informatics intersect. Healthcare is an information-intensive field, and the information comes in various forms and from disparate sources with the central aim of creating health knowledge and improving the practice of medicine as well as general operations. From biological data repositories, genomic data, patient registries, to electronic healthcare records, complex health-related data, and the systems to manage them drive the work of many informaticians.

Vast amounts of literature and other information resources are equally critical to the advancement of health science and the practice of medicine, and the tools methods of searching these fall within the scope of IR. Hersh [5] distinguishes between primary literature, consisting of original research and inquiry published in journal articles, conference proceedings, etc. and, secondly, knowledge-based information resources that include reviews, books, or other forms of condensing and synthesizing primary literature. A good example of this might be in the consumer/patient literature where findings in various health areas are synthesized, or various small manuals and guides [5].

Bibliographic information is available through libraries, publishing companies, and other organizers of information. Most notably, the National Library of Medicine (NLM) offers access to the largest collection of health and biosciences literature, with over 36 million citations and abstracts (https://pubmed.ncbi.nlm.nih.gov).

4.4 Information Behavior and Information Seeking

Information science is not only focused on how information is managed in computing systems, but also on the implications of the information for human beings as they seek and utilize information in navigating through a complex information society. The concept of *information behaviors* (IB) is overarching and subsumes a variety of actions. These would include both *intentional* (actively seeking information) and *unintentional* (serendipitous or passive information exposure) or other information-related behaviors including purposeful *information avoidance*, which might occur for any number of reasons [1].

IB involves several component concepts. First, *information need* generally refers to the recognition of a gap between what one knows and wants to know [2]. A need can be conscious or subconscious and may or may not be well articulated by the individual. Moreover, even a recognized need does not necessarily result in subsequent information actions. The primary action we tend to look at is *information seeking*, which refers to the purposive acquisition of information from selected information carriers or sources to satisfy a recognized gap or need [9]. We often find, however, that individuals will not seek information to fill a need, or even actively avoid information [6]. Not seeking information can come in various forms, particularly in health contexts, such as information avoidance, blunting, coping, or dissonance. For instance, if a person feels they may have a genetic predisposition to a certain disease for which there are no known treatments or cures, this may cause discomfort and fear that could lead to disinclination to seek out information confirming whether or not they have or will have it (genetic testing or screening, for instance). Another concept, *information use,* relates to how information gained through information seeking is used to close a gap or otherwise lead to other information actions or a decision [2]. Other actions might also be considered following *information acquisition*, such as *information sharing* within one's personal or social network. This, too, is often seen in health contexts such as across patient support or advocacy groups online.

4.4.1 Models and Theories

As with any human behaviors, information actions are highly individualized and so it is difficult to make any generalizations. As Line noted, we are all individuals and will seek and use information in different ways, "...There is no such thing as a homogenous body of information users" [7]. This makes studying information behaviors challenging, and partly explains the many theories and models that have emerged in IB. However, if we hope to learn more about what motivates or impedes certain types of IB, and how we might use such knowledge to better inform the development of systems, services, and information interventions, then these can help guide investigations.

Information behavior theories and models help frame our understanding and perspectives, guide research questions, and are used to build a body of knowledge that is ultimately useful in practice. The term theory, in information science and other social sciences, suggests some level of developed understanding, or an explanation, for how we believe things operate. This includes the assumptions and hypotheses that we may have, or will test, that help strengthen and fine-tune this framework of understanding. We might start by drawing from theories from other disciplines to help study phenomenon in information science since it is inherently interdisciplinary. There are many theories that relate to IB alone, though it is outside the scope of this chapter to detail all these. For an excellent review, however, see Fisher, Erdelez, and Mechenzie's book, *Theories of Information Behavior* [8].

Models help us explore processes and test our hypotheses as we construct a theory. They are popular in that they help us represent, often using graphics, the relationships among core concepts and elements [9]. There are many in IB, particularly in health contexts. These can be categorized depending on their structure and use, and range from more descriptive models (e.g., Wilson's Model of Information Seeking), to process models that show causal relationships across factors in a process (such as Johnson's Comprehensive Model of Information Seeking, or CMIS [10]), to cognitive and complex models that integrate additional environmental or contextual elements and may be much more detailed and elaborate [2].

Models should reflect an idea of processes and relationships, among factors influencing information behaviors, to explore and explain IB in certain contexts and across groups. For instance, the CMIS has been empirically tested, and has been used as a framework for investigating information seeking in cancer contexts [10–12]. The CMIS represents antecedent factors and characteristics or information carriers/channels that may impact information-seeking actions. It has been recommended for use in understanding health and cancer information-seeking behaviors.

Health information seeking has been a focus of study for informatics, information science, and communication researchers focused on health contexts and behaviors. As Johnson and Case note, "... information seeking is a key facilitator for promoting, maintaining, and returning to health as broadly conceived" [9]. People's interaction with health information enables them to be more engaged in decisions related to their own care, better adjust to changes in their health status, and to engage in behaviors that could lead to early detection and prevention and other health outcomes [11]. Health information seeking, then, is a salient example of the power information actions can have and, therefore, consumer health informatics and related areas seek to advance the design, implementation, and evaluation of tools and interventions that can impact health information actions.

4.5 Organization and Classification of Information

Addressing the information problem implies that information is organized in such a way that it is retrievable. Each of us organizes information in our personal and professional lives every day, whether informally or according to some proscribed set of standards or protocols. From our personal documents to files or images on our phones, to our books or video collections, we apply some type of organizing system to the things in our lives (both digital and physical) to facilitate our interactions with them [13]. As a society, humans have more formally organized and classified information for hundreds of years. Information science emerged as a discipline in part to develop tools that support, formalize, and help in the progress related to how we might organize information for retrieval.

Of specific interest to this discussion are the methods of information organization, also referred to as knowledge organization. In information science, the focus of information organization is how to represent information objects in all formats in order to facilitate user interaction with them; that is *retrieval, access,* and *use*. This often involves a variety of specialized tools and standards to classify concepts logically to also support access, retrieval, and maintenance. Of interest to modern information organization practitioners is how traditional approaches have been adopted and modified into modern uses. Below, we look only at a few of the more common approaches used to organize the information world around us.

4.5.1 Metadata

The term *Metadata* is commonly defined as "data about data." A definition from the Oxford English Dictionary, which is a bit more descriptive, defines it, "data whose purpose is to describe and give information about other data." The latter suggests that metadata are structured data about information objects. Metadata might involve a range of approaches given the need, context, and information object of interest. For instance, traditional library catalog records (the card catalog) are formalized descriptions and representations (the catalog record) of an information object (say, a book). But metadata can be an index record, digital or print, or the embedded information for a digital document in a coding scheme such as XML [2]. What is important to recognize here is that metadata collectively constitutes a surrogate representation of the actual item. These may vary in structure and detail but are nevertheless a representation of an information object designed to help locate it in a collection.

There are many metadata schemes and standards developed for different reasons and using both manual and automated approaches. Metadata schemes could be some variation on traditional bibliographic control, for instance, with the goal of creating bibliographic surrogates of books, articles, and similar items in a standardized way to enable retrieval from diverse systems. Other metadata approaches are driven by the need to support information sharing of online or digital resources of all sorts. These may be integrated, of course, as access and use of information is increasingly done online [2].

The traditional bibliographic approach can be separated into two main categories, *descriptive metadata* and *subject metadata*. Descriptive metadata is used to describe who created the work (author), what it is called (title), the size, where it is located, and other characteristics. Subject metadata refers to its *aboutness* or the topics that are discussed in the document or item. The extent of description and level of detail or granularity will vary greatly for different objects (a small webpage versus some in-depth text or other information resource). Moreover, the standards for what is allowable in each element vary depending on the metadata scheme employed. The subject description will include either keywords selected by the creator of the metadata file, or some controlled terminology as is described in greater detail in Chap. 25.

The traditional and more formal approaches have a long tradition and are extensively standardized in their development and implementation. The most common one comes from libraries, the Machine Readable Catalog (MaRC) record (https://www.loc.gov/marc/). This standard was developed decades ago in the early period of computing and is an exemplar of interoperability of bibliographic and related information across libraries and information agencies. MaRC was prescient in seeking to develop a flexible and extensible standard to enable the creation of bibliographic surrogates (catalog records that library systems are based on) that can be shared across various institutions and enabling bibliographic control within a collection.

4.5.2 Indexing

Indexing records are another form of traditional bibliographic metadata schemes. *Indexing* is generally used to describe citations for journal articles and similar information objects. Historically, these were originally in print, of course. Overtime, standards to better enable search and retrieval have evolved along with evolving computing and network technologies. For instance, *Index Medicus* was created in the late nineteenth century and was an extensive resource for seeking out articles on certain topics in biomedicine. This served as the basis for the online version, MEDLARS and eventually MEDELINE, which is the most extensive online database for biomedical literature and available for free via PubMed by the National Library of Medicine (NLM) [5]. A brief look at a typical PubMed (MEDLINE) record (Fig. 4.3) shows the various descriptive and subject elements that collectively form the metadata informing us what the article is, where it is published, what it is about, who wrote it, etc.

As resources on the Internet and WWW have grown, including many created by individual people and not from traditional creators and publishers of information, the need for metadata schemes emerged. Dublin Core (DC) is one of the most common and popular. It was developed to be simple enough for any web content creator to use (e.g., non-catalogers). The idea is that if

```
PMID- 16059425
OWN - NLM
STAT- MEDLINE
DCOM- 20051025
LR  - 20181113
IS  - 1536-5050 (Print)
IS  - 1558-9439 (Electronic)
IS  - 1536-5050 (Linking)
VI  - 93
IP  - 3
DP  - 2005 Jul
TI  - Avoiding versus seeking: the relationship of information seeking to avoidance,
      blunting, coping, dissonance, and related concepts.
PG  - 353-62
AB  - QUESTION: How have theorists and empirical researchers treated the human tendency
      to avoid discomforting information? DATA SOURCES: A historical review (1890-2004)
      of theory literature in communication and information studies, coupled with
      searches of recent studies on uptake of genetic testing and on coping strategies
      of cancer patients, was performed. STUDY SELECTION: The authors' review of the
      recent literature included searches of the MEDLINE, PsychInfo, and CINAHL
      databases between 1992 and summer of 2004 and selective, manual searches of
      earlier literature. Search strategies included the following subject headings and
      key words: MeSH headings: Genetic Screening/psychology, Decision Making,
      Neoplasms/diagnosis/genetics/psychology; CINAHL headings: Genetic Screening,
      Genetic Counseling, Anxiety, Decision Making, Decision Making/Patient; additional
      key words: avoidance, worry, monitoring, blunting, cancer. The "Related Articles"
      function in MEDLINE was used to perform additional "citation pearl" searching.
      MAIN RESULTS: The assumption that individuals actively seek information underlies
      much of psychological theory and communication practice, as well as most models
      of the information-seeking process. However, much research has also noted that
      sometimes people avoid information, if paying attention to it will cause mental
      discomfort or dissonance. Cancer information in general and genetic screening for
      cancer in particular are discussed as examples to illustrate this pattern.
      CONCLUSION: That some patients avoid knowledge of imminent disease makes
      avoidance behavior an important area for social and psychological research,
      particularly with regard to genetic testing.
FAU - Case, Donald O
AU  - Case DO
AD  - School of Library and Information Science, University of Kentucky, 502 King
      Library, South Lexington, Kentucky 40506, USA. dcase@uky.edu
FAU - Andrews, James E
AU  - Andrews JE
FAU - Johnson, J David
AU  - Johnson JD
FAU - Allard, Suzanne L
AU  - Allard SL
LA  - eng
PT  - Historical Article
PT  - Journal Article
PL  - United States
TA  - J Med Libr Assoc
JT  - Journal of the Medical Library Association : JMLA
JID - 101132728
SB  - IM
CIN - J Med Libr Assoc. 2006 Oct;94(4):375. PMID: 17082826
MH  - Adaptation, Psychological
MH  - *Attitude to Health
MH  - Cognitive Dissonance
MH  - *Defense Mechanisms
MH  - History, 19th Century
MH  - History, 20th Century
MH  - Humans
MH  - Information Storage and Retrieval/*history
MH  - Library Services/*history
MH  - Patient Compliance
MH  - Patient Education as Topic/*history
MH  - United States
PMC - PMC1175801
EDAT- 2005/08/02 09:00
MHDA- 2005/10/26 09:00
PMCR- 2005/07/01
CRDT- 2005/08/02 09:00
PHST- 2005/08/02 09:00 [pubmed]
PHST- 2005/10/26 09:00 [medline]
PHST- 2005/08/02 09:00 [entrez]
PHST- 2005/07/01 00:00 [pmc-release]
PST - ppublish
SO  - J Med Libr Assoc. 2005 Jul;93(3):353-62.
```

Fig. 4.3 Example of a MEDLINE record

more people might adopt this metadata standard, information would be more accessible on a global scale (e.g., interoperability which will be discussed further in later chapters of this book). Beyond simplicity and interoperability, DC was designed based on international consensus, and also to be extensible so that it could accommodate various types of metadata needs.

4.6 Summary

A commonality between information science and health informatics is that both go beyond the mere application of information and computing technologies to broader information issues. They are complex disciplines that seek to understand and affect the interactions among people, information, and technology within a given domain. At the core of each discipline is to understand information in and of itself, and to focus on the communities within which it is created, stored, communicated, disseminated, and ultimately its value to those who need it to make decisions or create new knowledge.

The tools and foundations of information science are common across other information fields, including health informatics. Obviously, however, the specific focus of these efforts is driven by the context. Challenges in such areas as information storage and retrieval share many essential features across these diverse information contexts and will benefit from new discoveries and tools that continue to emerge to make these processes more efficient and effective. Part of the role of information professionals, then, is to understand the people and communities creating and using information in all its forms, and to create models and theories to help guide future appreciation for their needs and actions. The heavy focus on humans and their interactions with information and technology is, indeed, the distinguishing feature of information science in comparison to other technology-focused fields. This emphasis fits well with health informatics, given its focus on the health and well-being of people.

References

1. Case DO, Given LM, editors. Looking for information: a survey of research on information seeking, needs, and behavior. 4th ed. UK: Emerald Group Publishing Limited; 2016.
2. Bawden D, Robinson L. Introduction to information science. 2nd ed. Facet Publishing; 2022.
3. Baeza-Yates R, Ribeiro-Neto B. Modern information retrieval. 2nd ed. Addison-Wesley; 2011.
4. Korfhage RR. Information storage and retrieval. Wiley; 1997.
5. Hersh W. Information retrieval. In: Shortliffe EH, Cimino JJ, Chiang MF, editors. Biomedical informatics: computer applications in health care and biomedicine. 5th ed. Springer; 2021.
6. Case DO, Andrews JE, Johnson JD, Allard SL. Avoiding versus seeking: the relationship of information seeking to avoidance, blunting, coping, dissonance, and related concepts. J Med Libr Assoc. 2005;93(3):353–62.
7. Line MB. Designing libraries round human beings. Aslib Proc. 1998;5(8):221–9.
8. Fisher KE, Erdelez S, McKechnie LEF. Theories of information behavior. Medford: Information Today; 2005.
9. Johnson JD, Case DO. Health information seeking. Peter Lang; 2012.
10. Johnson JD. Cancer-related information seeking. Cresskill: Hampton Press; 1997.
11. Andrews JE, Applequist J, Ward HL, Fuzzell LN, Vadaparampil ST. Cancer-related information behavior among black and hispanics in an NCI-designated comprehensive cancer center catchment. Patient Educ Couns. 2023;114:107812.
12. Andrews JE, Johnson JD, Case DO, Allard S, Kelly K. Intention to seek information on cancer genetics. Inf Res. 2005;10(4):238.
13. Glushko RJ. The discipline of organizing. 4th ed. Berkeley Press; 2016.

5 Computer Science Review: The Basics

Stephen E. Bronsburg and Vanessa D'Amario

Foundational Domains

This chapter addresses the following AMIA Foundational Domains: F2—Information Science and Technology, F4—Health Information Science and Technology.

Learning Objectives

1. Describe computer technology infrastructure, hardware, and software.
2. Summarize the characteristics of data communications and networking.
3. Articulate how the fundamentals of computer programming concepts are applied in health informatics.

5.1 Introduction

Computer science is a broad area covering computers, hardware, software, network design, data transmission, computing, data modeling, programming, and artificial intelligence [1]. The field of computer science is an important foundational component of health informatics. This chapter cannot cover every area of computer science, so it focuses on universal fundamental basics from the specific health informatics point of view. Despite the vastity of computer science and intersections among areas in this field, the structure of this chapter follows the characterization of CHHIMS (fourth ed), 2022. This states that the basics of the computer environment are hardware, software, and network (see Fig. 5.1). As it will become clearer along this chapter, it is hard to draw a neat line among the three areas. Across this chapter, several concepts including hardware, software, basic computer networking, digital data, and computer programming will be introduced. These foundational concepts are part of the critical knowledge and background that health informatics professionals are expected to know.

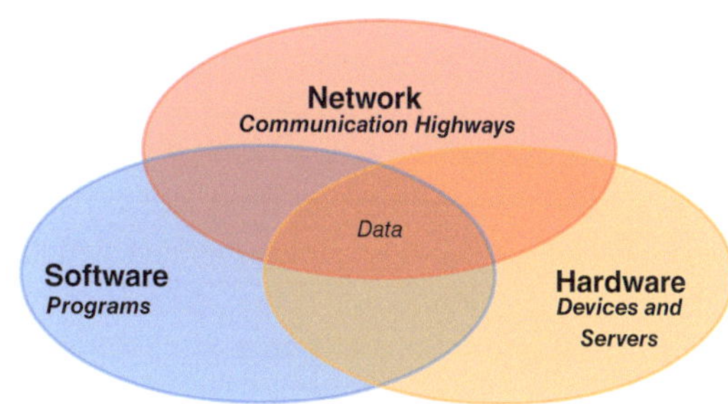

Fig. 5.1 Basic computer environment. Note: This figure depicts the relationship of the network, software, hardware, and data environment. Created by the chapter's authors

Stephen E. Bronsburg and Vanessa D'Amario contributed equally to this work.

S. E. Bronsburg (✉) · V. D'Amario
Department: Health Informatics, Nova Southeastern University, Fort Lauderdale, FL, USA
e-mail: bronsbur@nova.edu; vdamario@nova.edu

C. Eldredge et al. (eds.), *Introductory Textbook in Health Informatics*, Health Informatics,
https://doi.org/10.1007/978-3-032-16657-9_5

5.2 Hardware

Computer hardware has gone through major changes over the last half century. The first-generation computers 1940–1956 were based on vacuum tubes and were large and bulky, the size of a classroom [2]. Since then, technological advancements had led to the current stage where hardware is heavily optimized to perform multiple operations at the same time.

Computers are an electronic device capable of capturing, storing, and processing data as well as to perform mathematical calculations. As such, while computer architectures can be very different (laptop, desktop, clusters), some key characteristics are shared.

The key element of a computer is its *Central Processing Unit* (CPU) which has several functions. The Arithmetic and Logic Unit (ALU) performs calculations, the control unit (CU) is responsible for data flow control, and the memory registers perform data storage and processing. The CPU houses the control unit and logic unit. An additional computational unit is the Graphical Processing Unit (GPU). GPUs were originally developed to render graphics because of their ability to manage many calculations at the same time and have been more recently adopted in several Artificial Intelligence (AI) applications.

Since computation is performed on data, another fundamental element in a computer is data storage in memory. A computer has two major forms of memory: *primary memory* and *secondary memory*. Primary memory is fast-access and mostly short-term, easily accessible for operations from the CPU but gone as the computer is turned off. Random Access Memory (RAM) is the main primary memory. Read Only Memory (ROM) is also a primary memory which makes an exception by being permanently encoded to disk [3], but easily accessible through CPU. Secondary memory is slower to access and typically much larger than primary memory. Examples of secondary memory include Solid State Drive (SSD) and hard-disk drive.

Hardware also includes a set of other physical components for interfacing with the user such as *input units* (keyboard, mouse, scanner, and joystick) and output units (terminal, laptop, speaker, monitor) [4].

5.3 Software and Applications

Software programs instruct or command hardware to perform an operation. The two types of software are *application* and *systems software*. Application software performs specific functions such as opening and editing a document (e.g., MS Word), streaming content (e.g., Spotify), or browsing the Internet (e.g., GoogleChrome). Systems software, on the other hand, runs in the background and manages the computer itself and its utilities. Operating Systems (OS) are an example of system software. Popular OSs include Microsoft Windows, macOS (Macintosh Operating System), and Linux open-source OS. Smartphone operating systems include iOS for iPads and iPhones, and Android for smartphones.

Software can be further distinguished as *open-source* or *proprietary*. Open-source means that the source code is available on the Internet, and the community can modify and test it. Examples of open-source software are Linux and Firefox. Proprietary software is owned by a company, and the source code is only available to the organization's programmers. Examples of proprietary software are Windows and Skype.

Applications in Healthcare. Clinical applications encompass specialized software programs including those for administration, clinical care support, and picture archiving and communication systems (PACS) (CPHIMS 2021). Focusing on health informatics, the primary software programs used include *electronic health records* (EHR), *electronic medical records* (EMR), and *personal health records (PHR)*. This is discussed at length in Chap. 10.

Firmware is another piece of the computer system responsible for lower-level functions of the computer and sits in the computer's memory "software for hardware". Firmware is the critical link between hardware and software ensuring reliable device operations and supports updates for improved functionality.

5.4 Communications and Networking

There are two primary conceptual frameworks for network communications used to understand how data stored in a computer is transferred from one device to another: the Open Systems Interconnection Reference (OSI) Model and the Transmission Control *Protocol/Internet Protocol* (TCP/IP).

Both the OSI and TCP/IP models are theoretical and are sets of layers, which depict how computer systems communicate using network-specific protocols. Protocols outline the transmission of data from one area to another. Both models help to understand the processes or steps in the network architecture so if something goes wrong or there is an issue those managing the system such as network engineers can pinpoint what part of the computer communication process is being affected. Prior to 1984 computer-to-computer communications were not standardized [5].

The OSI Model consists of seven layers compared to the TCP/IP model which has four layers. Both models are compared in Fig. 5.2. Notice in Fig. 5.2 how data changes as it transmits through the OSI model starting at the physical layer with raw data or bits.

Layer 1 of the OSI Model is the Physical Layer. The physical layer transmits unstructured raw data (0 s and 1 s), encodes it, and decides where it is going including how many bits per second, what voltage is used as well as the connectors and cable used. Layer 2 of the OSI Model is the Data Link Layer. The data link layer takes the data (bits) from the physical link layer and packages them into frames to be digitally transmitted. Frames are checked for errors and corrections are made if needed. *Switches* operate in the data link layer performing error checking and transferring data to its destination. Layer 3 of the OSI Model is the Network Layer. The network layer determines the best route to send the packets to the appropriate computer.

Layer 4 of the OSI Model is the Transport Layer. The transport layer handles network end-to-end issues. It manages logical connections, eliminates duplication, and performs error control. Layer 5 of the OSI Model is the Sessions Layer. The sessions layer manages computer sessions by establishing connections, maintaining connections, terminating the session, transferring files, and doing security. Layer 6 of the OSI Model is the Presentation Layer. The presentation layer formats the data to be used by the application layer. Layer 7 of the OSI Model is the Application Layer. The application layer is what the end user accesses. The two noticeable differences in the models are that the TCP/IP model layer 1 performs the functions of the OSI Model layers 1, 2, and 3. Layer 4 of the TCP/IP model performs the functions of the OSI Model layers 6 and 7.

A *network* is the component which allows computers to transmit, receive, and share information. Networks are characterized by several elements, among those, nodes, links, topologies, and communication standards. *Nodes* are physical devices, like laptops and tablets, which send, receive, and store data. On a larger scale are servers which are capable of storing and processing much larger amounts of data. These nodes are

Sending

Data	OSI Model Layers	TPC/IP Model Layers
Data	7 Application	4 Application
	6 Presentation	
	5 Session	
Segment	4 Transport	3 Transport
Packets	3 Network	2 Network
Frames	2 Data Link	1 Network Interface
Bits	1 Physical	

Receiving

Fig. 5.2 OSI and TCP/IP models. Note. How data flows through both the OSI and TP/IP models. Created by the chapter's authors

interconnected by *links* using transportation modes that include wire and/or wireless system to communicate [5]. The third piece is the *topology* of a network, which describes how the nodes are physically connected, the presence of a hierarchy, etc. Lastly, there is a *communication standard*, which dictates the rules of how information is transmitted or received. One major example of networking is the *Internet.*

5.4.1 Network Types and Definitions

Networks may span over short distances or be more expansive. A *Local Area Network (LAN)* may consist of an office floor or campus [6]. A *Wide Area Network (WAN)* covers a much larger area and may connect smaller networks to each other [6]. A *body area network (BAN)* operates within a few meters range. An example of this is using remote patient monitoring devices to collect blood pressure, glucose levels, and heart rate.

There are four main types of networks: Internet, intranet, extranet, and Virtual Private Network (VPN). The Internet is public. An Internet service provider (ISP) such as Sprint or AT&T connects with each other moving enormous amounts of data through high-speed broadband technologies. The intranet is a private network allowing individuals and organizations to share data and information within the Health Care Organization (HCO). An extranet extends an intranet incorporating strong security requiring username and password. A VPN provides strong security for users of an HCO to transmit data through encrypted tunnel blocking. Providers can access patient data securely [7].

Case Study: Implementing a Digital Medical Record, San Cristobal, Galapagos (Ecuador)

The case study is an ongoing academic project and is a demonstration of how health informatics plays a key role in this medical outreach trip, by digitalizing a paper-based medical record.

During a medical outreach trip, a variety of data including demographic information, vital signs, diagnosis, and medications. A paper-based record-keeping system is riddled with multiple issues including legibility, lost pages, missed documentation, and security, and maintaining a medication inventory is excessively time-consuming. This medication inventory is necessary to identify shortages which would prompt administration to purchase them to replenish stock for the next day.

Given all these limitations, several attempts were made to digitalize this process with limited or no results. The major obstacle was that the internet connection was limited, and bandwidth was spotty. In 2023, access to the internet was expanded through satellite connection in the Galapagos. This provided an opportunity to create an online digital data collection instrument, to capture data at check-in, triage, visit content at multiple provider stations, pharmacy, and discharge. The tool selected was an existing academic secure web application which allows for customizable data capture.

Medical students and healthcare providers used laptops and tablets to digitally access the forms. Once data was collected and recorded in the digital forms, it was automatically available to all providers, thus, eliminating any duplication of efforts such as data collection, procedures, or medications. This equated to better-informed caregivers about the overall health of the population they were working with. Time and effort were streamlined in several areas such as medical service workstation to workstation, patient data and information transfer, identification of health care needs, and dispensing of medication and medication inventory. Further, this critical information is now digitally available for training purposes including analysis, evaluation of the population's needs, and preparation for future outreach trips.

5.5 Data and Storage in a Computer

Data is the general collection of quantities, facts, and statistics, that can assume the form of text, images, and numbers. Computers are built to handle and store data. At their core, computers operate through binary computation, utilizing *bits* as the basic units of digital information [8]. In traditional computing systems, bits can be assumed between one of two possible states: "0" or "1", which can also be interpreted as True or False. Every piece of data within a computer is translated into and stored as a sequence of these binary values. Since binary is not a natural format for human comprehension, computers are designed to interact with humans in more understandable forms [9].

A prime example of this adaptation is the *ASCII (American Standard Code for Information Interchange) system* [10]. ASCII incorporates a wide array of standard characters used in text writing. It works by assigning a unique 7-bit binary string to each symbol in its repertoire (see Fig. 5.3). For instance, the character "A" is represented by the binary sequence 1,000,001, while "a" is represented by 1,000,011, and so forth. Although these binary codes are the actual format in which information is stored and processed within a computer, they are seamlessly translated into familiar characters and symbols.

Building on the concept of binary computation, it is important to understand that all types of digital information—not just text—are encoded as well. The smallest measurable unit of an image or a video is a pixel, which encodes the intensity of colors through specific binary sequences.

When we discuss data, a key attribute to consider is the amount of storage they occupy. A standard metric is the byte, which is defined as a string of 8 bits. A byte can represent 2^8 or 256 possible values. Being aware of the amount of memory data occupied is crucial for identifying the storage capacity of hardware, as well as the

Bits				b_7 b_6 b_5 →	0 0 0	0 0 1	0 1 0	0 1 1	1 0 0	1 0 1	1 1 0	1 1 1
b_4 ↓	b_3 ↓	b_2 ↓	b_1 ↓	Column → / Row ↓	0	1	2	3	4	5	6	7
0	0	0	0	0	NUL	DLE	SP	0	@	P	`	p
0	0	0	1	1	SOH	DC1	!	1	A	Q	a	q
0	0	1	0	2	STX	DC2	"	2	B	R	b	r
0	0	1	1	3	ETX	DC3	#	3	C	S	c	s
0	1	0	0	4	EOT	DC4	$	4	D	T	d	t
0	1	0	1	5	ENQ	NAK	%	5	E	U	e	u
0	1	1	0	6	ACK	SYN	&	6	F	V	f	v
0	1	1	1	7	BEL	ETB	'	7	G	W	g	w
1	0	0	0	8	BS	CAN	(	8	H	X	h	x
1	0	0	1	9	HT	EM	)	9	I	Y	i	y
1	0	1	0	10	LF	SUB	*	:	J	Z	j	z
1	0	1	1	11	VT	ESC	+	;	K	[	k	{
1	1	0	0	12	FF	FS	,	<	L	\	l	|
1	1	0	1	13	CR	GS	—	=	M	]	m	}
1	1	1	0	14	SO	RS	.	>	N	^	n	~
1	1	1	1	15	SI	US	/	?	O	_	o	DEL

Fig. 5.3 ASCII Table. Note. ASCII standard characters used in text writing. Created by an unknow employee of the United States government

Table 5.1 Data dimensions are expressed as multiples of bits and bytes

Unit	Conversion	Example
1 byte [B]	8 bites	ASCII characters
1 kilobyte [KB]	1024 B	A paragraph in a document
1 megabyte [MB]	1024 kB	An image
1 gigabyte [GB]	1024 MB	A video
1 terabyte [TB]	1024 GB	All the X-rays in a hospital
1 petabyte [PB]	1024 TB	4000 mammograms per day, over an entire life
1 exabyte [EB]	1024 PB	A videocall longer than 200,000 years
1 zettabyte [ZB]	1024 EB	All information streamed through internet globally [Xu, Z. W. [11]]
1 yottabyte [YB]	1024 ZB	1 B for each star in the universe [12]

Note. Data dimensions are expressed as multiples of bits and bytes. Created by the chapter's authors

capacity to process and transform data. Memory is typically expressed as denoted in Table 5.1.

5.6 Computer Programming Overview

The versatility of computer systems spans a vast list of functionalities. Indeed, the case study above shows us the integration of computer technology into the clinical routine at different stages. The flexibility and complexity of computer operations, which include the generation of systems of data collection, the ability to connect to networks, and the possibility of manipulating data, stems from the capability of programmers to build instructions for machines. In this section, we introduce concepts of logic and computer programming.

5.6.1 Programming

Programming can be compared to the process of architectural design. Just as architect plans and details all the aspects in a building, from the foundation to the roof, considering both functionality and aesthetics, a programmer must detail all the components of the code, structuring the steps logically, and anticipating potential issues to ensure the realization of a functional computer program.

In this process, programmers engage with computational thinking on multiple levels. In the initial phase, the programmer defines the program's objectives and identifies the specific goals to be achieved. The next stage requires the choice of appropriate computational tools and the identification of methods and logical steps to reach these goals. Assessing the complexity of a program is crucial, as it influences the execution time and resource required.

After these considerations, programmers must assess the operational environment for the program. This phase involves designing comprehensive tests to ensure the program's correct functionality across scenarios. Once this phase is completed, the program is ready to be implemented. This is not a solo effort, and it requires extensive planning and collective effort.

5.6.2 Overview of Programming Languages

Communicating with computers necessitates specific syntax—a programming language that translates human-readable instruction into machine-executable binary code. Computer programs operate using languages that are distinctly different from human language, characterized by their precision and lack of ambiguity. Unlike the nuanced and often multi-interpretable nature of human communication, programming languages are designed to be equivocal, ensuring that each instruction is interpreted in only one way by the computer.

Numerous programming languages exist, each with its unique features and capabilities. They are characterized by paradigms, as functional [13], object-oriented [14], and logic [15]. A detailed description of those goes beyond the scope of this chapter. Nonetheless, it is worth noting that each paradigm offers a unique way of thinking about how to structure and execute the code, and those sometimes complement each other. For this rea-

Table 5.2 Programming languages and applications

Language	Language level	Example of usage in healthcare
SQL	High level	Querying patient databases, electronic health records management.
Python	High level	Data analysis, clinical analysis, AI in medical imaging, and natural language processing.
R	High level	Statistical modeling for clinical and research studies.
MATLAB	High level	Signal processing of physiological measures.
Java	High-level	Backend development for hospital management systems.
C	Intermediate	Embedded in some medical products with limited memory.
C++	Intermediate	Embedded in many medical imaging software.
C#	High-level	Used for image and communication standards.
JavaScript	High-level	Interactive visualization in web applications.
Ruby	High-level	For web platforms for telemedicine and health data portals.
Bash	Low-level	Automating data pipelines for operations on large health datasets.
Assembly	Low-level	Firmware development for medical devices like pacemakers.

Note. Common programming languages and examples of application in the healthcare field. Created by the chapter's authors

son, depending on the specific requirements and the nature of the application, certain languages may align more closely with a programmer's needs than others. Table 5.2 contains a small selection of some programming languages among the many options available.

High, Intermediate, and Low-Level Languages This distinction clarifies the extent to which programming languages rely on strong abstractions: they become more comprehensible to humans but further from computational operations at a machine level [16]. *Low-level programming languages*, such as Assembly, are less intuitive for humans due to their resemblance to machine code. This proximity to machine code allows for faster execution times on the computer's part. On the other hand, *high-level programming languages* like Python or R are designed to mirror more closely natural language and be user-friendly. This typically comes with a trade-off in execution speed since these languages must undergo a process of translation, or interpretation, into machine code, which can be complex and time-consuming. *Intermediate-level languages*, such as C, strike a balance by offering quicker execution times than higher-level languages without being as cryptic as low-level languages. They do so by having a syntax that is more challenging than high-level languages but still more accessible than low-level languages. Notably, high-level languages like Python can achieve optimized performance by incorporating routines written in C, leveraging its faster execution capability.

Execution Programming languages can be divided into three ways of execution: compiled, interpreted, and hybrid [9]. In compiled programs, the code gets translated by a program called *compiler* from the high-level language to binary code and becomes highly specific on the computer architecture. The compiling process can be split in chunks depending on the complexity of the program. With interpreted execution, a system that parses the code and executes it line by line. This makes the code portable but requires the installation of an interpreter on the machine where it must be run. Lastly, the hybrid approach is based on a translation of the high-level code into an intermediate-level code, followed by interpretation.

5.7 Case study: Programming in Health Informatics

Despite the variety of standard programming languages, it is noteworthy that these languages often exhibit many commonalities. Figure 5.4 shows an example of an application of two mainstream programming languages, Python on

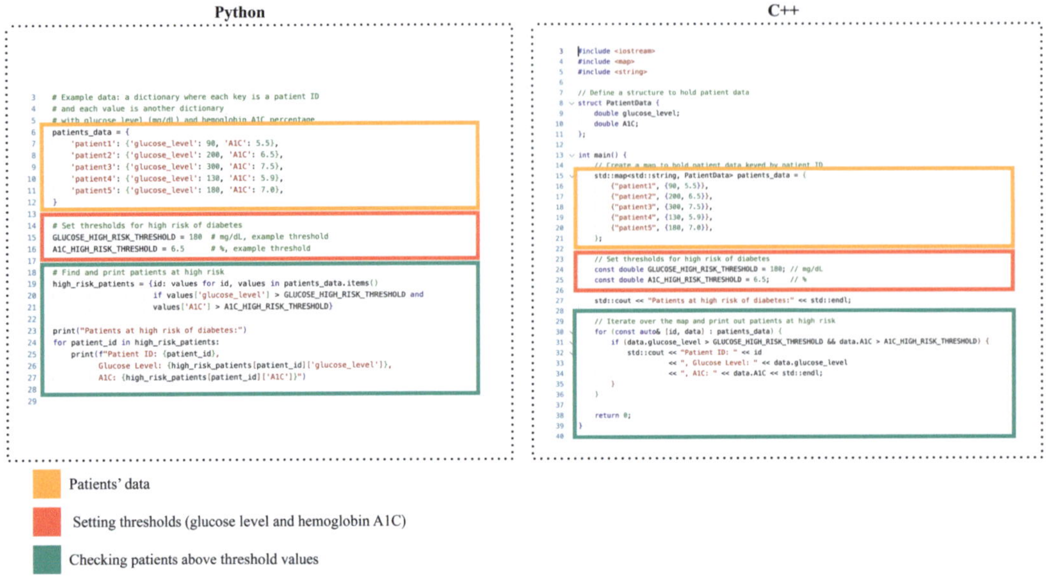

Python

```python
3  # Example data: a dictionary where each key is a patient ID
4  # and each value is another dictionary
5  # with glucose level (mg/dL) and hemoglobin A1C percentage
6  patients_data = {
7      'patient1': {'glucose_level': 90, 'A1C': 5.5},
8      'patient2': {'glucose_level': 200, 'A1C': 6.5},
9      'patient3': {'glucose_level': 300, 'A1C': 7.5},
10     'patient4': {'glucose_level': 130, 'A1C': 5.9},
11     'patient5': {'glucose_level': 180, 'A1C': 7.0},
12 }
13
14 # Set thresholds for high risk of diabetes
15 GLUCOSE_HIGH_RISK_THRESHOLD = 180  # mg/dL, example threshold
16 A1C_HIGH_RISK_THRESHOLD = 6.5      # %, example threshold
17
18 # Find and print patients at high risk
19 high_risk_patients = {id: values for id, values in patients_data.items()
20                       if values['glucose_level'] > GLUCOSE_HIGH_RISK_THRESHOLD and
21                       values['A1C'] > A1C_HIGH_RISK_THRESHOLD}
22
23 print("Patients at high risk of diabetes:")
24 for patient_id in high_risk_patients:
25     print(f"Patient ID: {patient_id},
26           Glucose Level: {high_risk_patients[patient_id]['glucose_level']},
27           A1C: {high_risk_patients[patient_id]['A1C']}")
28
29
```

C++

```cpp
3  #include <iostream>
4  #include <map>
5  #include <string>
6
7  // Define a structure to hold patient data
8  struct PatientData {
9      double glucose_level;
10     double A1C;
11 };
12
13 int main() {
14     // Create a map to hold patient data keyed by patient ID
15     std::map<std::string, PatientData> patients_data = {
16         {"patient1", {90, 5.5}},
17         {"patient2", {200, 6.5}},
18         {"patient3", {300, 7.5}},
19         {"patient4", {130, 5.9}},
20         {"patient5", {180, 7.0}},
21     };
22
23     // Set thresholds for high risk of diabetes
24     const double GLUCOSE_HIGH_RISK_THRESHOLD = 180; // mg/dL
25     const double A1C_HIGH_RISK_THRESHOLD = 6.5;     // %
26
27     std::cout << "Patients at high risk of diabetes:" << std::endl;
28
29     // Iterate over the map and print out patients at high risk
30     for (const auto& [id, data] : patients_data) {
31         if (data.glucose_level > GLUCOSE_HIGH_RISK_THRESHOLD && data.A1C > A1C_HIGH_RISK_THRESHOLD) {
32             std::cout << "Patient ID: " << id
33                       << ", Glucose Level: " << data.glucose_level
34                       << ", A1C: " << data.A1C << std::endl;
35         }
36     }
37
38     return 0;
39 }
40
```

Patients' data

Setting thresholds (glucose level and hemoglobin A1C)

Checking patients above threshold values

Fig. 5.4 Identifying high-risk diabetic patients in Python and C++. *Note* This image shows the realization of a code in Python (left) and C++ (right) to perform a basic screening of the patients that might be at risk of diabetes, based on their glucose level and hemoglobin A1C

the left and C++ on the right, in the context of health informatics. In both cases, the code aims at identifying high-risk diabetic patients given their blood glucose level and their hemoglobin A1 C value. Note that in real-world scenarios, diabetes diagnosis is based on a multi-faceted evaluation of the patient and this example is an over-simplification. The example shows how the overall logic and sequence of operations performed using two different syntaxes are identical.

In each example, data for five patients, which include their blood glucose level and hemoglobin A1 C, are stored in a data structure (line 6–12 in Python, line 15–21 in C++). The risk thresholds are internally set up by the programmer with a glucose value of 180 mg/dL and A1 C of 6.5 (line 15–16 in Python, line 24–25 in C++). The final part of the code identifies and displays the patients considered at elevated risk based on the threshold parameters. In Python, high-risk patients are first identified among all patients, based on the threshold values (line 19–21). For all patients in this group (line 24), their ID is printed (line 25) with the respective blood glucose level and A1 C (line 26–27). In C++, for each patient (line 30), those with values above threshold are identified (line 31), and their ID and values are printed (line 32–34).

5.8 Conclusions

This chapter introduced the fundamentals of computer science. While computer science is an intricate field, this chapter offered a dictionary of terms and a set of core concepts essential for anyone working in health informatics. Leveraging on this knowledge is crucial to understand how healthcare technology can rely on computational resources, including hardware, software, and network to deliver new solutions.

Nonetheless, the essence of healthcare informatics goes beyond the theoretical and practical principles of computer science. The use of computer science skills and concepts is the first step toward the organization of raw data into structured and meaningful information that can be interpreted in the clinical setting, and which is at the very heart of the health informatics field.

Knowledge Check Questions

1. One of the three components of a computer is:
   (a) Hardware
   (b) Monitor
   (c) Speakers
   (d) Internet
2. The OSI Model is a theoretical concept which includes guidelines to be implemented using network-specific protocols.
   (a) True
   (b) False
3. Among the main types of networks are the internet, the extranet, and a virtual private network
   (a) True
   (b) False
4. How many bits are necessary to specify a character in ASCII?
   (a) 3
   (b) 8
   (c) 10
   (d) 22
   (e) 144
5. A low-level and high-level language are:
   (a) Python and C++
   (b) R and Python
   (c) Assembly and Python
   (d) Java and Python
6. An image needs approximately one megabyte of space. How much is that in terabytes?
   (a) 10 TB
   (b) 0.1 TB
   (c) 0.001 TB
   (d) 0.000001 TB
7. Which of the following is not a component in building a computer program:
   (a) Design
   (b) Implementation
   (c) External Marketing
   (d) Testing

Answers

1. (a)
2. (a)
3. (a)
4. (b)
5. (c)
6. (d)
7. (c)

References

1. Donham P. Introduction to computer science. 1st. ed. San Diego: Cognella Academic Publishing, Elsevier; 2019.
2. Ionescu A. Categories and generations of computers. Eur J Comput Sci Inf Technol. 2015;3(1):15–42.
3. Wilson K. Exploring computer hardware—2022 edition: the illustrated guide to understanding computer hardware, components, peripherals, and networks (exploring networks). Elluminet Press; 2022.
4. Wolf M. Computers as components: principles of embedded computing systems design (the Morgan Kaufmann series in computer architecture and design). 5th ed. San Francisco: Morgan Kaufmann; 2022.
5. Fitzgerald J, Dennis A, Durcikova A. Business data communications and networking. 13th ed. Hoboken: Wiley; 2017.
6. West J, White J. Data communications and computer networks: a business users approach. 9th ed. Boston: Cengage Learning; 2022.
7. Sewell, J. (2019). Informatics and nursing: opportunities and challenges 6th ed. Lippincott Williams and Wilkins, Philadelphia.
8. Buchholz W. Planning a computer system: project stretch. McGraw-Hill, Inc; 1962.
9. Sebesta RW. Concepts of programming languages. Pearson Education, Inc.; 2012.
10. Gorn S, Bemer RW, Green J. American standard code for information interchange. Commun ACM. 1963;6(8):422–6.
11. Xu ZW. Cloud-sea computing systems: towards thousand-fold improvement in performance per watt for the coming zettabyte era. J Comput Sci Technol. 2014;29(2):177–81.
12. The European Space Agency. Science and exploration: how many stars are there in the universe? The European Space Agency; 2024. Retrieved March 30, 2024, from https://www.esa.int/Science_Exploration/Space_Science/Herschel/How_many_stars_are_there_in_the_Universe.

13. Hughes J. Why functional programming matters. Comput J. 1989;32(2):98–107.
14. Bruegge B, Dutoit AH. Object–oriented software engineering. Using UML, patterns, and java. Learning. 2009;5(6):7.
15. Kowalski RA. The early years of logic programming. Commun ACM. 1988;31(1):38–43.
16. Horowitz E. Fundamentals of programming languages. Springer Science & Business Media; 2012.
17. Greenes, R. A., & Del Fiol, G. (2023). Clinical decision support and beyond: Progress and opportunities in knowledge-enhanced heath and healthcare 3rd ed. Academic, Elsevier.
18. Healthcare Information and Management System Society. The CPHIMS review guide. 4th ed. Chicago: Routledge; 2021.

Basics of Data Science: A Case Study

6

Katie A. McCarthy

Foundational Domains

This chapter addresses the following AMIA Foundational Domain: F4—Health Information Science and Technology.

Learning Objectives

By the end of this chapter, you will be able to:

1. Define data science, artificial intelligence, and data storytelling.
2. Identify and describe the four types of data analysis.
3. Describe the typical data science process.
4. Compare and contrast data science tools.
5. Summarize key challenges in data science.

6.1 Introduction

To illustrate the concepts within this chapter, we will use a hypothetical case study that focuses on Chen, who is a nurse practitioner within a primary care clinic. The clinic is part of a large healthcare system that includes 10 hospitals and several hundred clinics. One of the hospitals is an academic medical center aligned with the region's largest research university.

K. A. McCarthy (✉)
Sullivan School of Business, Engineering, and Technology, Carroll University, Waukesha, WI, USA
e-mail: kamccart@carrollu.edu

One day, while eating lunch in the break room, Chen has a conversation with several other clinicians about the anxiety levels their patients are reporting, especially between 10 and 16 years of age. More of these patients are reporting isolation, trouble sleeping, and inability to focus or concentrate, and clinicians are concerned that the age of patients reporting these concerns is getting younger.

Chen asks the group how they can understand the situation and intervene. Malia, who is a primary care physician, shares that she is currently working with a research team at the academic medical center. This team includes Sarah, a data scientist, who knows the best ways to gather and analyze data. Malia volunteers to contact Sarah to see if she can help the clinicians investigate the anxiety levels their patients are reporting.

6.2 What Is Data Science?

Malia reaches out to Sarah, who agrees to meet with the clinicians. Malia requests that Sarah start the meeting by explaining what data science is, her role as a data scientist, and the data science process.

In the meeting, Sarah explains that healthcare organizations can capture data on every aspect of their work including patient care, finances, and service. To be useful, though, these data need to be transformed into insights, which are conclusions

C. Eldredge et al. (eds.), *Introductory Textbook in Health Informatics*, Health Informatics,
https://doi.org/10.1007/978-3-032-16657-9_6

drawn from the analysis of these data. From these insights, healthcare organizations can recommend:

- Personalized treatments for patients
- Improvements in access to care
- Improve quality of care
- Reduce errors, disparities, and cost

Sarah explains that data science is the study of extracting meaningful insights from data, which requires a multidisciplinary approach [1, 2]. Data science combines principles and practices from fields including informatics, mathematics, statistics, and computer science to analyze data and transform this analysis into actionable insights [1, 3–5]. This analysis answers questions like what has happened, what is currently happening, why did something happen, what is predicted to happen, and what is the optimal outcome [1, 6].

For example, data science in healthcare has been used to:

- Predict the 5-year life expectancy of patients 50 years of age and older. This model could be used by clinicians to personalize cancer screening guidelines for each patient [7].
- Predict a pediatric patient's likelihood of acute kidney injury (AKI) after cardiac surgery. AKIs increase the risk for early mortality, chronic kidney disease, and end-stage renal disease, so clinicians could use this information to improve patient outcomes [8].

6.2.1 What Jobs Exist in Data Science?

Next, Sarah explains the variety of roles and titles within data science, with the most common being *data analyst*, *data scientist*, and *data engineer*.

Data analysts often focus on gathering data and finding trends and patterns within data. They try to identify interesting insights that organizations can use to make data-driven decisions [9]. To do this work, they may need an undergraduate degree in informatics, data analytics, mathematics, or engineering. They must be able to work with databases, communicate analysis results, and use analytics software or programming languages.

Data scientists design and develop new systems that can automate the processing and analysis of data, especially for large amounts of data. To perform this work, data scientists may have a graduate degree and training in multiple fields (such as statistics, computer science, data mining, and information science) [9, 10].

Data engineers establish the technological foundation for the work completed by data analysts, data scientists, and computer scientists. They ensure that data are received, transformed, and stored so that they are accessible to project teams. They build and optimize databases, data tools, and *data pipelines* [11]. (For more information about databases, data tools, and data pipelines, refer to the data management chapter in this textbook.)

Chen asks, "so how do these roles work together in healthcare?" To answer, Sarah provides an example of a team that is concerned about frequent failures of laboratory testing devices, which are causing patients to wait longer for their test results. A project team is assigned to investigate this problem, and the team includes a data analyst, data scientist, and data engineer.

The data analyst and data scientist work with the team to identify the questions that need to be answered about the devices. They help determine what data are (and are not) available to answer these questions, and they develop a step-by-step process for gathering data. As part of this process, the data engineer sets up a database that will be used to store the data they collect.

Initially, the team decides to focus on gathering data for a device in one laboratory. The data analyst captures the data for this device, stores the data within the database, and then analyzes the data to look for patterns and trends. The analyst identifies that the machine tends to fail 2 or 3 weeks before scheduled maintenance is due.

The team is unclear, though, if this same pattern is occurring in other laboratories. As a next step, the data scientist automates the collection of data from all the laboratory testing devices and stores the data within a larger database created by the data engineer. Then, based on these data, the data scientist performs a deeper analysis and determines that machines tend to fail after 100 test runs (a threshold that is typically reached 2–3 weeks prior to scheduled maintenance).

With this insight, the team recommends that the laboratories change their schedules to perform preventative maintenance 3 weeks earlier than usual. The team monitors the devices and finds that the failures are reduced by 80% after implementing this change. As a result of this work, patients are receiving their laboratory testing results more quickly.

6.2.2 What Makes Data Science Different?

Before continuing, Sarah asks if the team has any questions. Malia asks, "how do informaticists, data analysts, data scientists, and data engineers work together?" And Chen asks, "How is artificial intelligence different from data science?"

To answer Malia's question, Sarah states that informaticists, data analysts, data scientists, and data engineers work together in healthcare organizations, and each role has a different focus. They collaborate to meet the needs of their organizations and communities.

Informaticists understand clinical and administrative processes and work closely with clinicians, leaders, and staff. They are skilled in communicating information to a variety of stakeholders and translating needs and wants into solutions. In the laboratory testing device example, an informaticist may have initially identified the delay in test results and worked with laboratory personnel to determine potential causes. In addition, informaticists could work with the data analyst, data scientist, and data engineer to explain how the devices work, the data they collect, and other relevant information. Finally, an informaticist may explain the clinical implications of delays in receiving test results.

To answer Chen's question, Sarah responds that *artificial intelligence* focuses on creation of computer programs (e.g., algorithms) that can perform tasks that typically require human intelligence such as analyzing, understanding, and interpreting complex data [12]. In the laboratory testing device example, a computer scientist working in artificial intelligence could create a computer algorithm (program) to automatically schedule a technician to perform preventive maintenance when 95 test runs are complete. With this algorithm, the scheduling occurs automatically (before 100 test runs are reached) so that failures can be prevented.

6.2.3 What Is the Typical Data Science Process?

Based on this information, the clinician team wants to work with Sarah to investigate the anxiety levels that their patients are reporting. Sarah explains that there is a typical data science process that they will follow during the project. This process includes the following:

- Identifying key questions
- Gathering and storing data
- Cleaning and understanding data
- Analyzing data
- Communicating the data analysis results

Sarah explains that this process is iterative (i.e., repetitive). For example, while determining the sources of data they will use, they may identify an additional key question. Or, while they are cleaning data, they may realize they need to store data differently to make analysis easier. This iteration is expected as the project continues.

Finally, Sarah explains that the data science process is most effective and efficient when individuals with different roles and responsibilities are included. Chen, Malia, and Sarah agree to work on this project and focus on the patients within their primary care clinic as a starting point. They identify a data analyst, a data engineer, an informaticist, and several additional clinicians to participate in the project, and invite them to participate in future meetings.

6.3 Identifying the Key Questions

During the first team meeting, Chen and Malia share their concerns about the symptoms of anxiety and depression they are seeing within their patients between 10 and 16 years of age, and the team identifies the goal for this project:

The goal of this project is to investigate the levels of anxiety being reported by patients between 10 and 16 years of age for the last 3 years at the primary care clinic and to identify factors that may be influencing these levels.

Based on this goal, the team identifies key questions for the project, including the following:

- For each of the last 3 years, what was the average anxiety level that was reported?
- Is there a statistically significant difference in anxiety levels reported each year? If so, is there a pattern in the levels (such as decreasing or increasing)?
- Are any demographic factors correlated with anxiety levels (identified gender, age, home address, school attended, etc.)?
- Are any lifestyle factors correlated with anxiety levels (nutrition, exercise, time outdoors, social media use, etc.)?
- For each of the last 3 years, how many patients in this age group have had referrals for mental health services?

To answer these questions, the team begins identifying potential sources of data. Chen and Malia explain that, during annual wellness visits, patients (or their guardians) complete a standard questionnaire about the patient's mental health. Ivan, the informaticist, states that the Informatics team implemented a note template about a year ago that clinicians can complete as they assess a patient's mental health during the visit. Finally, several clinicians on the team indicate that they refer patients to mental health services based on the results of their assessment.

Based on this information, the team agrees that the data from the mental health questionnaires could be useful in answering the key questions. Diane, the data analyst, states that she can get a report of the number of mental health referrals for patients over the last 3 years. Although information captured using the notes template may be helpful, the template has only been in use for a year, so the team decides not to use this information for now.

Finally, the team reaches out to the Compliance Department and the Institutional Review Board (IRB). Initially, the questionnaires and referrals were used to care for individual patients (the primary use of the data). Now, the team is planning to aggregate the data to find better treatments for a patient population (a secondary use of the data). The IRB is a committee that has been formally designated by the organization to review and monitor research involving human subjects (such as patients). The purpose of having IRB review is to assure that the appropriate steps are taken to protect the rights and welfare of individuals who participate in research, which includes the use of an individual's data; therefore, the team needs review and approval by the IRB before they continue [13]. The team receives appropriate approvals to use the data in the project if they store the data within a secured server and database. In addition, they are instructed to use de-identified and aggregated (i.e., summary) data if they decide to present or publish information about this project.

6.4 Gathering and Storing Data

With the help of Ericka, the data engineer, the team spends several weeks determining the best way to collect and store the data for the project.

The data will be collected from a variety of sources (questionnaires and reports). In addition, each of the team members will need access to the data. Based on these requirements, Ericka recommends using one of the secure virtual servers available within the healthcare organization. In addition, she works with a database administrator and determines that the data should be stored within a relational database, which is structured well for data analysis and reporting. Ericka reviews this plan with the team, and they agree to the approach. Ericka and the database administrator work together to set up the server, database, and security for the team members, as well as ensure that the requirements of the Health Insurance Portability and Accountability Act (HIPAA) are met (For more information about HIPAA, refer to the health information privacy chapter in this textbook.)

Next, Diane pulls a report from the electronic health record (EHR) system to identify the mental health referrals for the last 3 years. She only includes referrals for patients who are 10–16 years of age and originating from the primary care clinic. She places this data on the secure server for the team.

Then the team reviews the mental health questionnaires that are completed during annual wellness visits, and they discover several problems.

- First, patients (or their guardians) complete paper questionnaires. While most questions are answered using checkboxes, several questions require handwritten answers, which can be difficult to read.
- Second, when complete, the questionnaires are scanned into the EHR system and stored as images, which means that the data are not available as individual fields and values.
- Finally, although Sarah has written computer algorithms to get data from similar documents before, these algorithms have not been successful in correctly identifying handwritten answers.

After discussing these challenges, the team decides that Sarah will write a computer program to get the "checkbox" answers from the scanned questionnaires. Then, the team will manually abstract the handwritten answers to the three questions most relevant to the goal of the project. As part of this process, they will also review the data obtained from running the computer program to ensure the data is accurate.

Within 1 month, the team has collected and reviewed all the data and stored it within the database on the secure server.

6.5 Cleaning and Understanding the Data

Once the initial data collection and review is complete, Ericka and Sarah run several checks on the data to determine if any potential issues or errors exist.

When the project team identified the data to be collected from the questionnaires, they also identified a set of "rules" to determine what data are valid. For example, the level of anxiety was reported using a scale of 1–5 (with 1 being low anxiety and 5 being high anxiety). Now that the data has been gathered, Ericka and Sarah run some automated checks based on these rules, and potential issues are flagged for further investigation by the team. In addition, Diane, Ericka, and Sarah begin looking for other issues within the database such as missing values or blanks, potential data entry errors, and other potential problems.

With the potential issues identified for investigation, the team works to review the issues and resolve them appropriately. During this data cleaning process, they review each potential issue and compare the flagged information to the original source, which can be challenging because the original data may come from multiple sources. As they work through each issue, they correct or remove the data (as appropriate). Each team member documents their investigation within a shared document so that they all have access to this information in the future. Although this process is time-consuming and requires attention to detail, Sarah and Ivan emphasize the importance of data cleaning to ensure any future analysis is built on accurate and valid data.

Once the data cleaning is complete, Diane begins exploring the data to look for outliers or other patterns that may indicate problems with the data. For example, she confirms that the data includes patients 10–16 years of age and that the identified genders are consistent with that patient population from the primary care clinic. She discovers, though, that a large number of patients are 16 years of age—more than are typically seen within the primary care clinic—which could indicate there are outliers within the dataset. As she investigates further, she determines that the clinic performed wellness exams for one of the local high schools as part of their health classes and the questionnaires were included as part of these exams. Most of the students within these classes were 15 or 16 years of age. Because these records were not created during typical wellness exams completed within the clinic, they are considered outliers in the dataset. The team discusses this issue and decides to remove any records from the dataset that were created as part of the wellness exams for the health classes. They document the investigation and their decision in the shared document for future reference.

6.6 Analyzing the Data

Based on this work, the team is ready to analyze the data. Ivan, Diane, and Sarah work together to answer the key questions using four types of analysis: descriptive, diagnostic, predictive, and prescriptive.

6.6.1 What Is Descriptive Analysis?

Diane and Ivan start by performing some *descriptive analysis* with the goal of answering questions about what has happened or is happening. They use techniques such as basic statistics (e.g., counts, averages, and percentages), as well as visualizations (such as bar charts).

One of the key questions is, "for each of the last 3 years, what was the average anxiety level that was reported?" To answer this question, they separate the level of anxiety data by year and calculate an average per year. In addition, they create bar charts showing the number of responses for each level (1 through 5). Based on these results, anxiety levels are increasing each year.

Other key questions are based on patient demographics like identified gender, age, home address, and school attended, so they identify the number of patients within each category. For example, they find that 85% of patients within the dataset live within 20 miles of the clinic and attend one of several schools within the area.

Diane also works to analyze lifestyle information including nutrition, exercise, time outdoors, and social media use. Although she can calculate statistics for most of these factors, nutrition information is challenging. Within the questionnaire, several questions gather this information such as "How many servings of fruits and vegetables do you eat each day?" and "How often do you each fast food each week?" The clinicians on the team review these data and recommend analyzing the responses to each question and then creating a new variable that assesses the overall "quality" of nutrition. Chen and Malia work with Ivan, Diane, and Sarah to define this new variable and its calculation.

Based on these data, Diane and Ivan find that the biggest increases in anxiety level are occurring in patients from 10 to 13 years of age who attend two of the local middle schools. In addition, patients reporting higher anxiety levels report high levels of social media use; no or minimal time spent outdoors; and low levels of nutrition.

Diane and Ivan share their findings with the team. The team confirms that this information is consistent with their experience and the data collected.

6.6.2 What Is Diagnostic Analysis?

Next, Diane, Ivan, and Sarah perform *diagnostic analysis*, which answers questions about why something happened. They use techniques such as correlation analysis, hypothesis testing, and cluster analysis with the goal of identifying patterns that are statistically significant.

From this analysis, they find several statistically significant patterns and correlations including the following:

- Patients who are 10–13 years of age report higher anxiety levels than patients who are 14–16 years of age.
- Patients who live within 10 miles of the clinic reported the highest anxiety levels in the past 3 years.
- Over the last 3 years, patients who are 10–11 years of age have reported the highest increases in anxiety levels.
- Over the last 3 years, anxiety levels have increased each year for patients attending two local middle schools.
- As the time spent using social media increases, anxiety levels increase.
- As the time spent outdoors increases, anxiety levels decrease.
- As the number of fast-food meals in a week increases, anxiety levels increase.
- The number of mental health referrals has increased each year over the past 3 years.

Diane, Ivan, and Sarah did not find any significant correlations between anxiety level and identified gender, socioeconomic status, race, ethnicity, or overall nutrition quality.

Finally, they performed a *cluster analysis* (a technique that is used to group data points that are similar) and identified several clusters including the following:

- Patients with the highest anxiety levels spent more than 2 h per day using social media; spent 0–10 min outdoors daily; and ate fast food meals at least three times per week.
- Patients with the lowest anxiety levels spent 0–30 min per day using social media; spent 30–45 min outdoors daily; and ate fast food less than once per week.

From this analysis, they have confirmed that anxiety levels have increased over the past 3 years and which populations have seen the highest increases. In addition, they have confirmed that the number of referrals to mental health services has increased. And they have found several factors that are correlated to anxiety levels.

6.6.3 What Is Predictive Analysis?

As a next step, Ivan, Diane, and Sarah meet with the team to discuss these patterns. Specifically, they ask the clinicians on the team to help identify factors that they feel are most important for predicting anxiety levels based on these correlations and clusters.

Although a correlation was found between anxiety levels and home address (within 10 miles of the clinic), the clinicians indicate that this finding may be correlated with the school that patients attend (the two local middle schools). Therefore, for further analysis, they recommend using school attended, social media use daily, time spent outdoors daily, and number of fast-food meals per week.

Sarah uses this recommendation to perform *predictive analysis*, which answers questions about what is likely to happen in the future. In this type of analysis, she uses historical patterns and techniques such as classification and regression to create a predictive model. Then, using this model, she attempts to predict a patient's anxiety level.

In creating a predictive model, the first step is identifying the factors that are most likely to impact the outcome being predicted. In this case, Sarah has four factors that have been identified to impact anxiety level. Then, she tries several techniques to create a model with the most accurate predictions.

When she has created a fairly accurate predictive model, Sarah shares her findings with the team. All four factors have been identified as significant in predicting anxiety levels. She does warn the team, though, to avoid assuming it always provides the correct "answer." Simply because something was historically true does not mean it will continue to be true in the future.

6.6.4 What Is Prescriptive Analysis?

The team discusses these concerns and decides not to use the predictive model to predict anxiety levels for individual patients. Instead, they want to use this model to determine the optimal levels of social media use, time outdoors, and fast-food meals to reduce anxiety levels.

To determine these optimal levels, Sarah uses *prescriptive analysis*, which answers questions about how to achieve the best outcome. Then, based on this analysis, the team can identify potential interventions to help their patients or decision support that could be built into the EHR to identify patients who may be at highest risk for increasing anxiety.

From the prescriptive analysis, Sarah identifies that the following factors result in the lowest anxiety levels:

- Less than 20 min per day are spent on using social media.
- At least 40 min per day are spent outdoors.
- No more than three fast food meals are eaten per month.

6.7 Communicating the Results

Sarah meets with the team to discuss her findings and next steps. The team agrees that something needs to be done to address the anxiety levels for their young patients; and the findings should be communicated with clinicians in the primary care clinic. Clinic leadership asks that results be presented during the next department meeting.

In planning their presentation, the team uses best practices within data storytelling, which is communicating the insights they identified using visualizations and a strong narrative [14, 15]. First, they consider the needs of each member of their audience. For clinicians, the team needs to share key factors influencing patient anxiety levels. For staff, the team needs to focus on the importance of continuing the questionnaires during visits. And, for leaders, the team needs to focus on potential outreach within the community.

Next, they create a clear "story" of their project so that everyone could follow the insights they discovered. Finally, they develop a simple PowerPoint presentation that focuses on the most important insights and the need to intervene to improve patient anxiety levels.

The team shares their insights during the next department meeting, and everyone engages in a discussion about next steps. They decide to work with the two local middle schools where the anxiety levels were the highest and create an after-school program that includes time in a community garden, cooking classes, and a social media challenge to reduce time using social media daily.

The project team reaches out to senior leaders within the healthcare system, who agree to fund a pilot intervention from the healthcare system's community foundation. With funding in place, clinic leaders and clinicians meet with individuals from both middle schools, who agree to try the interventions for the next 30 days with students who are 10–11 years of age. The project team captures data before and after the intervention to determine what impacts (if any) there are on student anxiety levels.

6.8 What Tools Are Used in Data Science?

As the end of the pilot intervention approaches, Chen discusses the next steps with Sarah. He has enjoyed his time on the project and is interested in doing some of the analysis of the data from the pilot. He asks Sarah if she can share some of the tools she uses when doing data science so that he can learn about them and try to use a few.

Sarah explains that many tools can be used within data science, so she provides the following information to Chen about the most common tools and their uses (Table 6.1).

When the pilot intervention is complete, Chen, Diane, and Sarah work together to analyze the data. They find that anxiety levels for the intervention participants decreased for those who worked within the community garden and who reduced their social media use. For participants in the cooking classes, the results are less clear—some anxiety levels decreased, while others remained the same. The most significant reductions occurred for students who participated in all three interventions. For all students who partici-

Table 6.1 Common data science tools

Tool	Use
Microsoft excel	Spreadsheet software that can be used to format, organize, and perform calculations on data. Part of the Microsoft Office suite of products [16]. Most common software for data analysis within healthcare organizations. Typically used for data collection, cleaning, descriptive analysis, and diagnostic analysis
IBM SPSS statistics	Software used for advanced statistical analysis, machine learning, and text analysis [17]. Commonly used for social sciences research and includes functionality for descriptive, diagnostic, and predictive analysis
SQL	Structured query language. Programming language for store, update, remove, search, and retrieve information from relational databases [18]. Often used to obtain data from databases and combine these data into a single storage structure (database, data warehouse, etc.)
Microsoft power BI	Desktop application, online software, and mobile apps that can be used to build reports and visualizations [19]. The desktop application is included within Microsoft Office 365 but more advanced features such as sharing data and more powerful analytics require additional subscriptions or licensing
Tableau	Analytics software used to prepare and analyze data and create visualizations and dashboards [20]. Tableau uses a drag-and-drop interface, which can be easy to learn. The software can be costly, though, and is typically limited to descriptive analysis and visualization
Python	An open-source programming language often used to automate data science tasks (data cleaning, analysis, visualization, etc.) [21]. Very powerful, free, and requires significant programming and data science knowledge to use effectively
R	An open-source programming language built for statistical computing and graphics [22]. Very powerful, free, and requires significant programming, statistics, and data science knowledge to use effectively

pated, they either reported decreased anxiety levels or no change—no one reported increased levels.

The team reports these results to the clinic, and everyone is hopeful that this type of program can help patients. Clinic leaders share the results with senior leaders in the healthcare system and the community foundation, and they agree that the pilot interventions were successful and need to continue. Senior leaders agree to support ongoing work to provide these interventions to more schools and patients. And they agree that data needs to continue to be captured to ensure these interventions are having the intended effects.

6.9 What Challenges Exist in Data Science?

The project team is thrilled with the results and continued support of the healthcare system. Sarah cautions them, though, that several challenges are likely to occur as they extend these interventions and continue to capture and analyze data.

First, as more clinics and schools participate in the intervention program, the sources of data will increase, and the team will need to integrate multiple data sources into a single database [23–25]. Each clinic that participates may capture patient anxiety levels differently, so the team will need to integrate all these sources into a single database/source. This integration can be challenging and time-consuming. Currently, Sarah is the only data scientist and Ericka is the only data engineer within the healthcare system, so additional staff are needed to move this project forward.

The second challenge is identifying individuals who can do this work [23–25]. Data science is a rapidly evolving field, and a gap exists between the number of open positions for this work and the number of individuals with appropriate training [26]. And existing data analysts and scientists may struggle to keep up with new and evolving software, technologies, and techniques. Therefore, a skills gap exists, so senior leaders within the organization begin identifying existing employees who could be trained to assist with this project.

A third challenge is ensuring the privacy and security of the data they collect and analyze [23–25]. As more patients participate in the intervention, more and more data will be collected. And, as the team grows to support this work, more people will need access to the data. Because the team is committed to ensuring the patient data remains private and secure, they decide to reach out to the Compliance Department and the Institutional Review Board (IRB) again for direction.

Finally, the cost of this project will increase due to expenses related to the interventions, the additional employees needed to help with the project, and the technical infrastructure to support more data (including storage and analysis tools) [24, 25]. They also agree that team members (such as Chen) who are interested in learning more may need financial support for professional development. Based on this challenge and the other challenges identified, they agree to ask senior leaders to assign a "point person" who will lead this effort moving forward and develop a timeline and budget.

6.10 Summary

By the end of their work, Chen, Malia, and Sarah have identified interventions to help reduce anxiety levels in young patients within the primary care clinic.

With Sarah's direction and a team of individuals from different backgrounds and perspectives, they have followed the data science process to understand why anxiety level may be increasing. They identified key questions, gathered data, cleaned the data, analyzed the data, and communicated the results. Once they communicated these results to the primary care clinic, they could identify and implement pilot interventions to address the factors correlated to higher anxiety levels.

Individuals who participated in the interventions reported the same or lower anxiety levels. As a result, leaders within the healthcare system have approved implementing this data-driven process in more clinics to hopefully help more patients. And, as Sarah explained to the team in their first meeting, that is the point of data science—extracting meaningful insights from data to improve health and healthcare.

6.11 Resources

See Table 6.2 for a list of data science resources.

Table 6.2 Data science resources

Resource	Website (Link)
Data science courses available online	Datacamp (https://www.datacamp.com/)
Website for sharing and collaborating on data science projects	Github (https://github.com/)
Information about careers in data science	Data analyst on indeed (https://www.indeed.com/career/data-analyst) Data engineer on indeed (https://www.indeed.com/career/data-engineer) Data scientist on indeed (https://www.indeed.com/career/data-scientist)
Data science software and tools	IBM SPSS statistics (https://www.ibm.com/spss) Microsoft excel (https://www.microsoft.com/en-us/microsoft-365/excel) Microsoft power BI (https://www.microsoft.com/en-us/power-platform/products/power-bi) Orange data mining software (https://orangedatamining.com/) Python programming language (https://www.python.org/) R programming language (https://www.r-project.org/) Salesforce tableau (https://www.tableau.com/) SQL (https://mode.com/sql-tutorial)

Knowledge Check Questions

1. *Define "data science."*
2. *Compare and contrast data science and artificial intelligence.*
3. *Identify and explain the four types of data analysis. Provide an example of each type of analysis.*
4. *Describe the steps in the data science process.*
5. *Why is data science an iterative process?*
6. *Identify and describe some common tools within data science.*
7. *Describe and provide examples of two challenges within data science.*

Answers

1. Data science is the field that focuses on extracting meaningful insights from data. Data science uses principles and practices from fields including informatics, mathematics, statistics, and computer science.
2. Data science is the field that focuses on extracting meaningful insights from data. Artificial intelligence is the field that focuses on creation of computer programs (algorithms) that can perform tasks that typically require human intelligence. Therefore, data science may be used to identify to identify an insight from data (such as a laboratory testing instrument requires preventive maintenance before 100 testing runs are completed). With this information, the laboratory may create a computer algorithm (artificial intelligence) to automatically schedule a technician to perform preventive maintenance when 95 testing runs are completed (before 100 runs is reached).
3. Descriptive analysis answers questions about what has happened or what is happening. An example is identifying the number of patients under the age of 16 years old in a dataset.
   Diagnostic analysis answers questions about why something happened. An example is identifying that a dataset includes a large number of 16-year-old patients because the data was collected during a high school health class.
   Predictive analysis answers questions about what is likely to happen in the future based on a set of factors. An example is predicting the anxiety level that will be reported by patients based on the school they attend, social media use daily, time spent outdoors daily, and number of fast-food meals per week.
   Prescriptive analysis answers questions about how to achieve the best outcome based on a set of factors. An example is predicting the lowest (best) anxiety levels including less than 20 min per day spent on using social media; at least 40 min per day spent outdoors; and no more than three fast-food meals eaten per month.
4. The typical data science process includes identifying key questions; gathering and storing data; cleaning and understanding data; analyzing data; and communicating results.
5. Data science is an iterative process because new or updated information from one step in the process may require changes in a previous step in the process. For example, when data are analyzed as part of the process, issues may be identified that require additional data to be gathered.
6. Some common tools within data science include:
   - Microsoft Excel: Spreadsheet software that can be used to format, organize, and perform calculations on data. Part of the Microsoft Office suite of products. Most common software for data analysis within healthcare organizations. Typically used for data collection, cleaning, descriptive analysis, and diagnostic analysis.
   - IBM SPSS Statistics: Software used for advanced statistical analysis, machine learning, and text analysis. Commonly used for social sciences research and includes functionality for descriptive, diagnostic, and predictive analysis.
   - SQL: Structured query language. Programming language for store, update, remove, search, and retrieve information

from relational databases. Often used to obtain data from databases and combine these data into a single storage structure (database, data warehouse, etc.).
- Microsoft Power BI: Desktop application, online software, and mobile apps that can be used to build reports and visualizations. The desktop application is included within Microsoft Office 365, but more advanced features such as sharing data and more powerful analytics requires additional subscriptions or licensing.
- Tableau: Analytics software used to prepare and analyze data and create visualizations and dashboards. Tableau uses a drag-and-drop interface, which can be easy to learn. The software can be costly, though, and is typically limited to descriptive analysis and visualization.
- Python: An open-source programming language often used to automate data science tasks (data cleaning, analysis, visualization, etc.). Very powerful, free, and requires significant programming and data science knowledge to use effectively.
- R: An open-source programming language build for statistical computing and graphics. Very powerful, free, and requires significant programming, statistics, and data science knowledge to use effectively.

7. (Answer can include any two of the following challenges.)

   As the number of data sources increases, so does the complexity of the data science project. For example, a data science project involving data for one clinic is significantly less complex and time consuming than a similar data science project involving 100 clinics.

   A gap exists between the number of open data science positions and the number of individuals who are appropriately trained in data science. For example, an organization may only have one person focusing on data science and may have problems hiring a second person because of a lack of applicants with appropriate training.

   A significant challenge is ensuring the privacy and security of the data used in data science projects. For example, the data may include patient names and birthdates, which must be protected and appropriately secured based local laws.

   The cost of data science projects can be significant. For example, costs may need to include additional employees and new/updated technical infrastructure to support more data and analysis work.

Glossary of Terms

Term	Definition
Artificial intelligence	Focuses on creation of computer programs (algorithms) that can perform tasks that typically require human intelligence such as analyzing, understanding, and interpreting complex data
Classification	A predictive analysis technique used to predict a class or category.
Cluster analysis	An analysis technique that separates data into groups (clusters) that have similar characteristics.
Data cleaning	Process of identifying issues within a dataset and resolving these issues appropriately.
Data engineering	Provides the technological foundation for the work completed within data science. Ensures data are received, transformed, and stored appropriately by building and optimizing databases, data tools, and data pipelines.
Data exploration	Process of understanding a dataset (size, outliers, distribution, etc.) using basic statistics and visualizations.
Data mining	Process that uses statistical and mathematical techniques to extract information and patterns from a dataset.
Data pipeline	A method used to obtain data from a variety of sources, transform the data, and then load the data into the appropriate storage location (such as a database) [27].
Data science	Field that focuses on extracting meaningful insights from data. Uses principles and practices from fields including informatics, mathematics, statistics, and computer science.
Data storytelling	A process of sharing data insights using narratives and visualizations.
Descriptive analysis	Type of analysis that answers questions about what has happened or is happening. Techniques include basic statistics and visualizations.

Term	Definition
Diagnostic analysis	Type of analysis that answers questions about why something happened. Techniques include correlation analysis, hypothesis testing, and cluster analysis.
Predictive analysis	Type of analysis that answers questions about what is likely to happen. Uses historical patterns to predict outcomes. Types of techniques include classification and regression.
Prescriptive analysis	Type of analysis that answers questions about how to achieve the best outcome. Identifies the "optimal" inputs to obtain a desired outcome.
Regression	A predictive analysis technique used to predict a numeric value.
Statistics	A field focusing on methods for collecting, analyzing, and interpreting data.
Visualization	A graphical representation of data such as charts and graphs.

References

1. Amazon AWS. What is data science? https://aws.amazon.com/what-is/data-science/.
2. Provost F, Fawcett T. Data science for business: what you need to know about data mining and data-analytic thinking. O'Reilly Media, Inc.; 2013.
3. Biswal A. What is data science: lifecycle, applications, prerequisites and tools. 2023. https://www.simplilearn.com/tutorials/data-science-tutorial/what-is-data-science.
4. IBM. What is data science? https://www.ibm.com/topics/data-science.
5. Shmueli G, Bruce PC, Gedeck P, Patel NR. Data mining for business analytics: concepts, techniques and applications in python. Wiley; 2020.
6. Cochran JJ, editor. INFORMS analytics body of knowledge. Wiley; 2019.
7. Mathias JS, Agrawal A, Feinglass J, Cooper AJ, Baker DW, Choudhary A. Development of a 5 year life expectancy index in older adults using predictive mining of electronic health record data. J Am Med Inform Assoc (JAMIA). 20(e1):e118–24. https://doi.org/10.1136/amiajnl-2012-001360.
8. Zeng X, Shi S, Sun Y, et al. A time-aware attention model for prediction of acute kidney injury after pediatric cardiac surgery. J Am Med Inform Assoc (JAMIA). 2023;30(1):94–102. https://doi.org/10.1093/jamia/ocac202.
9. Indeed Editorial Team. Data analyst vs. Data scientist (Key differences to consider). 2023. Accessed 20 Sept 2023. https://ca.indeed.com/career-advice/finding-a-job/data-analyst-vs-data-scientist.
10. U.S. Bureau of Labor Statistics. Data scientists. Occupational outlook handbook. 2023. https://www.bls.gov/ooh/math/data-scientists.htm.
11. Dataquest. Data engineer, data analyst, data scientist – what's the difference. 2021. Accessed 5 Feb 2024. https://www.dataquest.io/blog/data-analyst-data-scientist-data-engineer/?utm_source=google&utm_medium=&matchtype=&device=c&utm_campaign=ai_launch_sale&campaignid=20758249356&adgroupid=&adid=&utm_content=&gad_source=5&gclid=EAIaIQobChMIysq78aGUhAMVRmVHAR2h3g7AEAAYBCAAEgIMU_D_BwE.
12. Cohen K. Comparing data science and artificial intelligence. 2023. Accessed 5 Feb 2024. https://www.iu.org/blog/programme-comparison/ai-vs-data-science/#area-737110.
13. U.S Food & Drug Administration (FDA). Institutional review boards frequently asked questions: guidance for institutional review boards and clinical investigators. 2025. https://www.fda.gov/regulatory-information/search-fda-guidance-documents/institutional-review-boards-frequently-asked-questions.
14. Nussbaumer KC. Storytelling with data: a data visualization guide for business professionals. Wiley; 2015.
15. Cote C. Data storytelling: how to effectively tell a story with data. 2021. https://online.hbs.edu/blog/post/data-storytelling.
16. Gillis AS. Excel. 2021. https://www.techtarget.com/searchenterprisedesktop/definition/Excel.
17. IBM. Why IBM SPSS software? https://www.ibm.com/spss.
18. AWS. What is SQL (structured quality language)? https://aws.amazon.com/what-is/sql/.
19. Microsoft. What is power BI? https://learn.microsoft.com/en-us/power-bi/fundamentals/power-bi-overview.
20. Salesforce. What is Tableau? https://www.tableau.com/why-tableau/what-is-tableau.
21. Yan E. Beginner's Python tutorial: learn Python. 2023. https://python.land/python-tutorial.
22. The R Foundation. What is R? https://www.r-project.org/about.html.
23. Vyas R. 6 data science challenges and how to address them. 2023. https://indatalabs.com/blog/data-science-challenges.
24. Kumar N. Challenges and opportunities of data science. 2023. https://www.analyticsinsight.net/challenges-and-opportunities-of-data-science/.
25. Nguyen T. Overcome the 10 most common data science challenges. 2023. https://www.neurond.com/blog/data-science-challenges.
26. Janssen N. The data science talent gap: why it exists and what businesses can do about it. 2022. https://www.forbes.com/sites/forbestechcouncil/2022/10/11/the-data-science-talent-gap-why-it-exists-and-what-businesses-can-do-about-it/?sh=71f314442398.
27. Stryker C. What is a data pipeline? IBM. https://www.ibm.com/think/topics/data-pipeline.

7 Medical Decision-Making and Decision Analysis

Athanasios Tsalatsanis

Foundational Domains
This chapter addresses the following AMIA Foundational Domains: F4—Health Information Science and Technology, F6—Social and Behavioral Aspects of Health.

7.1 Introduction

Medical decisions affect the well-being of individuals and the greater public. Often, these decisions involve multiple stakeholders, including patients and their families, healthcare providers, administrators, and public health officials. They are complex and entail trade-offs such as health risks and benefits, potential costs, and the decision-maker's preferences and values. Nonetheless, from routine patient consultations to intricate policy development proceedings, medical decisions have the potential to impact a person's life and public health in a significant way.

Medical decisions are made by a patient, a healthcare provider, or other stakeholders. They include choices regarding lifestyle changes (i.e., smoking, exercise, alcohol consumption, stress), preventive care (i.e., screening, vaccinations), managing chronic conditions (i.e., adherence to medications and lifestyle changes), treatment options (i.e., surgery vs. physical therapy), choices between treatments after examining expected outcomes, risks, side effects, and end-of-life planning (i.e., advance directive: living will and durable power of attorney).

These decisions, particularly when they occur in a clinical setting, are part of a broader process known as medical decision-making. Formally, *medical decision-making* is defined as "the process by which a diagnosis or treatment plan is formulated from the available test information, often with incorporation of known patient preferences [1]. It involves evaluating clinical data, considering risks and benefits, and tailoring medical interventions to individual patients". Studying and understanding medical decision-making helps us appreciate the complexity associated with medical decisions, which can directly affect an individual's health and quality of life. To illustrate this complexity, consider the following case related to the treatment of a sore throat. We will be using this case throughout this chapter to demonstrate theoretical topics.

Example Case Study 1: Sore Throat Treatment A patient visits their primary care provider complaining of a sore throat that started two days ago and is worsening. The pain is moderate, especially when swallowing. After a physical examination, the clinician notices redness and swelling of the throat and enlarged lymph nodes. The clinician suspects the patient has a bacterial

A. Tsalatsanis (✉)
Morsani College of Medicine, University of South Florida, Tampa, FL, USA
e-mail: atsalats@usf.edu

C. Eldredge et al. (eds.), *Introductory Textbook in Health Informatics*, Health Informatics,
https://doi.org/10.1007/978-3-032-16657-9_7

infection (acute pharyngitis) and considers the following treatment alternatives:

1. Treat the suspected bacterial infection with antibiotics.
2. Wait and see: Manage the symptoms with over-the-counter medication, and if they worsen, schedule a follow-up visit.
3. Perform a diagnostic test to confirm and treat the bacterial infection as needed.

Each alternative presents tradeoffs that should be considered:

1. While antibiotics provide immediate treatment for a bacterial infection, they will not be effective if the infection is viral. Early antibiotic treatment can prevent the spreading of the infection; however, antibiotics can cause several side effects, such as digestive issues and allergic reactions.
2. The waiting and see alternative avoids unnecessary antibiotics but increases the risk of complications related to the infection.
3. A diagnostic test can confirm if the infection is bacterial, but diagnostic tests are not perfect and may return false positive results.

Other examples of medical decisions include the following:

1. Considering a knee replacement when the pain from arthritis affects one's quality of life. The implant is expected to reduce pain and improve mobility, but the procedure could result in infections or implant failure in short/long term.
2. C-section vs. vaginal birth. The C-section is preferred in high-risk pregnancies but has a longer recovery time than vaginal birth and may present an increased risk of infections.
3. Palliative care vs. aggressive curative treatment for a terminally ill patient. Palliative care focuses on improving comfort and quality of life but could reduce the patient's remaining lifespan.
4. Electing prophylactic mastectomy (removal of both breasts) and/or oophorectomy (removal of both ovaries) on a patient with BRCA1 gene mutation (a mutation that could indicate the development of breast cancer). The operations significantly reduce the risk of developing breast/ovarian cancer, but the surgeries carry risks such as infections, bleeding, and complications. In addition, the removal of breasts and/or ovaries may affect the patient physically and emotionally.
5. Performing total or partial prostatectomy on a patient diagnosed with prostate cancer after testing for the presence of a prostate-specific antigen. A total prostatectomy may increase the risk of side effects, while a partial prostatectomy may increase the risk of cancer recurrence.

While the conditions and circumstances outlined in the examples above vary, they all follow a similar decision-making process that includes some aspect of diagnosis, testing, and/or treatment. Initially, the clinician assesses the patient's symptoms and/or clinical presentation to establish a diagnosis. Diagnostic tests may be used to confirm or exclude competing diagnoses. Then, the clinician discusses the available treatment options with the patient and recommends the most suitable with the information they have at that time. It is important to note that lab tests may provide additional information that might alter the decisions already made.

From the cases above, it is evident that medical decisions must be made, often without every detail of information. In an ideal scenario, clinicians would diagnose patients based on their symptoms and clinical presentation and prescribe the appropriate treatment. However, reality introduces significant uncertainty at every stage of this process. For instance, uncertainty may stem from misinterpreting the patient's symptoms, incomplete or inaccurate patient history, or incomplete information about the patient that could be the result of the lack of interoperability between health information systems (see Chap. 22 on interoperability). Diagnostic tests are not perfect and often yield false positive or false negative results. Treatments are associated with trade-offs between benefits and potential harms/

side effects, and optimal treatment choices vary depending on patient preferences and risk tolerance. To address these and other uncertainties in medical decisions, a systematic (i.e., structured and methodological) approach is needed to help describe and analyze all available data, information, choices, and trade-offs to reach the optimal treatment decision for a patient.

One of these systematic approaches is *decision analysis*, defined as the "formal, mathematical approach to analyzing difficult decisions faced by clinical decision makers (i.e., patients, clinicians, policy-makers)" [2]. It is a "quantitative approach to medical decision-making" [3], and a "systematic, explicit, quantitative way of making decisions in health care that can lead to both enhanced communication about clinical controversies and better decisions". [4] Notice that all these definitions emphasize the importance of formal, systematic, and quantitative approaches.

Decision analysis falls within the realm of decision theories, which include normative, descriptive, and prescriptive approaches to decision-making [5–7]. *Normative* theories [5–7] aim to identify the most rational decision, assuming the decision maker is fully aware of all available evidence. They focus on how individuals "should" be making decisions. *Descriptive* theories [5–7] examine how people are "actually" making decisions, acknowledging the psychological and cognitive factors that affect choices. *Prescriptive* theories [5–7]bridge the gap between normative and descriptive theories by providing decision-makers with guidance through decision aids, algorithms, guidelines, etc., to improve the decision-making process.

It is crucial for individuals pursuing a career in the field of health informatics to gain an understanding of decision-making theories, particularly decision analysis. Health informatics professionals are tasked with developing or implementing tools to support clinical decisions to improve the quality of care, patient outcomes, patient safety, and overall efficiency of care delivery. Understanding how healthcare providers and patients make decisions enables health informatics professionals to design systems that are easy to use, available at the point of care, compatible with clinical workflows, driven by the latest clinical evidence, and utilize appropriate methods to derive optimal choices in various healthcare settings.

To demonstrate these principles, we explain how decision analysis concepts are applied in medical decision-making using the example case provided earlier, in the following section.

7.2 Decision Analysis

As was mentioned earlier, decision analysis is used to solve medical decision-making problems systematically and quantitatively. To that end, decision analysis utilizes decision trees [3] to depict strategies under consideration and their outcomes and then calculates the best strategy based on a decision model. Some decision models that can be used in decision analysis include expected utility theory [8], prospect theory [9], and expected regret theory [10–12]. The expected utility theory model assumes that individuals are rational and will choose the strategy that leads to the maximum expected utility (i.e., a measure associated with how good or preferable an outcome is) [8]. The prospect theory model assumes that individuals prefer strategies with more certain outcomes and are likely to prefer strategies that avoid losses over strategies that risk gaining outcomes [9]. The regret theory model assumes that individuals prefer strategies that will bring the least amount of regret if, in retrospect, these strategies are incorrect [10–12]. Let's see how decision trees, in conjunction with expected utility theory, are implemented in decision analysis.

7.2.1 Decision Trees

A decision tree is a graphical representation of a clinical problem. It includes nodes representing the available choices (or strategies) and their consequences (outcomes), probabilities representing the likelihood of an outcome to occur, and the decision-maker's valuations of each outcome (i.e., how preferable an outcome is). Solving the decision tree derives the optimal solution for the specific decision maker.

Consider the example case study of sore throat treatment above, where the clinician is contemplating three treatment alternatives, not knowing at the time whether the patient suffers from a bacterial infection or not:

1. *Treat the suspected bacterial infection with antibiotics.*
2. *Wait and see: Manage the symptoms with over-the-counter medication, and if they worsen, schedule a follow-up visit.*
3. *Perform a diagnostic test to confirm and treat the bacterial infection as needed.*

Suppose the clinician decides to treat with antibiotics (treatment alternative 1). Because at the time of the exam, it is uncertain whether the patient has a bacterial infection, this decision may result in beneficial treatment if the patient has a bacterial infection (i.e., treatment with disease) or unnecessary treatment if the patient does not have a bacterial infection (i.e., treatment without disease). Similarly, the wait and see strategy (treatment alternative 2) may result in withholding treatment from a patient suffering from a bacterial infection (i.e., no treatment with disease) or withholding treatment from a patient who does not have a bacterial infection (i.e., no treatment with no disease).

The diagnostic test strategy (treatment alternative 3) adds one more layer of uncertainty related to the diagnostic test accuracy (i.e., the ability of the diagnostic test to identify the presence of a disease). Diagnostic accuracy is typically measured in terms of sensitivity and specificity, which quantify how well a test identifies true positive and true negative results. This added uncertainty substantially reduces the uncertainty around the patient's bacterial infection status by a factor of test sensitivity and specificity. Because diagnostic tests are not perfect, test results may still be incorrect (i.e., false positive or false negative). Thus, a patient may still receive unnecessary treatment if the test result is false positive, similar to treatment alternative 1, or not receive beneficial treatment if the test result is false negative, similar to treatment alternative 2.

All of this discussion can be represented graphically in the decision tree depicted in Fig. 7.1, which outlines all the choices and the consequences associated with the example case.

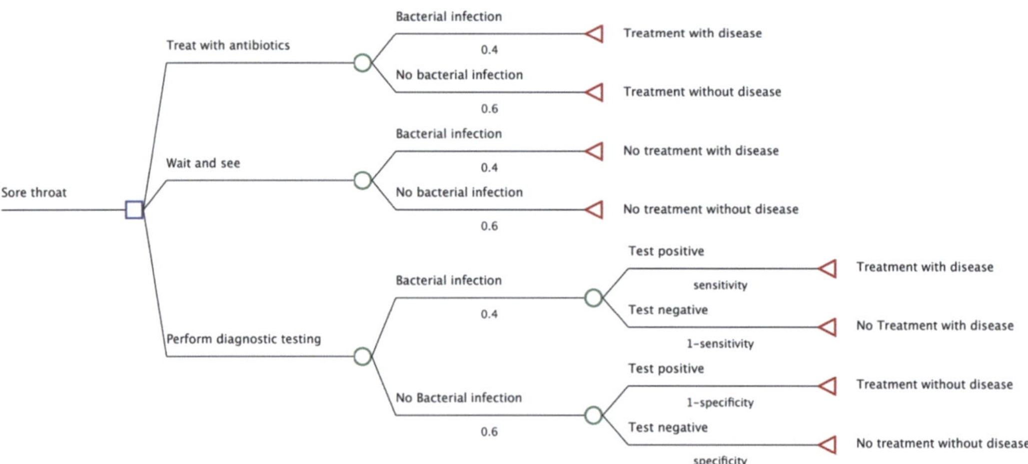

Fig. 7.1 Decision tree depicting all choices associated with treating a sore throat. The decision node is depicted as a square, the chance nodes as circles, and the terminal nodes as triangles. The values under each branch correspond to the probability of the event on the branch occurring. The probability of a patient having a bacterial infection is 40% and not having an infection is 60%. The probability of a positive test result for a patient with a bacterial infection is the test's sensitivity. The probability of a negative test result for a patient with no bacterial infection is the test's specificity. Figure created by A. Tsalatsanis

The decision tree begins on the left with a *decision node*, represented by a square. The lines starting from the decision node represent the alternative treatment options to manage sore throat (i.e., treat with antibiotics, wait and see, perform diagnostic testing). Each line leads to a *chance node* represented by a circle. A branch leaving the chance node represents an event whose outcome is up to chance (i.e., having a disease—in our case, bacterial infection—or not). A triangle in the decision tree is called a *terminal node* and represents the outcome of an event (i.e., treatment with disease or treatment without disease).

With all the choices, events, and outcomes drawn on the decision tree, we use *probabilities* to quantify the uncertainty of each event (i.e., each branch leaving a chance node). Probability is a measure of the likelihood that an event will occur. It is expressed with values between 0 and 1, where 0 denotes an impossible event, and 1 denotes an event that will certainly occur. A probability value of 0.5 indicates that the likelihood of the event occurring is equal to the likelihood of the event not occurring. In the sore throat example, we need to estimate the following probabilities:

1. The patient has a bacterial infection.
2. The diagnostic test sensitivity and specificity.

The clinician can estimate the probability of a patient having a bacterial infection based on several sources of information, including observation of the patient's characteristics (i.e., age, gender), patient symptoms and clinical presentation, local or global health trends (i.e., flu season), and medical literature and research. The test sensitivity and specificity can be found in medical literature. For demonstration, let's assume the probability values are as follows:

1. The patient has a bacterial infection, $p = 0.4$ or 40%. This implies that the patient's probability of not having a bacterial infection is $p = 0.6$ or 60%.
2. The test sensitivity is 0.8, and the test specificity is 0.7.

The probabilities are placed in the decision tree below the respective branches, ensuring that the sum of probabilities in each chance node is equal to 1 (Fig. 7.1). The probability of a test returning a positive result if the patient has a bacterial infection is equal to the test sensitivity. The probability of a test returning a negative result if the patient did not have a bacterial infection is equal to the test specificity.

The final item of information needed to complete the decision tree is a value, or *utility*, that is used to quantify how desirable each outcome is. Formally, the utility represents the decision maker's valuation of a specific health state or outcome. For simplicity, we assume that the utility of positive outcomes is 1, while the utility of adverse outcomes is 0. For example, the utility of the outcome "*treatment with disease*," indicating that the antibiotic treatment is beneficial, is *1, and "treatment without disease,"* indicating that the antibiotic treatment was unnecessary, is 0. Conversely, the outcome "*no treatment with the disease," indicating treatment was withheld incorrectly, is 0, and "no treatment without disease*," indicating that treatment was withheld correctly, is 1. These utilities are placed next to the end nodes. The decision tree in Fig. 7.2 depicts the branches with their probabilities and the end nodes with the utilities of each outcome.

The process for solving the tree and identifying the optimal decision is called *averaging out* [4] the tree. It relies on basic probability operations to calculate the *expected value* of each outcome's utility. The process begins at the right side of the tree and involves multiplying the utility of an outcome with the probability of the event that led to this outcome. The result of this calculation is then summed for each chance node, yielding a partial expected utility for the specific chance node. The process is repeated until the first chance node of every decision choice is reached. The choice with the highest expected utility is the optimal decision. In example 1, the expected utility of the alternative "treat with antibiotics" is $1 * 0.4 + 0 * 0.6 = 0.4$ and the expected utility of the alternative "wait and see" is $0 * 0.4 + 1 * 0.6 = 0.6$. The expected utility of the

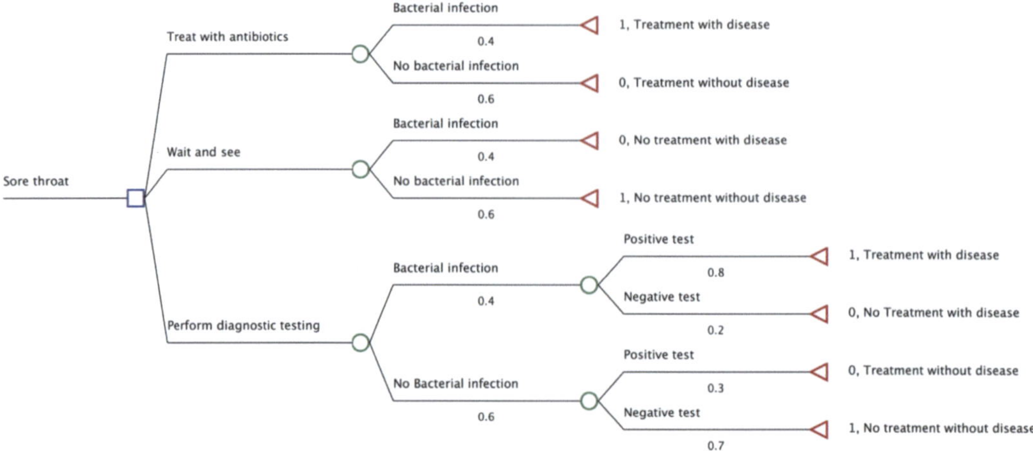

Fig. 7.2 The decision tree depicts all choices associated with the treatment of sore throat, including the probabilities of each event and the utilities of each outcome. The utility of the "treatment with disease" and "no treatment without disease" outcomes is 1 and the utility of the "treatment without disease" and "no treatment with disease" is 0. Figure created by A. Tsalatsanis

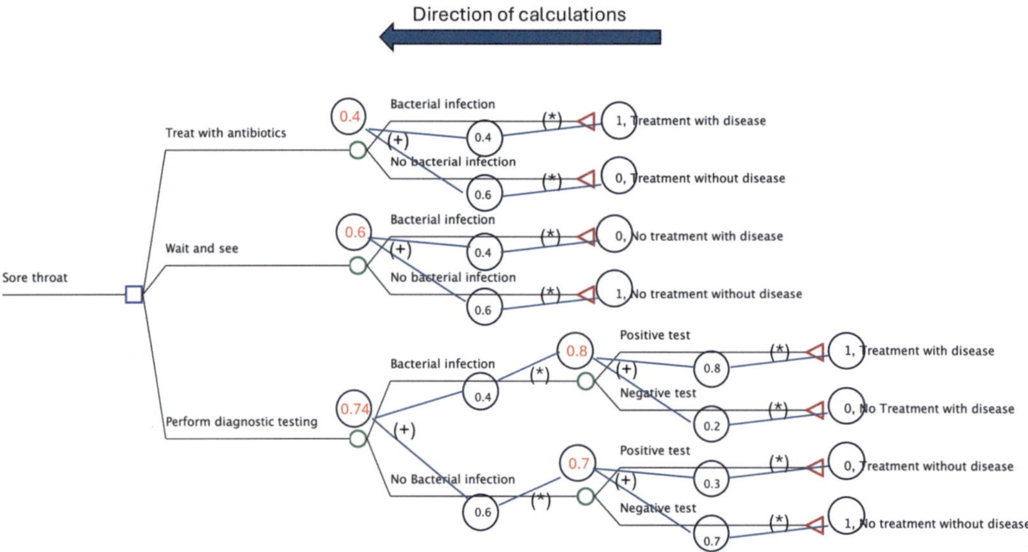

Fig. 7.3 The optimal decision for example case is to perform diagnostic testing before treating with an expected utility of 0.74. (The figure was created by the author)

alternative "perform diagnostic testing" is (1 ∗ 0. 7 + 0 ∗ 0.3) ∗ 0.6 + (1 ∗ 0.8 + 0 ∗ 02) ∗ 0.4 = 0. 74. Figure 7.3 shows the solved tree with the expected values for each choice and the partial expected values of chance nodes. The optimal solution is to perform a diagnostic test with an expected utility of 0.74.

7.2.2 Populating the Decision Tree with Evidence—Evidence-Based Medicine

The structure of a decision tree can grow quite large as the complexity of modeled medical decision increases. Decision trees may include multiple competing treatments, several diagnostic tests, combinations of treatment/ diagnostic strategies, considerations for treatment effectiveness, and/or a variety of outcomes such as cost, life expectancy, survival, and quality of life. Regardless of how complex a tree is or how accurately it maps the alternative choices and their outcomes, it will most certainly fail to identify the optional decision if the data used to populate it are flawed or invalid.

It was mentioned earlier that estimates of probabilities used in a decision tree, such as the probability of bacterial infection or the performance characteristics of a diagnostic test, can be retrieved from the medical literature. It is not uncommon that there is more than one published study available researching the estimates we are interested in. Often, these studies may have conflicting results. How do we decide which study's estimates to pick? Assessing the quality and validity of evidence found in literature falls in the realm of *Evidence-Based Medicine (EBM)*.

EBM is defined as "the conscientious, explicit, judicious and reasonable use of modern, best evidence in making decisions about the care of individual patients". [13, 14] It supports medical decision-making by integrating clinical experience and patient values with the best available evidence [15]. Under the EBM framework, evidence is ranked according to a *hierarchy of evidence* or *pyramid of evidence*, as the one depicted in Fig. 7.4. Different study designs are positioned at different levels of the pyramid. The higher the level, the better the quality of evidence produced by the study. At the bottom, we find case reports that represent the weakest form of evidence, and at the highest level, we find systematic reviews and meta-analyses that produce the highest level of evidence. This is because case reports are limited in scope and generalizability, while systematic reviews and meta-analyses synthesize data from multiple studies to create high-level evidence for a topic. A description of each of the study designs shown in the figure is below.

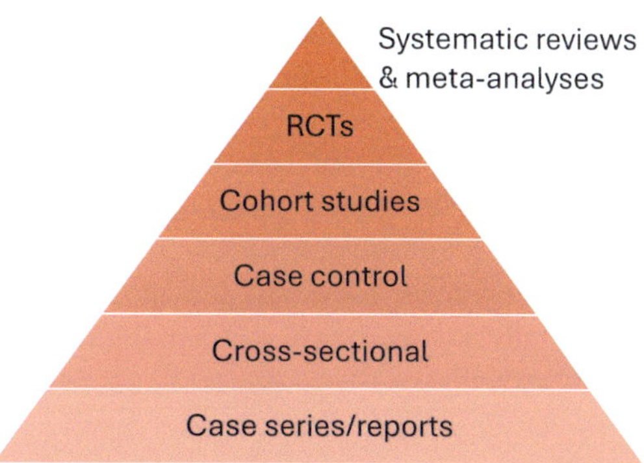

Fig. 7.4 Hierarchy of evidence. Case reports represent the weakest form of evidence. Systematic reviews and meta-analyses produce the highest level of evidence, above Randomized controlled trials (RCTS). (The figure was created by the author from the original that appeared in [15])

- Systematic reviews and Meta-analyses. Systematic reviews [16, 17] use a structured process to identify all studies performed to answer a specific research question, appraise the methods used in each study, select the studies of acceptable quality, and summarize and present results and limitations. Meta-analyses studies extend systematic reviews by mathematically combining the results of the studies in the systematic review.
- Randomized controlled trials [18] (RCTs) divide patients into two or more groups at random. One group receives the intervention of interest, and subsequent groups receive alternative treatments or no treatment (placebo). Due to the randomization process, RCTs minimize biases related to known and unknown prognostic factors.
- Cohort studies [19] follow a group of patients with common characteristics over a period of time to assess how exposure to a risk factor affects a health outcome.
- Case-control studies [20] compare how exposure to a risk factor affects two groups of similar patients. One group has the outcome of interest, and the other does not (i.e., having a disease or not).

- Cross-sectional studies [21] aim to describe population-level outcomes at a given time point.
- Case reports [22] and case series are studies that describe atypical features identified in patients.
- Ideas, opinions, editorials, and anecdotes are typically informational in scope rather than research.

Given the above hierarchy, one may think the best evidence on a subject comes from systematic reviews and/or meta-analyses. In the absence of systematic reviews, the best evidence comes from the next level, RCTs, and so on. While this is understandable, it is not necessarily correct. In fact, the highest level of evidence [23] on a subject comes from the study design that matches the question domains of treatment, diagnostic accuracy, prognosis, cost, etc. For example,

- Questions on how a treatment or intervention affects a patient outcome are best answered using the RCT study design or a systematic review and meta-analyses of multiple RCTs. In the absence of RCTs, treatment effectiveness questions can be answered using cohort or case-control study designs.
- Questions on how prognostic or risk factors are associated with an outcome are best answered using a cohort study design followed by a case-control design.
- Questions on diagnostic accuracy are best answered using a cross-sectional analytic study design followed by a case-control study design or a systematic review and meta-analyses of multiple cross-sectional/case-control studies. These studies assess the test's performance in correctly identifying the presence or absence of a disease using statistical terms such as sensitivity and specificity.
- Questions on cost associated with a treatment/intervention are best answered with economic analyses. These studies typically compare different strategies in terms of cost and effectiveness and report net cost-benefit, return on investment, and/or incremental cost-effectiveness ratio.

When searching the literature for the evidence necessary to populate a decision tree, it is crucial to use search engines that categorize search results using the hierarchy of evidence. Examples of such search engines include PubMed [24] clinical queries and Trip database [25]. These engines allow for search queries specific to therapy, diagnosis, prognosis, etc., and filter the resulting articles based on study design.

For the example case, the search for "acute pharyngitis" and "diagnosis" in the Trip database returns a systematic review of studies assessing the diagnostic accuracy of rapid tests for streptococcal infections in people with a sore throat [26]. If the clinician considers a rapid test to diagnose the bacterial infection, the study [26] will inform them that the test's sensitivity (ability to detect the presence of a disease) varies from 67.9 to 100% and its specificity (ability to detect the absence of a disease) ranges from 73.3% to 100%. The same search in PubMed produced a systematic review and meta-analysis of the accuracy of two scoring systems used to diagnose pharyngitis in patients presenting to secondary care [27]. The study concluded that neither of the scoring systems is accurate in predicting the risk of pharyngitis.

7.2.3 Assigning Values to Outcomes

Earlier in the chapter, we described *utility* as the means of assigning a value to an outcome, where 1 denotes a desirable outcome (e.g., survival) and 0 denotes an undesirable outcome (e.g., death). However, utility is a multifaceted concept that goes beyond a binary system. Utilities can be expressed in terms of various quantitative outcomes, such as *life expectancy* and *cost*; qualitative outcomes, such as *patient satisfaction and quality of life; and* a combination of quantitative and qualitative outcomes, such as *life expectancy and quality of life*. More interestingly, utilities can be used to quantify the decision maker's value judgments regarding the harms vs. the benefits of a decision and, therefore, incorporate the decision maker's preferences in the decision process. Some of the techniques that have been used to elicit patient preferences for outcomes include the rating scale or feeling thermometer, standard gamble, and the time trade-off [4].

When using a rating scale, we ask the decision maker to rate an outcome with a value that ranges from 0 to 100. For example, "On a scale from 0 to 100, where 0 represents no pain, and 100 represents the worst pain you have ever felt, what number would describe your current level of pain?". We ask similar questions for each outcome we want to consider in our model.

The standard gamble technique is a much more complicated than the rating scale and it aims to quantify how much risk of death a person would accept to improve their health with a series of questions. For example, consider we are interested in assessing a patient's valuation of a health state (e.g., living with some level of pain). The gamble scenario will be presented as "There is a pill that will cure your pain but has a 50% chance of causing death. Would you take it?" If they say "no," we lower the chance of death and the chance of full recovery, "What if the chance the pill would cause death was 1%, but the chance for full recovery was 99%? Would you take the pill?" If they say "yes," we ask again, "What if the chance of death was 25% and the chance of full recovery was 75%?". We continue these questions until both choices feel the same. Then, the utility of the outcome we wanted to measure is the probability of permanent relief.

The time trade-off technique estimates the utility of a health state by asking how much survival time one would give up to improve the health state. For example, assuming a patient in their 40 s has a life expectancy of another 40 years, we ask, "There is a pill that will cure your condition, but it will reduce your life expectancy to 20 years. Would you take it"?, if they say no, we ask again, "What if it would reduce your life expectancy to 39 years"? and continue asking until taking the pill or not feels the same (i.e., 36 years). The utility of the health state would be equal to the ratio of reduced life expectancy over the starting life expectancy (i.e., 36/40).

7.3 Summary

In this chapter, we discussed the complexities of medical decision-making, which involves decisions made under uncertainty with trade-offs between risks and benefits. We introduced decision analysis to model and solve decision problems via decision trees representing all treatment alternatives and their consequences. We learned about the hierarchy of evidence, which is useful when we search for data to populate the decision trees, and about techniques to elicit decision-maker preferences on the modeled outcomes. All in all, this chapter provided a starting point for health informatics professionals to understand the mechanisms of medical decision-making and enable them to build and implement clinical decision support systems available at the point of care.

References

1. Whang W. Medical decision-making. In: Gellman MD, Turner JR, editors. Encyclopedia of behavioral medicine. New York: Springer New York; 2013. p. 1209–10.
2. van der Velde G. Clinical decision analysis: an alternate, rigorous approach to making clinical decisions and developing treatment recommendations. J Can Chiropr Assoc. 2005;49(4):258.
3. Sox HC, Higgins MC, Owens DK, Schmidler GS. Medical decision making. Wiley; 2024.
4. Hunink MM, Weinstein MC, Wittenberg E, Drummond MF, Pliskin JS, Wong JB, Glasziou PP. Decision making in health and medicine: integrating evidence and values. Cambridge University Press; 2014.

5. Bell DE, Raiffa H, Tversky A. Decision making: descriptive, normative, and prescriptive interactions. Cambridge University Press; 1988.
6. Kahneman D, Tversky A. Choices, values, and frames. Am Psychol. 1984;39(4):341.
7. Tang V, Otto K, Seering W, Tang V, Otto K, Seering W. Decision theories and methodologies. In: Executive decision synthesis: a sociotechnical systems paradigm; 2018. p. 63–105.
8. Hellinger FJ. Expected utility theory and risky choices with health outcomes. Med Care. 1989;27:273–9.
9. Kahneman D, Tversky A. Prospect theory: an analysis of decision under risk. In: Handbook of the fundamentals of financial decision making: Part I. World Scientific; 2013. p. 99–127.
10. Bell DE. Regret in decision making under uncertainty. Oper Res. 1982;30(5):961–81.
11. Tsalatsanis A, Barnes LE, Hozo I, Djulbegovic B. Extensions to regret-based decision curve analysis: an application to hospice referral for terminal patients. BMC Med Inform Decis Mak. 2011;11:1–13.
12. Tsalatsanis A, Hozo I, Vickers A, Djulbegovic B. A regret theory approach to decision curve analysis: a novel method for eliciting decision makers' preferences and decision-making. BMC Med Inform Decis Mak. 2010;10:1–14.
13. Sackett DL. Evidence-based medicine. Spine. 1998;23(10):1085–6.
14. Sackett DL, Rosenberg WM, Gray JM, Haynes RB, Richardson WS. Evidence based medicine: what it is and what it isn't. British Medical Journal Publishing Group; 1996. p. 71–2.
15. Masic I, Miokovic M, Muhamedagic B. Evidence based medicine–new approaches and challenges. Acta Informatica Medica. 2008;16(4):219.
16. Cook DJ, Mulrow CD, Haynes RB. Systematic reviews: synthesis of best evidence for clinical decisions. Ann Intern Med. 1997;126(5):376–80.
17. Oxman AD, Cook DJ, Guyatt GH, Bass E, Brill-Edwards P, Browman G, Detsky A, Farkouh M, Gerstein H, Haines T. Users' guides to the medical literature: VI. How to use an overview. JAMA. 1994;272(17):1367–71.
18. Setia MS. Methodology series module 4: clinical trials. Indian J Dermatol. 2016;61(4):393–402.
19. Setia MS. Methodology series module 1: cohort studies. Indian J Dermatol. 2016;61(1):21–5.
20. Setia MS. Methodology series module 2: case-control studies. Indian J Dermatol. 2016;61(2):146–51.
21. Setia MS. Methodology series module 3: cross-sectional studies. Indian J Dermatol. 2016;61(3):261–4.
22. Sayre JW, Toklu HZ, Ye F, Mazza J, Yale S. Case reports, case series–from clinical practice to evidence-based medicine in graduate medical education. Cureus. 2017;9(8)
23. Aslam S, Georgiev H, Mehta K, Kumar A. Matching research design to clinical research questions. Indian J Sex Transm Dis AIDS. 2012;33(1):49–53.
24. Pubmed. Clinical queries. Bethesda, MD: National Library of Medicine; 1946. [cited 2024]. Available from: https://pubmed.ncbi.nlm.nih.gov/clinical/
25. Montori VM, Ebbert JO. TRIP database. BMJ Evid Based Med. 2002;7(4):104.
26. National Institute for Health and Care Excellence (NICE). Rapid tests for group A streptococcal infections in people with a sore throat Diagnostics Guidance [DG38]). 2019.
27. Kanagasabai A, Evans C, Jones HE, Hay AD, Dawson S, Savović J, Elwenspoek MM. Systematic review and meta-analysis of the accuracy of McIsaac and Centor score in patients presenting to secondary care with pharyngitis. Clin Microbiol Infect. 2024;30:445.

Human Factors, Ergonomics (HFE), and Systems Thinking

8

Onur Asan, Bijun Wang, and Linghan Zhang

Foundational Domains

This chapter addresses the following AMIA Foundational Domain: F5—Human Factors and Socio-technical Systems.

Learning Objectives

1. Define the field of human factors.
2. Describe the principles of human factors methodologies.
3. Summarize the application of human factors in healthcare and HIT.
4. Describe the systems thinking process and how it is related to HF principles.
5. Explain how people fit into socio-technical systems.

Definitions

Human factors engineering: Human factors engineering is the application of knowledge about human capabilities and limitations to design systems, products, and environments that are safe, effective, and easy to use.

Systems thinking: Systems thinking is a problem-solving approach that examines how the parts of a system interact and influence each other.

8.1 Human Factors and Ergonomics (HFE): Domain, Goals, and Considerations

Human factors, situated at the crossroads of psychology and engineering, is committed to crafting every facet of a work system to enhance human performance and ensure safety. Human factors, also referred to as *ergonomics*, employ scientific approaches to enhance system performance and mitigate the risk of inadvertent harm. In the realm of healthcare, the objectives of human factors are dual: facilitating the cognitive and physical tasks of healthcare professionals [3] and fostering the delivery of high-quality, secure care for patients [4]. According to the International Ergonomics Association (IEA), ergonomics or human factors is defined as "The scientific discipline concerned with the understanding of interactions among humans and other elements of a system, and the profession that applies theory, principles, data and methods to design in order to optimize human well-being and overall system

O. Asan (✉)
Stevens Institute of Technology, Hoboken, NJ, USA
e-mail: oasan@stevens.edu

B. Wang
University of Nevada, Reno, Reno, USA
e-mail: bijunw@unr.edu

L. Zhang
Eindhoven University of Technology, Eindhoven, Netherlands
e-mail: l.zhang1@tue.nl

C. Eldredge et al. (eds.), *Introductory Textbook in Health Informatics*, Health Informatics,
https://doi.org/10.1007/978-3-032-16657-9_8

performance" (www.iea.cc). The IEA divides HFE into three categories:

1. *Physical ergonomics* primarily centers on the physical attributes of individuals. In the healthcare domain, specific examples include the design of hospital facilities, the layout of physical environments, patient handling equipment, patient room design, the creation of safer patient beds, the development of surgical instruments, the strategic placement of diagnostic equipment, and the design of ergonomic chairs or desks.
2. *Cognitive ergonomics* addresses the cognitive characteristics of individuals or users, focusing on optimizing the interaction between individuals and information, interfaces, or technology. Many patient safety concerns, such as medication errors in the patient safety domain, fall within the realm of cognitive ergonomics. Traditionally, this discipline involves understanding and enhancing cognitive processes such as perception, attention, memory, decision-making, and problem-solving to enhance the overall performance of systems. In healthcare, cognitive ergonomics plays a pivotal role in the design of systems, technologies, and environments that empower healthcare professionals to deliver safe and effective care. The design and implementation of various technologies in healthcare brought up many cognitive ergonomics issues, including the usability of technologies or medical devices. Some of the exemplary applications are (a) designing user-friendly interfaces for electronic health record systems or EHRs (discussed more in Chap. 10); (b) implementing communication systems that support effective information exchange among healthcare team members, reducing cognitive workload and the potential for miscommunication, (c) designing patient education materials using clear language, visuals, and interactive formats to enhance patient understanding, compliance, and self-management, taking cognitive factors into account, and (d) designing user-friendly interfaces for telehealth platforms and remote monitoring devices, considering cognitive aspects to facilitate seamless interactions between healthcare providers and patients.
3. *Organizational or macro ergonomics* deals with the overall *socio-technical system* in which the work is performed. In healthcare context, some of the application areas are workflow design, team coordination, job stress and burnout of workers, organizational culture and learning, teamwork, technology integration, work schedule, care transition and organizational design, patient-centered care, and policy development. By applying macro-ergonomics principles in healthcare, organizations can create systems and environments that enhance overall efficiency, improve patient outcomes, and contribute to the well-being of healthcare professionals. This holistic approach considers the complex interactions between various elements within the healthcare system.

HFE methods are applied in many domains, such as aviation, nuclear, transportation, and getting more attention in healthcare. In this chapter, we are focusing more on human factors in the healthcare domain. In the healthcare field, HFE possesses significant potential to enhance the design of various systems involving people, such as work systems and product/service systems. However, it also encounters challenges related to market readiness and the availability of high-quality applications. HFE is characterized by a unique blend of three essential features: (1) a systems approach, (2) a design-driven nature, and (3) a focus on two closely interconnected outcomes—performance and well-being. To effectively contribute to future system design, HFE must showcase its value more convincingly to the key stakeholders in system design [5]. While HFE already holds a robust value proposition, primarily centered around well-being, and engages with the stakeholder group of 'system actors' (doctors, nurses, patients, families, staff, technicians, designers, and administrative), there is a need to engage stakeholders, especially patients and families when a patient-centered healthcare system is intended to design.

Although HFE methodologies contributed to the design of processes, technologies, devices, physical environments, and other aspects of work systems, there are primary challenges that limit the potential use of HFE. These challenges can be listed as cultural differences between engineers and healthcare professionals, resource and expertise limitations, the organizational environment, fragmentation of the care process, and policy and market issues [8]. Some of these challenges can be solved with longitudinal programs to better introduce the value of HF methodologies to healthcare professionals. One primary misconception that needs to be corrected when it comes to HFE considerations, as explained by Russ et al. [6], is that "HFE is about eliminating human errors." Errors are inherent, and the pursuit of eradicating human imperfections in healthcare or any industry proves to be an unattainable objective. Therefore, human factors experts collect data on human characteristics and interactions within the work environment to formulate systems and tools that align with the physical and cognitive capabilities of humans and demonstrate resilience to unforeseen events. Additionally, adopting a human factors approach can cultivate a safety-oriented culture, foster a conducive learning environment, and promote the establishment of a culture where unintentional errors are reported without the fear of reprisal. The findings from these reports can then be utilized to enhance various components of the system, facilitating sustainable and positive changes. Therefore, the primary fact is *"Human factors is about designing systems that are resilient to unanticipated events."* [6].

8.2 HFE Considerations in Health Information Technologies

Health Information Technology refers to a broad array of technologies, hardware, software, and services that are designed for the collection, storage, access, updating, sharing, and data analysis of individuals' health information for healthcare providers, organizations, laypeople, patients, and caregivers [9]. These technologies are being increasingly deployed and is transforming healthcare to the next level with multiple potential benefits such as improving communication, patient-centered care, patient safety, and overall quality of healthcare. For ultimate value, these technologies should be designed to be perceived as useful and to be easy to use according to well established technology acceptance model [7]. On the other hand, poorly designed health information technologies might contribute to negative outcomes as well as a lack of adoption. Poor usability and other unmet human factor challenges associated with the implementation and evaluation of these health information technologies are the main factors that slow down and deter their adoption. Even worse, these challenges are reported to be the possible causes of errors in healthcare delivery, such as prescribing and administering medicines, clinical workflow and process, etc., which can eventually cause physician and clinician burnout [14] and preventable harm to patients. In 2021, certified EHRs were ubiquitously adopted in the United States by 96% of all non-federal acute care hospitals and around 80% of office-based physicians in 2021 [13]. It is predicted that the healthcare IT market size will be 358.5 billion in 2024 and keep increasing at the average rate of 15.24% in the next five years, reaching 728.63 billion in 2029 [18]. Given the significant beneficial/detrimental effects and prevalence of health information technologies in healthcare, it is necessary to optimize their implementation. Especially, we need systematic approaches to examine the entire socio-technical systems, from the perspectives of human factors and usability.

8.2.1 Using HFE Methods to Study HITs

Over the last few years, *SEIPS (Systems Engineering Initiative for Patient Safety)* was used to describe the key characteristics of three major components, i.e., the work system, processes, and outcomes, and the impacts of work system and processes on outcomes [8]. The SEIPS model is a conceptual framework developed to understand and improve the complex interactions between people, technology, tasks, and the overall work system within healthcare settings. It was created to enhance patient safety by addressing the intricate relationships and dynamics that influence the delivery of healthcare services. The work system has five components: person, tasks, tools and technologies, physical environment, and organizational conditions that interact with each other. Each of these components contains several elements. For example, the component "person" has elements like education, skills, and motivations; the component "organization" has elements like teamwork, coordination, and communication; the component "tools and technologies" has elements such as any type of technologies used or introduced to the healthcare system. The structure of this work system affects the processes of caring and other processes that support the caring processes (e.g., communication), which eventually decides the patient care outcomes (quality of care and patient safety) and employee and organizational outcomes. Additionally, the SEIPS model suggests that the outcomes of patient care and employee/organizational are related.

Studies used the SEIPS model to better understand the impact of any given health information technologies on other elements and patient outcomes. For instance, Martinez et al. used SEIPS 2.0 to understand the system variables that could affect patients' and clinicians' experiences with a consumer health IT application for blood pressure monitoring and management [17]. Another study utilized the SEIPS model to better understand how use of EHRs in clinics impacts doctor-patient communication and patient engagement/empowerment in clinic environment [1].

In summary, human factors methods should be considered in the entire development process of health information technologies, which can improve the design of the technologies, and eventually improve the experiences of patients, clinicians, and other involved parties in the work system. However, despite much effort from human factors experts in health information technologies, doctors often state that these technologies complicate their jobs and increase time spent on administrative tasks such as charting [15]. Therefore, there are still a lot of opportunities to apply human factors methods in the development of health information technologies.

8.3 Case Vignette: Application of HF Methodologies (Usability) in HIT Development

More than 85% of people globally own smartphones [10], and approximately 63% of adults in the United States have engaged with mobile health (mHealth) applications [16]. These mHealth apps serve diverse functions, such as monitoring health status, providing medical references, aiding medical decision-making, and regulating health behaviors. Despite their widespread use, most mHealth app developments lack substantial end-user inputs and feedback, typically undergoing only a single usability assessment, such as measuring time efficiency, during a specific development stage, like prototyping. Researchers assert that usability is a primary hindrance to the adoption and sustained use of mHealth apps [19], emphasizing the necessity to consider it both before and after the prototyping phase.

In response to this, Cho et al. adopt a theoretically driven methodological approach based on the Stratified View of Health Information Technology Usability Evaluation Framework [20] from human factors perspective. They devised a multi-level evaluation framework to be applied to the design, development, and evaluation of a mHealth app named mVIP [2]. The framework encompasses three levels: Level 1 focuses on user-task interaction, Level 2 examines task performance in laboratory settings, and Level 3 incorporates environmental factors in system evaluation.

Implementing each level for their mHealth application designed for symptom self-management in people living with HIV (PLWH), Cho et al. conducted a comprehensive evaluation. In Level 1, they utilized a card sorting technique to establish the information architecture based on existing literature before prototyping. PLWH end-users ranked index cards listing symptoms and self-management strategies, determining the information structure for the application. Moving to Level 2, usability was tested with both end-users and experts, evaluating tasks like log-in, password updates, and symptom-specific strategy retrieval. Task performance time, eye gaze tracking, and user experiences were compared among participants with and without difficulties using the application. Recommendations from end-users led to improvements in content, functionality, and interface. Experts provided heuristic ratings for the severity of usability problems, guiding further adjustments. In Level 3, Cho et al. assessed the feasibility of mVIP in improving symptoms for PLWH participants in their daily lives. An intervention group used mVIP with self-reported symptoms and self-management strategies, while a control group had access only to self-reported symptoms. Both groups found mVIP useful and easy to use, with suggestions for personalization based on initial HIV diagnosis, age, and conditions. In summary, this study underscores the importance of establishing app components before prototyping, emphasizing that good information architecture is crucial for developing intuitive and user-friendly technology, which will eventually improve the patient/user experience and long-term outcomes.

8.4 Systems Thinking Approach in Healthcare

The modern healthcare system is fundamentally complex, primarily due to the involvement of numerous stakeholders such as patients, healthcare providers, policymakers, and insurance companies reflecting the multifaceted challenges and demands of providing care in a diverse and ever-changing society. Each group has its shared and distinct goals, viewpoints, and impacts, contributing to the intricate nature of the healthcare environment. Although there is no universal definition, systems thinking addresses that interactions among varied systems create a dynamic and nonlinear network where actions and decisions in one area can propagate through the system, causing unpredictable results. Systems thinking, first conceptualized by Ludwig von Bertalanffy through his General Systems Theory in the 1930s, emphasizes the importance of understanding systems as a whole, considering the interrelations and interactions within [21]. This approach was later applied in healthcare in the late twentieth century. Peter Senge used systems thinking in organizational and healthcare contexts, advocating for a holistic view to understand complex systems better [28].

The application in healthcare has evolved significantly, with the World Health Organization integrating systems thinking into its strategies for strengthening health systems [22]. For example, in the realm of policymaking, a study by Rutter et al. [23] explored the incorporation of systems thinking to enhance public health policies by understanding complex systems and their impact on health outcomes, highlighting its potential for more effective health interventions. In the context of technological advancements, research by Zhang et al. [24] demonstrated how systems thinking, integrated with big data, can optimize personalized health strategies. This work illustrates the capacity of technology-driven system-thinking approaches to revolutionize healthcare delivery by enabling personalized, efficient care. Focusing on patient outcomes, a cross-sectional study by Sarhan et al. [26] investigates the impact of systems thinking on postoperative complications. The findings reveal that applying systems thinking principles in clinical settings can significantly enhance patient safety and outcomes, showing its practical benefits in direct patient care.

In conclusion, despite the absence of a universally accepted definition, systems thinking in healthcare is broadly recognized as an approach aimed at comprehensively understanding and addressing the complexities inherent in healthcare systems. It focuses on analyzing the relationships and interactions among all elements of the system—including patients, healthcare providers, administrative processes, and technological tools—to improve health outcomes and enhance the efficiency of healthcare delivery. By adopting systems thinking, healthcare practitioners and policymakers can develop more effective strategies that account for the interconnected nature of health services and patient care.

8.5 Systems Thinking Approach and HFE

In the context of human factors in healthcare, integrating systems thinking into today's complex healthcare systems addresses the complexity of human behavior, technology, and organizational workflows aimed at improving patient care and overall healthcare delivery. We propose a simplified framework to illustrate how human factors and systems thinking converge to influence and enhance healthcare delivery shown in Fig. 8.1. The "Human Factors" aspect focuses on optimizing the user experience, considering everything from ergonomic design to cognitive load, ensuring that the system is navigable and sensitive to the end-users' requirements. "Systems Thinking," on the other hand, ensures that the healthcare system is viewed and understood as a cohesive unit, where each part's role and influence are considered in the context of the whole.

In the healthcare framework, the interaction between Governance, Socio-Technical Systems, and Patient-Centered Care is foundational to the successful application of Human Factors and Systems Thinking. Governance and regulation support the deployment and operation of socio-technical systems. This ensures that such systems are not only technologically advanced but also adhere to ethical standards and regulatory compliances that are crucial for patient safety and privacy [31]. These regulations are dynamic, evolving in response to technological advancements to maintain relevant and robust oversight. The socio-technical systems, which represent a combination of technological tools and social processes, are pivotal in actualizing patient-centered care [11]. Leveraging advanced technology, socio-technical systems in healthcare facilitate personalized and humanized care. By prioritizing the user experience, these systems transform patient and provider feedback into actionable insights, leading to continuous

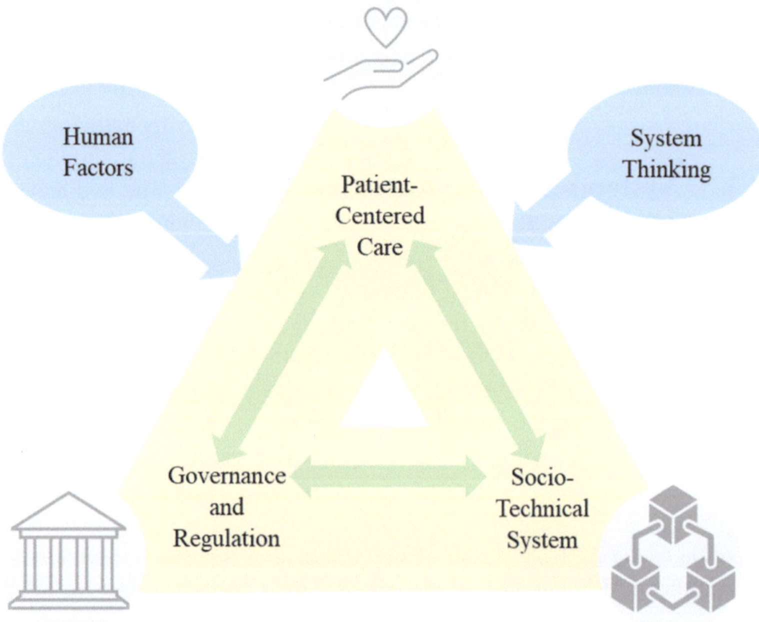

Fig. 8.1 Combination of systems thinking and human factors in healthcare

enhancements in both the design and function of healthcare delivery. The focus on the user experience drives improvements in system designs and functionalities, which in turn may prompt a re-evaluation and update of governance protocols to better serve patients' interests [30].

Case Vignette

In their 2016 empirical study, Bowie et al. endeavored to merge human factors principles with systems thinking to address the prevalent issue of inadequate *Significant Event Analysis (SEA)* in primary care [12]. The challenges in SEA are often linked to clinicians' emotional distress and a lack of systemic insight. The study aimed to enhance SEA's effectiveness by incorporating guiding tools grounded in human factors principles.

From the perspective of systems thinking at the individual practitioner level, the intervention introduced a personal handbook. This handbook was designed to mitigate emotional distress and facilitate human factors analysis following critical incidents. It sought to diminish self-blame and promote objective self-analysis by guiding practitioners through emotional challenges and elucidating systemic contributory factors. Empirical evidence demonstrated widespread acceptance, with participants acknowledging its utility in managing emotional challenges and improving understanding of critical incidents. This emphasizes the effectiveness of systems thinking in recognizing and addressing the intricate interplay between individual emotional responses and broader systemic factors, underscoring the importance of considering human factors within the systemic framework to enhance both personal well-being and systemic efficiency in healthcare settings.

Conversely, at the system level, the study introduced the Desk Pad tool and a structured Report Format. These tools aimed to guide team-based systemic analysis and provide a coherent format for reporting, respectively. They were designed to foster structured, systemic analysis during team discussions, encouraging comprehensive incident understanding, identification of learning opportunities, and actionable improvements. Post-intervention SEA reports predominantly reflected a systemic approach, showcasing the tools' effectiveness in shifting the focus from individual blame to systemic understanding. This contributed to fostering a culture of learning and systemic improvement. This case exemplifies the successful integration of human factors and systems thinking in healthcare, illustrating how well-crafted interventions can address both personal emotional well-being and systemic understanding, ultimately enhancing patient care and healthcare system efficiency.

8.6 Systems Approach Application in Modern Healthcare: The Case of Artificial Intelligence

Building on the principles of systems thinking, the Systems Approach in modern healthcare translates this conceptual framework into actionable strategies that incorporate advanced technologies like AI to enhance patient care and system efficiency. This methodology involves a comprehensive understanding of the healthcare environment as an interactive and evolving network where the importance of the interconnectedness of human-technology-governance interactions cannot be overstated. For example, incorporating AI into modern healthcare systems exemplifies the Systems Approach through a sequence of interconnected steps:

Identification of System Boundaries This step involves defining the reach and impact of AI within healthcare, which could vary from its role in a single unit to its integration across the entire health service delivery.

Mapping of Interactions It is crucial to map out how AI interfaces with patients, healthcare providers, and the organizational framework. This includes understanding how AI-driven decision support systems interact with clinical workflows and patient care.

Analysis of Feedback Loops The Systems Approach investigates the impact of AI on healthcare delivery, such as how machine learning algorithms' suggestions are utilized by healthcare professionals and how patient outcomes feedback into the AI's learning process.

Scenario Planning Anticipating various outcomes from the integration of AI, such as enhanced diagnostic accuracy or potential disruptions, helps in preparing for future states of the healthcare system.

Implementation of Interventions Using the insights from system analysis, healthcare systems can implement AI applications to optimize patient care, automate administrative tasks, and enhance decision-making processes.

Monitoring and Adjustment Post-implementation, the Systems Approach involves continuous monitoring of AI's impact on healthcare delivery and readiness to adapt based on feedback from the system's performance.

Figure 8.2 demonstrates a feedback loop within this context, where AI's role in healthcare is continuously refined through interactions with patients and care providers. AI's ability to process patient-generated data allows for more customized care, which in turn, informs care providers for better decision-making. This ongoing loop ensures that healthcare services are both adaptive and personalized.

Moreover, care providers act as a bridge between patients and governance, communicating patients' concerns and preferences, as well as advocating for their needs. This exchange of information is crucial in shaping policies that are both patient-centered and adaptable to the evolving healthcare landscape [27]. Another essential interaction is between AI and governance, as real-time data and analytics provided by AI inform policymakers, enabling them to make data-driven decisions and refine regulatory frameworks. In turn, governance guides the development and deployment of AI technologies, ensuring that ethical considerations and patient safety are at the forefront [25].

By applying systems approach to the study of these interactions, researchers and stakeholders can better comprehend how various elements of the healthcare system influence each other and identify best practices, potential challenges, and

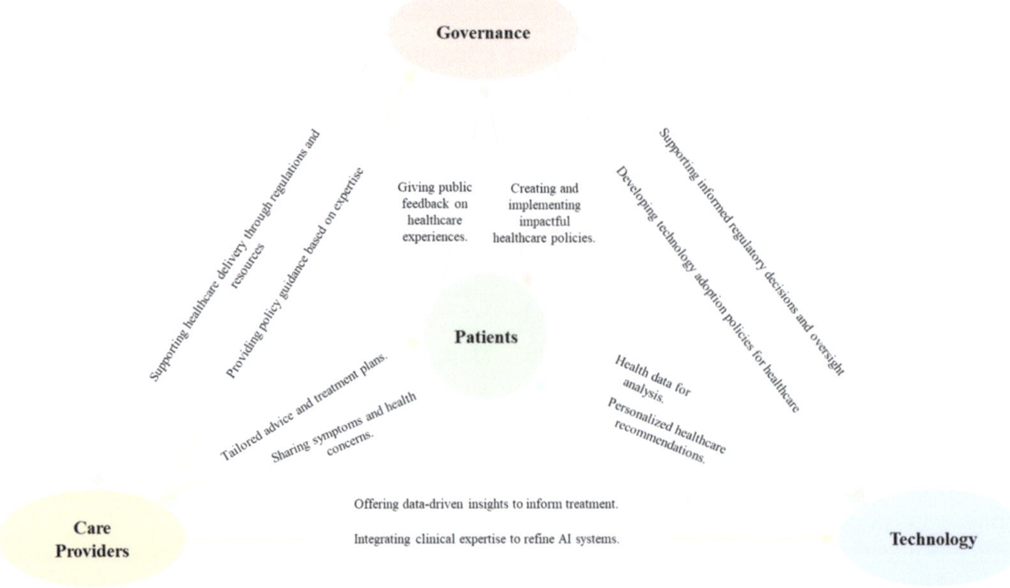

Fig. 8.2 Governance-AI-Technology interaction in patient-centered healthcare system

areas for improvement [29]. This holistic approach enables the development of more efficient, effective, and patient-centered healthcare systems by considering the broader context and the complex interplay between AI, care providers, and governance [25].

8.7 Conclusion

The potential of human factors and systems thinking approach to enhance patient safety, doctor-patient communication, and overall healthcare systems delivery is evident but not fully realized. Recognized and proven application areas encompass healthcare implementation, medication safety, team communication, patient-centered care, medical device design and usability, as well as workload analysis, clinician burnout, and complexity management. Despite these demonstrated benefits, challenges persist in expanding the scale, application, and impact of these methodologies. There has been a gradual development of systems thinking and human factors awareness in healthcare, which should be more widely cultivated. Engagement of more HFE/systems thinking approaches into the overall curriculum and research agenda of healthcare systems will eventually make our healthcare system safer and of higher quality.

Resource Table

Organization	Website URL
Human Factors and Ergonomics Society	www.hfes.org
International Ergonomics Association	www.iea.cc
Resources on usability testing	https://digital.gov/topics/usability/
Descriptions of many HF tools and tutorials	https://www.hf.faa.gov/

References

1. Asan O. Providers' perceived facilitators and barriers to EHR screen sharing in outpatient settings. Appl Ergon. 2017;58:301–7.
2. Cho H, Yen PY, Dowding D, Merrill JA, Schnall R. A multi-level usability evaluation of mobile health applications: a case study. J Biomed Inform. 2018;86:79–89.
3. Karsh BT, Holden RJ, Alper SJ, et al. A human factors engineering paradigm for patient safety: designing to support. Qual Saf Health Care. 2006;15 (Suppl 1):i59–65.
4. Saleem JJ, Russ AL, Sanderson P, et al. Current challenges and opportunities for better integration of human factors research with development of clinical information systems. Yearb Med Inform. 2009:48–58. https://doi.org/10.1055/s-0038-1638638. [pii] [Published Online First: Epub Date]. me09010048
5. Dul J, Bruder R, Buckle P, Carayon P, Falzon P, Marras WS, et al. A strategy for human factors/ergonomics: developing the discipline and profession. Ergonomics. 2012;55(4):377–95.
6. Russ AL, Fairbanks RJ, Karsh BT, Militello LG, Saleem JJ, Wears RL. The science of human factors: separating fact from fiction. BMJ Qual Saf. 2013;22:802.
7. Holden RJ, Asan O, Wozniak EM, Flynn KE, Scanlon MC. Nurses' perceptions, acceptance, and use of a novel in-room pediatric ICU technology: testing an expanded technology acceptance model. BMC Med Inform Decis Mak. 2016;16:1–10.
8. Carayon P, Wooldridge A, Hose BZ, Salwei M, Benneyan J. Challenges and opportunities for improving patient safety through human factors and systems engineering. Health Aff. 2018;37(11):1862–9.
9. Alsyouf A, Lutfi A, Alsubahi N, Alhazmi FN, Al-Mugheed K, Anshasi RJ, et al. The use of a Technology Acceptance Model (TAM) to predict patients' usage of a personal health record system: the role of security, privacy, and usability. Int J Environ Res Public Health. 2023;20(2):1347.
10. Bankmycell. How Many Phones are in the World. 2024. https://www.bankmycell.com/blog/how-many-phones-are-in-the-world
11. Borycki E, Kushniruk A. Towards an integrative cognitive-socio-technical approach in health informatics: analyzing technology-induced error involving health information systems to improve patient safety. Open Med Inform J. 2010;4:181–7. https://doi.org/10.2174/1874431101004010181.
12. Bowie P, Mcnaughton E, Bruce D, Holly D, Forrest E, Macleod M, Kennedy S, Power A, Toppin D, Black I, Pooley J, Taylor A, Swanson V, Kelly M, Ferguson J, Stirling S, Wakeling J, Inglis A, McKay J, Sargeant J. Enhancing the effectiveness of significant event

analysis: exploring personal impact and applying systems thinking in primary care. J Contin Educ Heal Prof. 2016;36(3):195–205. https://doi.org/10.1097/CEH.0000000000000098add.

13. Diaz N. 96% of US hospitals have EHRs, but barriers remain to interoperability, ONC says. Becker's Health IT. 2023, March 7. https://www.beckershospitalreview.com/ehrs/96-of-us-hospitals-have-ehrs-but-barriers-remain-to-interoperability-onc-says
14. Gardner RL, Cooper E, Haskell J, Harris DA, Poplau S, Kroth PJ, Linzer M. Physician stress and burnout: the impact of health information technology. J Am Med Inform Assoc. 2019;26(2):106–14.
15. Gawande A. Why doctors hate their computers. 2018, November 5. https://www.newyorker.com/magazine/2018/11/12/why-doctors-hate-their-computers
16. Insider Intelligence.Nearly two-thirds of US consumers are Mobile health app users. 2023. https://www.insiderintelligence.com/content/nearly-two-thirds-of-us-consumers-mobile-health-app-users
17. Martinez VI, Marquard JL, Saver B, Garber L, Preusse P. Consumer health informatics interventions must support user workflows, be easy-to-use, and improve cognition: applying the seips 2.0 model to evaluate patients' and clinicians' experiences with the conduit-hid intervention. Int J Human-Comput Interact. 2017;33(4):333–43.
18. Mordor Intelligence. Healthcare IT Market Size & Share Analysis—Growth Trends & Forecasts (2024–2029). 2024. https://www.mordorintelligence.com/industry-reports/global-healthcare-it-market-industry
19. Vuong AM, Huber JC Jr, Bolin JN, Ory MG, Moudouni DM, Helduser J, et al. Factors affecting acceptability and usability of technological approaches to diabetes self-management: a case study. Diabetes Technol Ther. 2012;14(12):1178–82.
20. Yen PY, Bakken S. Review of health information technology usability study methodologies. J Am Med Inform Assoc. 2012;19(3):413–22.
21. von Bertalanffy L. General system theory: foundations, development, applications. New York: George Braziller; 1968.
22. Adam T, de Savigny D. Systems thinking for strengthening health systems in LMICs: need for a paradigm shift. Health Policy Plan. 2012;27(suppl_4):iv1–3. https://doi.org/10.1093/heapol/czs084.
23. Rutter H, Savona N, Glonti K, Bibby J, Cummins S, Finegood DT, et al. Lancet. 2017;390(10112):2602–4.
24. Zhang Y, Padman R, Patel N. Paving the COWpath: Learning and visualizing clinical pathways from electronic health record data. J Biomed Inform. 2015;58:186–97.
25. Lipsitz LA. Understanding health care as a complex system: the Foundation for Unintended Consequences. JAMA. 2012;308(3):243–4. https://doi.org/10.1001/jama.2012.7551.
26. Sarhan M, Weatherburn G, Graham Y, Ling J. Enhancing the effectiveness of significant event analysis: exploring personal impact and applying systems thinking in primary care. Perm J. 2020;24. [1]
27. Yeung K. Regulation by Blockchain: the emerging Battle for supremacy between the code of law and code as law. Mod Law Rev. 2019;82(2):207–39. https://doi.org/10.1111/1468-2230.12399.
28. Yeo R. Revisiting the roots of learning organization. Learn Organ. 2005;12:368–82. https://doi.org/10.1108/09696470510599145.
29. Wang B, Xu S, Mansouri M. Modeling the emergence of COVID-19: a systems approach. In: 2020 IEEE 15th international conference of system of systems engineering (SoSE); 2020. p. 000445–50. https://doi.org/10.1109/SoSE50414.2020.9130555.
30. Wang B, Asan O, Mansouri M. What may impact trustworthiness of AI in digital healthcare: discussion from patients' viewpoint. In Proceedings of the international symposium on human factors and ergonomics in health care (vol. 12, no. 1, pp. 5-10). 2023, March SAGE CA: Los Angeles, CA: SAGE Publications.
31. Wang B, Asan O, Mansouri M. Patients' perceptions of integrating AI into healthcare: systems thinking approach. In: In 2022 IEEE international symposium on systems engineering (ISSE). IEEE; 2022, October. p. 1–6.

EHRs, PHRs, and Patient Portals

9

Sue Boren

Foundational Domains
This chapter addresses the following AMIA Foundational Domains: F4—Health Information Science and Technology, F5—Human Factors and Socio-technical Systems.

Learning Objectives

1. Understand the key components and functions of electronic health records (EHRs) and their role in improving patient care and healthcare efficiency.
2. Explore the advantages and challenges associated with EHR implementation, including privacy and security concerns, technical challenges, and the potential for healthcare provider burnout.
3. Understand the features of personal health records (PHRs), including the different types (standalone and tethered/connected), and how PHRs empower patients, enhance patient-provider communication, and assist in personal health management.
4. Identify the benefits and barriers of patient portals, including their role in patient engagement, communication with healthcare providers, and management of appointments and prescriptions.
5. Compare and contrast EHRs, PHRs, and patient portals, examining their integration within healthcare systems, interoperability issues, and the future direction of patient-centered technology in healthcare.

9.1 Introduction

Digital technology has significantly transformed the healthcare industry, introducing systems that enhance the way health information is recorded, stored, and accessed. Among these pivotal advancements are electronic medical records (EMRs), electronic health records (EHRs), personal health records (PHRs), and patient portals. Each plays a critical role in modern healthcare, offering unique features and benefits while sharing some overlaps and distinctions.

9.2 Definition and Overview of EHRs, PHRs, and Patient Portals

EHRs are defined as digital versions of patients' paper charts, accessible to authorized healthcare providers across various settings, and are essential for maintaining comprehensive health records [4, 6]. Unlike electronic medical records (EMRs), which primarily document a patient's medical history within a single provider's office,

S. Boren (✉)
University of Missouri, Columbia, MO, USA
e-mail: borens@health.missouri.edu

C. Eldredge et al. (eds.), *Introductory Textbook in Health Informatics*, Health Informatics,
https://doi.org/10.1007/978-3-032-16657-9_9

EHRs provide a more extensive perspective on a patient's health history, facilitating improved care and treatment outcomes through enhanced information sharing [17]. EHRs include the same information found in EMRs but are designed for sharing among multiple healthcare providers, enabling a broader view of a patient's care [17]. Personal health records (PHRs), however, are maintained by patients themselves, allowing for greater engagement in their own health management. This approach empowers patients to manage, track, and share their health data at their discretion, fostering an active role in their healthcare [54]. Patient portals are secure online platforms granting patients 24/7 access to their personal health information through a secure username and password [4, 6]. Typically integrated with EHRs, these portals offer functionalities such as messaging healthcare providers, scheduling appointments, and viewing lab results. They may also provide tools for managing PHRs, thereby enhancing patient engagement and participation in their healthcare [14, 39]. Overall, the interconnectivity and functionalities of EHRs, PHRs, and patient portals significantly contribute to developing patient-centered care models and improving health outcomes.

Table 9.1 illustrates the overlap and distinctions between EMRs, EHRs, and PHRs. This table shows EMRs as the foundation, EHRs as an expansion for broader healthcare integration, and PHRs as the patient-managed component, intersecting with EHRs through patient portals.

Historical Context The journey from paper-based records to digital health information systems began in the late twentieth century, with the introduction of EMRs. The evolution to EHRs, PHRs, and ePrescribing marked a shift toward a more interconnected and patient-centered approach to healthcare information management. The history of these systems reflects broader trends in healthcare, including enhanced data interoperability, improved medication management through ePrescribing, and the empowerment of patients in their own care processes.

Importance in Modern Healthcare The importance of electronic health records (EHRs), personal health records (PHRs), and patient portals in modern healthcare cannot be overstated. They collectively enhance the quality of care, improve patient safety, streamline ePrescribing, and increase the efficiency of healthcare delivery [56]. By providing a comprehensive and accessible view of patient health information, these digital health records support better clinical decisions, streamline workflows, and foster a more collaborative healthcare ecosystem [36, 51]. Moreover, by empowering patients through PHRs and patient portals, they promote more active patient engagement in healthcare processes, contributing to improved health outcomes [29, 35]. The integration of these digital records into healthcare practices effectively bridges the gap between patients and healthcare providers, ensuring that health information is accurately shared while enhancing the overall patient experience [24, 50, 55].

Table 9.1 Comparison of EMRs, EHRs, PHRs, and patient portals

Feature	EMR (electronic medical records) [25, 61]	EHR (electronic health records) [21]	PHR (personal health records) [48, 52]	Patient portals [13]
Definition	Digital version of a patient's paper chart in a clinician's office. Contains the medical and treatment history of the patients within one practice.	A more comprehensive record than an EMR. It contains all the medical and treatment history of the patients and is designed to be shared outside a single practice.	An electronic record of health information that is managed, shared, and controlled by the patient or consumer.	Online applications that allow patients to interact with their healthcare providers and access their health information.
Ownership	Owned and maintained by the healthcare provider.	Owned and maintained by the healthcare provider but designed to be shared with other providers across more than one healthcare organization.	Owned and maintained by the patient.	Typically maintained by the healthcare provider but accessed and used by patients.
Access	Primarily by the healthcare provider.	Shared access among authorized healthcare providers across different healthcare settings.	Controlled by the patient who can grant access to any healthcare provider.	Accessible to patients through a secure online platform, often with login credentials provided by the healthcare provider.
Purpose	To document, monitor, and manage the treatment of patients within one healthcare provider's practice.	To provide a comprehensive overview of a patient's health that can be accessed and used for better coordinated care and treatment across multiple healthcare settings.	To enable patients to maintain and manage their own health information in a private, secure, and confidential environment.	To facilitate communication between patients and healthcare providers, provide access to medical records, and manage appointments and prescriptions.
Portability	Limited to one practice or provider. Not designed to be shared outside of the practice without manual effort (e.g., printing or emailing records).	Designed for easy sharing across different healthcare providers to support coordinated care and treatment.	Highly portable as the patient controls who sees their health information.	Accessible from any internet-enabled device, providing patients with the ability to access their information from anywhere.
Data included	Detailed records of patient visits, diagnoses, treatments, and medical history as seen in one healthcare provider's practice.	Similar to EMR content but also includes information from all clinicians involved in a patient's care and can be integrated with a broader view of patient's health.	Can include data entered by the patient, health records from multiple providers, as well as wellness data tracked by the patient themselves (e.g., fitness trackers).	May include medical records, lab results, appointment schedules, prescription information, and communication tools for messaging providers.
Interoperability	Low. Primarily used within a single practice or organization.	High. Designed to be interoperable across different healthcare systems and practices.	Variable. Depends on the platform and the extent to which it can integrate data from various sources and share information with healthcare providers.	Generally high within the systems they are connected to but may vary in terms of integration with other health information systems.

9.3 Electronic Health Records

Electronic health records (EHRs) are comprehensive digital repositories that contain various components crucial for patient care and management [19]. These components typically include patient demographics, medical history, medication and allergy information, treatment plans, progress notes, laboratory data, imaging reports, and billing information [30]. Table 9.2 provides additional information on the components. EHRs play a pivotal role in improving patient care by providing enhanced access to critical health data and reducing medical errors [1]. The streamlined record-keeping and data analysis capabilities of EHRs contribute to enhanced data management and decision-making processes [18]. Moreover, EHRs increase efficiency in healthcare delivery by simplifying tasks such as prescription refills, appointment scheduling, and facilitating communication among healthcare providers. Examples of EHRs are provided in Table 9.3.

Advantages In the United States, the adoption of EHRs in hospitals has been a focal point, especially considering the COVID-19 pandemic, emphasizing the importance of digital health records in crisis management [47]. The transition from paper-based medical records to EHRs has been a significant shift in healthcare, with EHRs

Table 9.2 Components of an electronic health record

Component	Description
Patient demographics	Fundamental components of EHRs, including basic information such as the patient's name, birth date, gender, ethnicity, and contact details. This section also often contains emergency contact information and may include marital status, employment information, and insurance details. Accurate patient demographics are crucial for identifying patients, supporting healthcare delivery, and ensuring effective communication with patients and between healthcare providers.
Medical history	Comprehensive information about a patient's past health issues, surgeries, hospitalizations, and treatments. This component also covers family medical histories to identify genetic or hereditary conditions that might affect the patient's health. Detailed medical histories aid healthcare providers in diagnosing conditions, understanding patient risks, and devising effective treatment plans.
Medication and allergies	Records all medications prescribed to the patient, including dosages, administration instructions, and the prescribing doctor. It also documents allergies, particularly drug allergies, to prevent adverse drug reactions. This information helps healthcare providers manage and coordinate care, ensuring that prescriptions do not interact negatively and that patients are not exposed to allergens that can trigger serious reactions.
Treatment plans	Detailed outlines of the care approach for addressing a patient's condition, including medications, therapies, surgeries, and any other recommended healthcare services. This component may also include goals and timelines for recovery or management of chronic conditions. Effective treatment plans are tailored to the individual patient, taking into account their medical history, current condition, and personal preferences.
Progress notes	Written by healthcare providers to document the care delivered to a patient during a visit and the patient's response to the treatment. These notes include observations, clinical findings, and the rationale for decisions made regarding the patient's care. Progress notes serve as a communication tool among providers and are essential for tracking the patient's progress over time.
Laboratory data	Includes results from blood tests, urine tests, biopsies, and other diagnostic tests. This section of the EHR provides critical information about the patient's health status, including measurements such as blood glucose levels, cholesterol levels, and the presence of infections or diseases. Laboratory data helps in diagnosing conditions, monitoring the progress of diseases, and evaluating the effectiveness of treatments.
Imaging reports	Contains findings from radiological and other imaging studies, such as X-rays, CT scans, MRIs, and ultrasounds. These reports provide visual evidence of the patient's condition and are used to diagnose, monitor, and treat various health issues. The imaging section may include both the radiologist's written report and digital images.
Billing information	Includes details about the healthcare services provided to the patient, associated costs, and payment records. This component is crucial for the financial management of healthcare practices and for patients to understand the cost of their care. Billing information is also used to process insurance claims and ensure that healthcare providers are compensated for their services.

Table 9.3 Examples of electronic health records

EHR System	Description
Epic	One of the largest and most widely used EHR systems in the United States. Offers comprehensive applications for various healthcare settings, including interoperability features, patient portals, and data-driven insights to support clinical decision-making.
Oracle health	Provides a range of EHR solutions through its millennium platform, integrating clinical and administrative data. Designed for scalability, making it suitable for large hospital systems and smaller healthcare providers.
Altera digital health	Offers multiple EHR solutions, including TouchWorks EHR and professional EHR, supporting a variety of healthcare specialties. Known for customizable interfaces and comprehensive clinical and practice management tools.
NextGen healthcare	Focuses on ambulatory care, offering EHR solutions designed to improve clinical outcomes, patient engagement, and regulatory compliance. Features include customizable templates, efficient charting, and integrated practice management capabilities.
Athenahealth	Cloud-based EHR system with features for electronic prescribing, patient scheduling, billing, and practice management. Designed for ease of use, continuous updates, and interoperability with other healthcare systems.
Meditech	Provides EHR solutions for hospitals, ambulatory clinics, and home care, integrating clinical, administrative, and financial functions within a unified platform.
eClinicalWorks	A cloud-based EHR system commonly used by ambulatory care providers and smaller practices. Includes features for medical documentation, patient engagement, revenue cycle management, and telehealth services.
Greenway health	Offers prime suite, an EHR designed for ambulatory practices with tools for electronic prescribing, patient scheduling, and revenue cycle management. Supports customizable templates to improve practice efficiency and patient care.
Practice fusion	A cloud-based EHR system designed for small and medium-sized practices. Features include patient charting, scheduling, e-prescribing, and billing, with an emphasis on affordability and usability.

playing a central role in modernizing healthcare delivery and enabling joint decision-making between healthcare providers and patients [37]. The ability to share clinical data through EHR systems is crucial for improving healthcare delivery and patient outcomes [42]. However, challenges persist in the post-implementation phase of EHRs, particularly in low and middle-income countries where unique obstacles hinder the full realization of EHR benefits [2]. Studies have highlighted the impact and potential of EHRs in healthcare settings. For instance, research has shown that EHR adoption can lead to improved hospital performance over time, with benefits such as enhanced process adherence and patient satisfaction [26]. Additionally, the integration of EHRs with PHRs and the leveraging of cloud services can streamline treatment approval processes and enhance patient care [7]. Studies have also explored the use of EHR data for predicting outcomes related to work-related musculoskeletal disorders, demonstrating the value of EHRs in occupational health settings [60].

Challenges Despite their numerous advantages, EHRs also present challenges and limitations that need to be addressed for optimal utilization [23]. Privacy and security concerns are paramount, given the risks associated with data breaches and the need to comply with regulations such as the Health Insurance Portability and Accountability Act (HIPAA) [58]. The implementation costs of EHR systems, including initial expenses and ongoing maintenance and training costs, can be significant barriers for healthcare organizations [59]. Technical challenges and interoperability issues are prevalent, as integrating EHR systems across different providers can be complex due to variations in standards and formats [46]. Moreover, the association of EHRs with documentation burden can contribute to healthcare provider burnout, impacting the quality-of-care delivery [9].

Summary Electronic health records (EHRs) play a vital role in modern healthcare systems by centralizing patient information, improving care quality, and enhancing operational efficiency. While EHRs offer significant advantages such as improved patient care, enhanced data management, and increased healthcare delivery efficiency, addressing challenges related to privacy, security, implementation costs, technical issues, and provider burnout is essential for maximizing their benefits. By leveraging EHRs effectively and addressing these challenges, healthcare organizations can enhance patient outcomes, streamline processes, and improve overall healthcare delivery.

9.4 Personal Health Records

Personal health records (PHRs) are patient-centered platforms that aim to provide individuals with accessible and comprehensive health information [28]. These records can be categorized into standalone PHRs, which operate independently from healthcare providers' systems, and tethered/connected PHRs, which are linked to specific healthcare organizations and automatically update with information from electronic health records (EHRs) [12]. Electronic personal health records (PHRs) are becoming more accessible to patients through health plans, healthcare providers, employers, and independent vendors. These tools provide a range of features for acquiring, storing, and comprehending health information including (1) contact information for the patient and their family members, (2) a list of healthcare providers involved in the patient's care, (3) a list of diagnoses, (4) a list of medications, (5) a list of allergies, (6) immunization history, (7) lab and test results, (8) family medical history [57].

Examples Here are examples of PHRs:

1. *Apple Health*: Apple Health, known as the Health app on iOS devices, acts as a health data aggregator. It consolidates information from an iPhone, Apple Watch, and compatible third-party apps into a single view. The app includes activity tracking, heart rate monitoring, nutrition data, and medical records from participating healthcare institutions, making it a key component of a personal health record (PHR) strategy.
2. *Google Fit*: A health tracking platform that aggregates data from fitness trackers, health apps, and wearable devices. While primarily focused on activity tracking, it can contribute to a broader PHR system by integrating various health metrics.
3. *Microsoft HealthVault* (Discontinued): HealthVault was a standalone PHR that allowed patients to store and manage their health information in a centralized location. It supported data uploads from home health devices and personal medical records but was discontinued in 2019.

Benefits PHRs empower individuals by granting them direct access to their health data, fostering greater involvement in healthcare management, and enhancing their understanding of health conditions [22]. This empowerment leads to improved patient-provider communication, as PHRs facilitate the sharing of health information, aid in clinical decision-making, and enhance the quality of interactions between patients and healthcare providers [12, 49]. Research indicates that PHRs have the potential to improve health outcomes, enhance patient engagement, and reduce healthcare costs [41]. PHRs play a crucial role in personal health management by assisting individuals in tracking and monitoring chronic conditions, vaccinations, and medications, which is particularly valuable in emergencies [16, 20]. Personal health records can support diabetes self-management by incorporating self-care behaviors and addressing clinical quality-of-care measures [20]. Additionally, PHRs have the potential to enhance patient navigation interventions for individuals with serious mental illness and housing instability, leading to improvements in healthcare and self-management [33].

Barriers PHRs also face concerns and barriers that need to be addressed. Despite the benefits of PHRs, usability remains a significant barrier to patient adoption, highlighting the need for user-friendly interfaces and design considerations [43]. Privacy and security issues are also critical, given the sensitive nature of health information stored electronically [8]. Robust security measures are essential to mitigate risks associated with unauthorized access or breaches [45]. Patient engagement and literacy pose additional challenges, as widespread adoption and regular use of PHRs require digital literacy and a comprehensive understanding of health information.

Integration with Electronic Health Records Integrating PHRs with EHRs also presents difficulties, with interoperability issues affecting the efficiency and usefulness of these systems [40]. Concerns about the privacy implications of sharing personal health data on electronic health records can influence patients' intentions to engage with PHRs [11]. Understanding the determinants of privacy concerns and individuals' willingness to share health data is essential for promoting the adoption of PHRs [11].

Summary Personal health records (PHRs) offer a patient-centered approach to healthcare management, empowering individuals by providing direct access to their health information and facilitating communication with healthcare providers. While PHRs have the potential to improve personal health management and patient outcomes, challenges such as privacy concerns, patient engagement, and integration with electronic health records (EHRs) need to be addressed to maximize their effectiveness in healthcare delivery.

9.5 Patient Portals

Patient portals are essential tools in modern healthcare, offering patients various features to enhance their engagement and care. These portals typically provide access to health information, communication tools, appointment management, prescription refills, and billing and payment functionalities [34]. By granting patients easy access to their health data, patient portals empower individuals to actively manage their health conditions and gain a better understanding of their well-being [10]. The communication tools within patient portals facilitate improved interactions between patients and healthcare providers, enhancing the patient-provider relationship through timely information exchange and improved communication [31].

Examples Here are examples of patient portals used in various healthcare settings:

1. *Epic MyChart*: Epic MyChart is one of the most widely used patient portals across healthcare organizations in the United States. It allows patients to access their health information, communicate with their care team, request prescription refills, schedule appointments, and view test results. Many healthcare providers use MyChart, offering a unified patient experience across different facilities.
2. *FollowMyHealth*: FollowMyHealth is a universal health record platform that serves as a patient portal for individuals to access their medical records from different healthcare providers. It enables users to manage doctor appointments, view personal health records, renew prescriptions, and communicate with their healthcare providers through a secure platform.
3. *Healow*: Healow is a mobile patient portal app integrated with electronic health record (EHR) systems from eClinicalWorks. It enables patients to manage their health information, track personal health records, manage medications, schedule appointments, and integrate health data from wearable devices.
4. *Patient Fusion*: Patient Fusion allows patients to securely access their medical records, view lab results, review medications, and read doctors' notes post-appointment. The platform also supports appointment scheduling and secure messaging with healthcare providers.

Patient Portals in Various Settings Patient portals are utilized in various healthcare settings to enhance patient engagement and care. For instance, inpatient portals have been implemented to provide hospitalized patients and caregivers with access to health information and communication tools [34]. Research has shown that hospitalized patients desire access to portals during their hospital stay, indicating the importance of inpatient portal usage [15]. Additionally, portals like the Digital Alzheimer Center focus on providing support and information for patients with dementia and their caregivers, demonstrating the specialized use of portals for specific conditions [27]. Patient portals such as MyChart have been successfully implemented to increase patient engagement among HIV-positive individuals by offering functionalities like viewing laboratory results and communicating with healthcare providers [53]. These examples highlight the diverse applications of patient portals in healthcare, showcasing how these platforms are tailored to meet the specific needs of patients in different care settings. By providing access to health information, communication tools, and specialized support, patient portals play a crucial role in enhancing patient engagement and improving the overall quality of care across various healthcare environments.

Advantages and Challenges Managing appointments and prescriptions through patient portals contributes to increased convenience and efficiency in healthcare needs management, ultimately leading to better adherence to treatment plans and follow-up care [32]. Patient portals offer improved accessibility and convenience, providing patients with 24/7 access to their health information and reducing the need for phone calls and in-person visits for routine matters [38]. However, challenges related to data accuracy and privacy issues exist, as patient portals can enhance data accuracy while also raising concerns about privacy and security [3]. Additionally, the digital divide and accessibility for all patients pose challenges, with factors such as internet access, digital literacy, and language barriers potentially limiting the equitable use of patient portals [44].

Emerging Trends and Future Directions Looking ahead, patient portals are expected to integrate with mobile health applications and wearable technology, enhancing their functionality and reach. The use of artificial intelligence is also anticipated to provide personalized health recommendations and reminders through patient portals, further enhancing patient engagement and care [4, 6]. Moreover, the expansion of telehealth services through patient portals is expected to address global health challenges by increasing access to healthcare services remotely [5].

9.6 Conclusion

Electronic medical records (EMRs), electronic health records (EHRs), personal health records (PHRs), and patient portals function as interconnected components that collectively enhance patient care, provider efficiency, and health data accessibility. EHRs serve as the foundation, acting as comprehensive digital repositories that healthcare providers use to document, manage, and share patient information across multiple settings. Patient portals bridge the gap between providers and patients by offering a secure online interface where individuals can access their EHR data, schedule appointments, and communicate with their care teams. Meanwhile, PHRs extend patient engagement beyond provider-controlled systems by allowing individuals to track, manage, and share their own health information, including data from wearable devices and personal health apps. When these systems work together effectively, they create a seamless flow of information between healthcare professionals and patients, leading to improved care coordination, enhanced patient engagement, and better health outcomes. However, this level of integration is only possible through interoperability—the ability of different health IT systems to exchange, interpret, and use patient information across various platforms and providers.

Interoperability Interoperability is essential for seamless healthcare delivery, allowing patient information to be securely shared across EMRs,

EHRs, PHRs, and patient portals. When EHRs and patient portals are designed with interoperability in mind, they enable the efficient exchange of patient data, supporting coordinated care and reducing the risk of errors. However, challenges such as lack of standardization, incompatible system architectures, and data silos can hinder interoperability, limiting the effectiveness of these health IT solutions. Addressing these barriers is crucial for creating a truly connected healthcare ecosystem where patient data flows freely and securely between systems and providers.

The Future The future of healthcare technology is moving toward more integrated, patient-directed systems. A unified platform offering comprehensive functionalities could streamline healthcare delivery, improve patient outcomes, and enhance overall healthcare experiences. Several key trends and advancements are shaping this future. Technological advancements such as Artificial Intelligence (AI), Machine Learning, and the Internet of Medical Things (IoMT) are enhancing data analysis, predictive analytics, and personalized healthcare, as well as enabling continuous monitoring and data collection through connected medical devices. Enhanced patient engagement is being facilitated by mobile health applications that provide patients with convenient access to health information and management tools on their mobile devices, and virtual health assistants that offer personalized health advice and support through AI-driven chatbots and virtual assistants. Evolving healthcare delivery models, such as telehealth and remote care, are expanding access to healthcare services through virtual consultations and remote monitoring, while patient-centric care models focus on personalized, holistic care that places patients at the center of healthcare delivery. Additionally, policy and regulatory evolution is developing to support the integration and interoperability of digital health systems while ensuring privacy and security.

Recommendations To maximize the benefits of EMRs, EHRs, PHRs, and patient portals, several key recommendations should be considered. Enhanced interoperability through the development and implementation of standardized protocols and systems is crucial to ensure seamless data exchange between different healthcare providers and platforms. Robust security measures must be in place to protect patient data from breaches and unauthorized access. User-centric designs should focus on usability, accessibility, and patient engagement to encourage widespread adoption of these systems. Further research is needed to explore and address the impact of integrating AI and machine learning into EHRs, PHRs, and patient portals. Strategies to enhance patient engagement and digital literacy, particularly among vulnerable populations, must be developed. The effectiveness of emerging telehealth and remote care models in improving patient outcomes needs to be evaluated, along with policy frameworks and regulatory approaches to support the evolving landscape of digital health technologies.

Knowledge Check Questions

1. What are some key components of electronic health records (EHRs)?
   (a) Patient Demographics
   (b) Medication and Allergies
   (c) Appointment Management
   (d) Billing and Payment Management
2. What is a significant advantage of personal health records (PHRs)?
   (a) Enhancing data management in healthcare
   (b) Reducing implementation costs
   (c) Fostering patient involvement in healthcare management
   (d) Streamlining record keeping
3. Patient portals play a crucial role in:
   (a) Reducing medical errors
   (b) Enhancing patient-provider communication
   (c) Providing 24/7 access to healthcare providers
   (d) Monitoring chronic conditions and vaccinations

4. What is one of the challenges associated with patient portals?
   (a) Improved data accuracy
   (b) Empowering patients with direct access to their health information
   (c) Raising privacy and security concerns
   (d) Reducing the need for phone calls in healthcare
5. In the context of Comparative Analysis, which of the following statements is true about the future of EHRs, PHRs, and Patient Portals?
   (a) They will remain separate systems with no integration.
   (b) They will become less patient-centered.
   (c) The lines between them may blur with increased interoperability.
   (d) Their roles in healthcare will diminish.

Answers

1. (a) and (b)
2. (c)
3. (b)
4. (c)
5. (c)

References

1. Adler-Milstein J, Everson J, Lee S. EHR adoption and hospital performance: time-related effects. Health Serv Res. 2015;50(6):1751–71. https://doi.org/10.1111/1475-6773.12406.
2. Alanazi B, Butler-Henderson K, Alanazi M. Perceptions of healthcare professionals about the adoption and use of EHR in gulf cooperation council countries: a systematic review. BMJ Health Care Inform. 2020;27(1):e100099. https://doi.org/10.1136/bmjhci-2019-100099.
3. Alturkistani A, Greenfield G, Beaney T, Norton J, Costelloe C. Ethnicity, deprivation, and the use of patient portals in England's general practices 2018–2020. Eur J Public Health. 2022;32(Supplement_3) https://doi.org/10.1093/eurpub/ckac129.302.
4. Alturkistani A, Greenfield G, Greaves F, Aliabadi S, Jenkins R, Costelloe C. Patient portal functionalities and uptake: systematic review protocol. JMIR Res Protoc. 2020a;9(7):e14975. https://doi.org/10.2196/14975.
5. Alturkistani A. Patient portal registration and healthcare utilisation in general practices in England: a longitudinal cohort study. BJGP Open. 2023:BJGPO.2023.0106. https://doi.org/10.3399/bjgpo.2023.0106.
6. Alturkistani A, Qavi A, Anyanwu P, Greenfield G, Greaves F, Costelloe C. Patient portal functionalities and patient outcomes among patients with diabetes: systematic review. J Med Internet Res. 2020b;22(9):e18976. https://doi.org/10.2196/18976.
7. Al-Zubaidie M, Zhang Z, Zhang J. PAX: using pseudonymization and anonymization to protect patients' identities and data in the healthcare system. Int J Environ Res Public Health. 2019;16(9):1490. https://doi.org/10.3390/ijerph16091490.
8. Archer N, Fevrier-Thomas U, Lokker C, McKibbon K, Straus S. Personal health records: a scoping review. J Am Med Inform Assoc. 2011;18(4):515–22. https://doi.org/10.1136/amiajnl-2011-000105.
9. Budd J. Burnout related to electronic health record use in primary care. J Prim Care Community Health. 2023 Jan-Dec;14:21501319231166921. https://doi.org/10.1177/21501319231166921.
10. Casacchia N, Rosenthal G, O'Connell N, Bundy R, Witek L, Wells B, Palakshappa D. Characteristics of adult primary care patients who use the patient portal: a cross-sectional analysis. Appl Clin Inform. 2022;13(05):1053–62. https://doi.org/10.1055/a-1951-3153.
11. Cherif E, Bezaz N, Mzoughi M. Determinants of privacy concerns and intention to share personal health data on electronic health records--model. APA PsycNet. 2021; https://doi.org/10.1037/t82057-000.
12. Chérif E, Bezaz N, Mzoughi M. Do personal health concerns and trust in healthcare providers mitigate privacy concerns? Effects on patients' intention to share personal health data on electronic health records. Soc Sci Med. 2021;283:114146. https://doi.org/10.1016/j.socscimed.2021.114146.
13. Cifuentes M, Davis M, Fernald D, Gunn R, Dickinson W, Cohen D. Electronic health record challenges, workarounds, and solutions observed in practices integrating behavioral health and primary care. J Am Board Fam Med. 2015;28(Supplement 1):S63–72. https://doi.org/10.3122/jabfm.2015.s1.150133.
14. Coughlin S, Prochaska J, Williams L, Besenyi G, Heboyan V, Goggans S, et al. Patient web portals, disease management, and primary prevention. Risk Manag Healthc Policy. 2017;10:33–40. https://doi.org/10.2147/rmhp.s130431.
15. Creber R, Grossman L, Ryan B, Qian M, Polubriaginof F, Restaino S, Bakken S, Hripcsak G, Vawdrey DK. Engaging hospitalized patients with personalized health information: a randomized trial of an inpatient portal. J Am Med Inform Assoc. 2018;26(2):115–23. https://doi.org/10.1093/jamia/ocy146.
16. Dameff C, Clay B, Longhurst C. Personal health records. JAMA. 2019;321(4):339. https://doi.org/10.1001/jama.2018.20434.

17. Dendere R, Slade C, Burton-Jones A, Sullivan C, Staib A, Janda M. Patient portals facilitating engagement with inpatient electronic medical records: a systematic review. J Med Internet Res. 2019;21(4):e12779. https://doi.org/10.2196/12779.
18. Dorr D, Bonner L, Cohen A, Shoai R, Perrin R, Chaney E, Young A. Informatics systems to promote improved care for chronic illness: a literature review. J Am Med Inform Assoc. 2007;14(2):156–63. https://doi.org/10.1197/jamia.m2255.
19. Evans R. Electronic health records: then, now, and in the future. Yearb Med Inform. 2016;25(S 01):S48–61. https://doi.org/10.15265/iys-2016-s006.
20. Fisher-Grace K, Turk M, Anthony M, Chia L. Use of personal health records to support diabetes self-management. CIN Comput Inform Nurs. 2020;39(6):298–305. https://doi.org/10.1097/cin.0000000000000682.
21. Francois M, Obisike E. Accelerating the national implementation of electronic health records in Canada. Eur Sci J. 2016;12(15):65. https://doi.org/10.19044/esj.2016.v12n15p65.
22. Fylan F, Caveney L, Cartwright A, Fylan B. Making it work for me: beliefs about making a personal health record relevant and useable. BMC Health Serv Res. 2018;18(1) https://doi.org/10.1186/s12913-018-3254-z.
23. Gans D, Kralewski J, Hammons T, Dowd B. Medical groups' adoption of electronic health records and information systems. Health Affairs. 2005;24(5):1323–33. https://doi.org/10.1377/hlthaff.24.5.1323.
24. Hagström J, Blease C, Haage B, Scandurra I, Hansson S, Hägglund M. Views, use, and experiences of web-based access to pediatric electronic health records for children, adolescents, and parents: scoping review. J Med Internet Res. 2022;24(11):e40328. https://doi.org/10.2196/40328.
25. Hamadi H, Niazi S, Zhao M, Spaulding A. Single-vendor electronic health record use is associated with greater opportunities for organizational and clinical care improvements. Mayo Clin Proc Innov Qual Outcomes. 2022;6(3):269–78. https://doi.org/10.1016/j.mayocpiqo.2022.05.001.
26. Hammack-Aviran C, Brelsford K, McKenna K, Graham R, Lampron Z, Beskow L. Research use of electronic health records: patients' views on alternative approaches to permission. AJOB Empir Bioeth. 2020;11(3):172–86. https://doi.org/10.1080/23294515.2020.1755383.
27. Hattink B, Dröes R, Sikkes S, Oostra E, Lemstra A. (2016) evaluation of the digital Alzheimer center: testing usability and usefulness of an online portal for patients with dementia and their carers. JMIR Res Protoc 2016;5(3):e144. https://doi.org/10.2196/resprot.5040
28. Hawthorne K, Richards L. Personal health records: a new type of electronic medical record. Rec Manag J. 2017;27(3):286–301. https://doi.org/10.1108/rmj-08-2016-0020.
29. Hodgson J, Welch M, Tucker E, Forbes T, Pye J. Utilization of EHR to improve support person engagement in health care for patients with chronic conditions. J Patient Exp. 2022;9 https://doi.org/10.1177/23743735221077528.
30. Holroyd-Leduc J, Lorenzetti D, Straus S, Sykes L, Quan H. The impact of the electronic medical record on structure, process, and outcomes within primary care: a systematic review of the evidence: figure 1. J Am Med Inform Assoc. 2011;18(6):732–7. https://doi.org/10.1136/amiajnl-2010-000019.
31. Janssen A, Keep M, Selvadurai H, Kench A, Hunt S, Simonds S, Shaw T. Factors that influence use of a patient portal by health professionals. Int J Environ Res Public Health. 2021;18(4):1877. https://doi.org/10.3390/ijerph18041877.
32. Jeong C. Navigating the digital divide: factors influencing patient portal adoption by older adults during the pandemic. Innov Aging. 2023;7(Supplement_1):1086. https://doi.org/10.1093/geroni/igad104.3489.
33. Kelly E, Braslow J, Brekke J. Using electronic health records to enhance a peer health navigator intervention: a randomized pilot test for individuals with serious mental illness and housing instability. Community Ment Health J. 2018;54(8):1172–9. https://doi.org/10.1007/s10597-018-0282-4.
34. Kelly M, Coller R, Hoonakker P. Inpatient portals for hospitalized patients and caregivers: a systematic review. J Hosp Med. 2017;13(6):405–12. https://doi.org/10.12788/jhm.2894.
35. King G, Maxwell J, Karmali A, Hagens S, Pinto M, Williams L, et al. Connecting families to their health record and care team: the use, utility, and impact of a client/family health portal at a children's rehabilitation hospital. J Med Internet Res. 2017;19(4):e97. https://doi.org/10.2196/jmir.6811.
36. Kruse C, Bolton K, Freriks G. The effect of patient portals on quality outcomes and its implications to meaningful use: a systematic review. J Med Internet Res. 2015;17(2):e44. https://doi.org/10.2196/jmir.3171.
37. Levy D. Identifying and addressing barriers to implementing core electronic health record use metrics for ambulatory care: virtual consensus conference proceedings. Appl Clin Inform. 2023;14(05):944–50. https://doi.org/10.1055/a-2187-3243.
38. Mook P, Trickey A, Krakowski K, Majors S, Theiss M, Fant C, Friesen M. Exploration of portal activation by patients in a healthcare system. CIN: Computers, Informatics, Nursing. 2018;36(1):18–26. https://doi.org/10.1097/cin.0000000000000392.
39. Morimoto Y, Takahashi T, Sawa R, Saitoh M, Morisawa T, Kagiyama N, et al. Web portals for patients with chronic diseases: scoping review of the functional features and theoretical frameworks of telerehabilitation platforms. J Med Internet Res. 2022;24(1):e27759. https://doi.org/10.2196/27759.
40. Nat D, Huiskes V, Taks M, Bemt B, Onzenoort H. Barriers and facilitators for the usage of a personal health record for medication reconciliation: a quali-

tative study among patients. Br J Clin Pharmacol. 2022;88(11):4751–62. https://doi.org/10.1111/bcp.15409.
41. Niazkhani Z, Ton E, Cheshmekaboodi M, Georgiou A, Pirnejad H. Barriers to patient, provider, and caregiver adoption and use of electronic personal health records in chronic care: a systematic review. BMC Med Inform Decis Mak. 2020;20:153. https://doi.org/10.1186/s12911-020-01159-1.
42. Olley R, Hozynka J. The effectiveness of scenario-based training of clinicians in the use of electronic health records—a systematic literature review. Asia Pac J Health Manag. 2023; https://doi.org/10.24083/apjhm.v18i1.1711.
43. Pachunka E, Windle J, Schuetzler R, Fruhling A. Natural-setting PHR usability evaluation using the NASA TLX to measure cognitive load of patients. In: Proceedings of the 52nd Hawaii international conference on system sciences; 2019. https://doi.org/10.24251/hicss.2019.480.
44. Philpot LM, Ramar P, Roellinger DL, Njeru JW, Ebbert JO. individual level digital determinants of health and technology acceptance of patient portals: a cross-sectional assessment. JMIR Form Res. 2024;8:e56493. https://doi.org/10.2196/56493.
45. Price M, Bellwood P, Kitson N, Davies I, Weber J, Lau F. Conditions potentially sensitive to a personal health record (PHR) intervention, a systematic review. BMC Med Inform Decis Mak. 2015;15(1) https://doi.org/10.1186/s12911-015-0159-1.
46. Reegu F, Abas H, Gulzar Y, Xin Q, Alwan A, Jabbari A, Sonkamble RG, Dziyauddin R. Blockchain-based framework for interoperable electronic health records for an improved healthcare system. Sustainability. 2023;15(8):6337. https://doi.org/10.3390/su15086337.
47. Reeves J, Hollandsworth H, Torriani F, Taplitz R, Abeles S, Tai-Seale M, Millen M, Clay BJ, Longhurst C. Rapid response to covid-19: health informatics support for outbreak management in an academic health system. J Am Med Inform Assoc. 2020;27(6):853–9. https://doi.org/10.1093/jamia/ocaa037.
48. Rotenstein L, Cohen D, Marino M, Bates D, Edwards S. Association of clinician practice ownership with ability of primary care practices to improve quality without increasing burnout. JAMA Health Forum. 2023;4(3):e230299. https://doi.org/10.1001/jamahealthforum.2023.0299.
49. Ruhi U, Majedi A, Chugh R. Sociotechnical drivers and barriers in the consumer adoption of personal health records: empirical investigation. JMIR Med Inform. 2021;9(9):e30322. https://doi.org/10.2196/30322.
50. Sethness J, Golub S, Evans Y. Adolescent patient portals and concerns about confidentiality. Curr Opin Pediatr. 2023;35(4):430–5. https://doi.org/10.1097/mop.0000000000001252.
51. Shah S, Liebovitz D. It takes two to tango: engaging patients and providers with portals. PM&R. 2017;9(5S) https://doi.org/10.1016/j.pmrj.2017.02.005.
52. Shuaib K, Saleous H, Shuaib K, Zaki N. Blockchains for secure digitized medicine. J Pers Med. 2019;9(3):35. https://doi.org/10.3390/jpm9030035.
53. Sigler R, Kubát R, Lopez A, Newman J. Implementation of a standardised sign-up process to increase MyChart enrolment among HIV-positive patients. BMJ Open Qual. 2019;8(3):e000602. https://doi.org/10.1136/bmjoq-2018-000602.
54. Sun R, Korytkowski M, Sereika S, Saul M, Li D, Burke L. Patient portal use in diabetes management: literature review. JMIR Diabetes. 2018;3(4):e11199. https://doi.org/10.2196/11199.
55. Tai-Seale M, Rosen R, Ruo B, Hogarth M, Longhurst C, Lander L, et al. Implementation of patient engagement tools in electronic health records to enhance patient-centered communication: protocol for feasibility evaluation and preliminary results. JMIR Res Protoc. 2021;10(8):e30431. https://doi.org/10.2196/30431.
56. Tapuria A, Porat T, Kalra D, D'souza G, Sun X, Ćurčin V. Impact of patient access to their electronic health record: systematic review. Inform Health Soc Care. 2021;46(2):194–206. https://doi.org/10.1080/17538157.2021.1879810.
57. The Office of the National Coordinator for Health Information Technology. Personal health records: what health care providers need to know. 2019. https://www.healthit.gov/sites/default/files/about-phrs-for-providers-011311.pdf
58. Tsai C, Eghdam A, Davoody N, Wright G, Flowerday S, Koch S. Effects of electronic health record implementation and barriers to adoption and use: a scoping review and qualitative analysis of the content. Life. 2020;10(12):327. https://doi.org/10.3390/life10120327.
59. Uslu A, Stausberg J. Value of the electronic medical record for hospital care: update from the literature. J Med Internet Res. 2021;23(12):e26323. https://doi.org/10.2196/26323.
60. Wassell M. Electronic health records for predicting outcomes to work-related musculoskeletal disorders: a scoping review. J Occup Rehabil. 2024; https://doi.org/10.1007/s10926-024-10175-1.
61. Xu R. Electronic health records: patient care quality. Revue Interdisciplinaire Des Sciences De La Santé – Interdisciplinary Journal of Health Sciences. 2016;5(1):27–31. https://doi.org/10.18192/riss-ijhs.v5i1.1442.

Imaging Informatics 10

Cesar Lam, Satyam Ghodasara,
and Charles E. Kahn Jr.

Foundational Domains
This chapter addresses the following AMIA Foundational Domains: F4—Health Information Science and Technology, F5—Human Factors and Socio-technical Systems.

Learning Objectives
1. Define the field of Imaging Informatics.
2. Summarize the history of Imaging Informatics.
3. Describe imaging modalities.
4. Describe the PACS ecosystem.
5. Summarize the radiologist's workflow.

10.1 Introduction

Imaging informatics falls under the domain of biomedical and health informatics with an emphasis on the acquisition, storage, and display of images for the purposes of diagnosis and treatment of health conditions [15]. Imaging informatics also applies principles from human factors, medicine, and behavioral science to enhance patient care and improve diagnostician workflow. Finally, imaging informatics supports data analytics, research, machine learning, and Artificial Intelligence (AI) by acquiring and facilitating access of large sets of imaging data for digital processing. In fact, most medical specialties utilize imaging informatics in their daily practice which include radiology, pathology, cardiology, dermatology, orthopedics, and gastroenterology [2].

In this chapter, we will focus on imaging informatics in the field of radiology. If you ever had an X-ray, CT, ultrasound, or MRI performed, then you have experienced radiology imaging informatics. Radiology has made significant advances into digital conversion from its early roots in analog film applications. In fact, "radiology was the first medical specialty to computerize" [45] with a significant growth in imaging informatics for the past 30 years [7] evolving into today's digital powerhouse. This field has created many jobs which include network specialists, PACS specialists, and image research analysts.

C. Lam (✉)
Diagnostic Imaging and Interventional Radiology, Moffitt Cancer Center, Department of Oncologic Sciences, University of South Florida Morsani College of Medicine, Tampa, FL, USA
e-mail: Cesar.Lam@moffitt.org

S. Ghodasara
Department of Radiology, University of Pennsylvania, Philadelphia, PA, USA

C. E. Kahn Jr.
Department of Radiology, University of Pennsylvania, Philadelphia, PA, USA

Institute for Biomedical Informatics, University of Pennsylvania, Philadelphia, PA, USA

C. Eldredge et al. (eds.), *Introductory Textbook in Health Informatics*, Health Informatics,
https://doi.org/10.1007/978-3-032-16657-9_10

10.2 PACS: From Film to Computers

Early medical imaging consisted of film exposed by X-rays creating the first medical images. X-rays, discovered in 1895 by Wilhelm Conrad Röntgen [43], were first utilized in 1896 to evaluate skeletal structures [41]. In fact, X-rays were called "X" because they were "unknown" at the time [3]. It was not until 1918 that Eastman introduced commercial X-ray film [30] with a similar format still in use (as printed film) until the early 2000s [26]. And, while film was adequate for early medical image interpretation, digital imaging would require the next evolution in medical imaging using computer systems to view, store, and transmit images. This would be known as a PACS. *PACS or Picture Archiving and Communication System* development started in the 1970s and 1980s [16]; however, "mass adoption" of the modern PACS would not take place until the early 2000s [39]. The application of digital imaging allowed for large image manipulation, electronic image transport, and universal image accessibility which helped pave the way for a multitude of applications such as dose reduction algorithms, three-dimensional modeling, research applications, and teleradiology.

10.3 What Is PACS?

The *Picture Archiving and Communication System (PACS)* is a core element of the imaging informatics ecosystem and provides the means to *store, organize, retrieve, transport, and display* digital medical images [4]. PACS platforms allow for the fast secure transfer of digital images to multiple recipients while maintaining their original format and resolution [48]. Four essential PACS components include: (1) *Imaging modality*, (2) *Network*, (3) *Storage*, and (4) *Viewing workstation* [20]. These components utilize the DICOM (see definition below) imaging standard to transfer the images and the HL7 standard to transfer clinical data to and from the Electronic Health Record (EHR) (Table 10.1).

Table 10.1 PACS advantages and disadvantages [5]

PACS advantages	PACS disadvantages
• Instantaneous availability of images • Avoid unnecessary copies • Digital manipulation to improve image quality and use of radiation minimizing protocols • Cost savings in terms of film, development, and storage	• Increased infrastructure cost for network, software, and hardware • Need for specialized IT and PACS management personnel • Ongoing updates and maintenance • Specialized training • Cybersecurity risk

PACS PACS platforms offer several advantages over earlier film [5, 48]. Medical digital images are instantly available to multiple sites both within and outside of a medical system. For example a radiologist could be interpreting a study while a surgeon views the same images at a separate location. Due to the digital availability and storage of medical imaging patient's "films" are no longer shared or lost. The transition to digital imaging has saved costs previously associated with film processing storage space and film library personnel. Digital Image processing also allows for optimization of image quality and the ability to use lower radiation exposure techniques. Importantly the transmission of digital images over long distances paved the way for the teleradiology work model increasing efficiency and improving flexibility. Successful implementation of tele-radiologist services was seen during the COVID-19 pandemic.

For security and redundancy in the event of disasters, digital images are stored on onsite and offsite server facilities [9]. A significant advantage of digitized images involves its use for research, machine learning, and artificial intelligence (AI) [5].

Disadvantages of PACS include increased information technology (IT) costs such as hardware, networks, and the requirement of specialized IT (information technology) personnel for maintenance and support. Additional concerns regarding digital imaging include cybersecurity risks, downtime, and network issues [5]. Notably, in 2021 the Food and Drug Administration (FDA) reclassified the term PACS to MIMPS (Medical Image Management and Processing Systems) to comply with software definition changes of a medical device under the twenty-first Century Cures Act [36]. Nevertheless, the PACS acronym is still in use today.

Table 10.2 Imaging modalities and the imaging source required for image acquisition [10, 19, 24, 42, 47]

Imaging modality	Imaging source
Radiography (plain films, X-rays)	Ionizing radiation
CT (computed tomography)	Ionizing radiation
US (ultrasound)	Sound waves
MRI (magnetic resonance imaging)	Magnetic field
Nuclear medicine	Alpha, beta, and gamma radiation agent injected, ingested, or inhaled

10.4 Imaging Modalities

Medical imaging modalities are classified by the "method" in which images are produced [19]. Common modalities include radiography (plain films), computed tomography (CT), ultrasound (US), and magnetic resonance imaging (MRI). Of these, radiography and CT utilize ionizing radiation to create images [10]. Ultrasound uses the properties of sound to create medical images and evaluate physiologic properties such as vascular flow and tissue stiffness [47]. MRI utilizes the properties of radio-frequency shifts via a strong magnet to create medical images. One advantage of MRI over CT is the lack of X-rays or ionizing radiation in the process of image acquisition. This is especially helpful when imaging younger patients to decrease the amount of radiation exposure over their lifetimes [24]. While radiation experts believe the risk of cancer from medical imaging is low, these risks are cumulative over time. Importantly, children are more susceptible to ionizing radiation than adults; therefore, medical imaging tests utilizing ionizing radiation should only be performed when absolutely necessary [42]. Finally, nuclear medicine utilizes radioisotopes placed in the body via injection, inhalation, or oral ingestion to create images using cameras to capture the radioisotopes within the body (Table 10.2).

10.5 Network

A local network connects the imaging modality, storage server, and viewing workstations utilizing the DICOM (see definition below) communication standard to transfer the images between these components. Communication with the EHR (Electronic Health Record) occurs through a RIS interface (see definition below) utilizing the HL7 (Health Level Seven) communication standard. The HL7 standard is utilized to transfer elec-

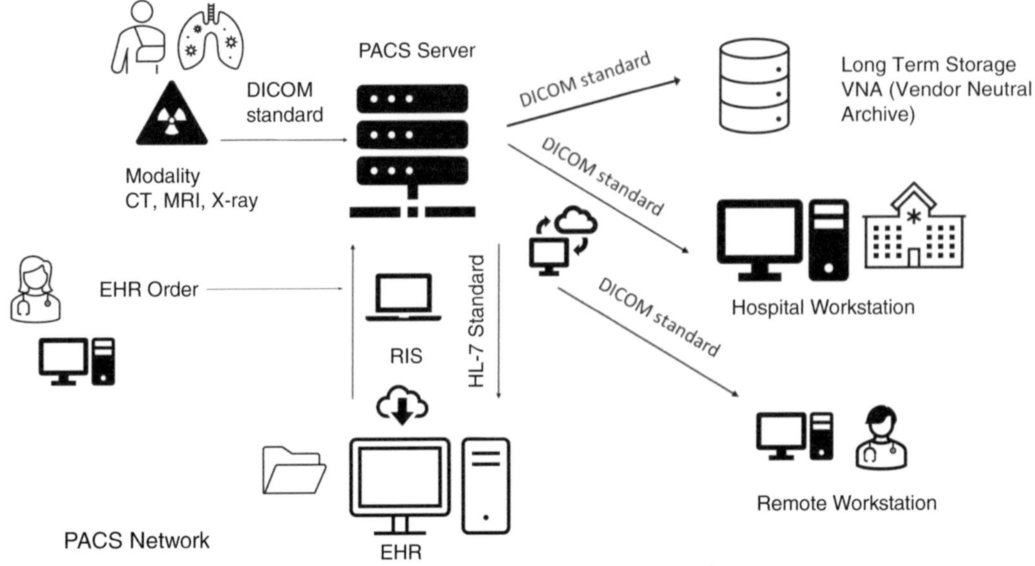

Fig. 10.1 PACS network diagram demonstrating Imaging flow from Modality to PACS to Radiologist Workstation

tronic health data between electronic health systems [17]. See Fig. 10.1.

When a clinical provider enters an imaging order into the *EHR (Electronic Health Record)*, the order is transmitted to the *RIS (Radiology Information System)* using the *HL-7 (Health Level 7)* standard which communicates with the modality. Once the images are acquired, the images are transmitted to the PACS server where the data is stored, cataloged, and immediately available for viewing and interpretation. Viewing workstations can be either local or remote. Remote (not located in the hospital) workstations allow for *teleradiology* services, a form of telemedicine, that allows images to be sent via a network to radiologists in a different city, a different state, or even a different country for interpretation. This online capability allowed for the scalability of teleradiology services during the COVID-19 pandemic [40].

10.6 DICOM Standard

DICOM (Digital Imaging and Communications in Medicine) is an international clinical messaging standard for medical images [11] and emerged out of the necessity to create a standard for image metadata annotation, communication, storage, and retrieval.

Due to vendor proprietary constraints, early modality and software communication interfaces were incompatible with different imaging modalities. Modality-specific images were printed on film or viewed at the work console (e.g., CT scanner console) and not intended to be viewed at a workstation. For images to be produced, viewed, transmitted, and stored across different systems, a vendor-neutral clinical image standard had to be created. In 1993, through a collaboration between the American College of Radiology (ACR) and the National Association of Electronic Manufacturers (NEMA), the *DICOM* standard was created [22]. The DICOM file is composed of a DICOM header and the corresponding image files. The header information is "encoded" with the DICOM file and cannot be separated from the image set. This feature ensures that a set of images is tied to a specific patient and cannot be accidentally linked to a different patient. *DICOM header* metadata contains patient information in the form of "tags" (i.e., pairs of identifiers and their specific values), which include patient and image-specific information such as: patient name, date of birth, unique patient identifier (e.g., medical record number), number of images and series, and amount of radiation exposure [44].

10.7 RIS Interface

The Radiology Information System or *RIS* is an important component of radiology operations which oversees radiology patient management including patient "registration, scheduling, and tracking" [35]. The RIS creates a radiology procedure accession number which links to the patient in the EHR. The RIS and *EHR* communicate through an international messaging standard called *HL7* which is a standard for the exchange of health information (see the chapter on standards in this textbook). Other RIS functions include billing, administrative tasks, report monitoring, and quality metrics. When a healthcare provider orders an imaging study through the EHR, a cascade of functions is triggered within the RIS (Fig. 10.2). The order creates a unique exam-specific *accession number*, which specifies the modality, exam type, and the exam date. Once the exam is completed, the accession number and other unique patient identifiers are encoded into the *DICOM header* and linked with the patient images. The completed exam is then sent to *PACS* using the DICOM standard. A radiologist inter-

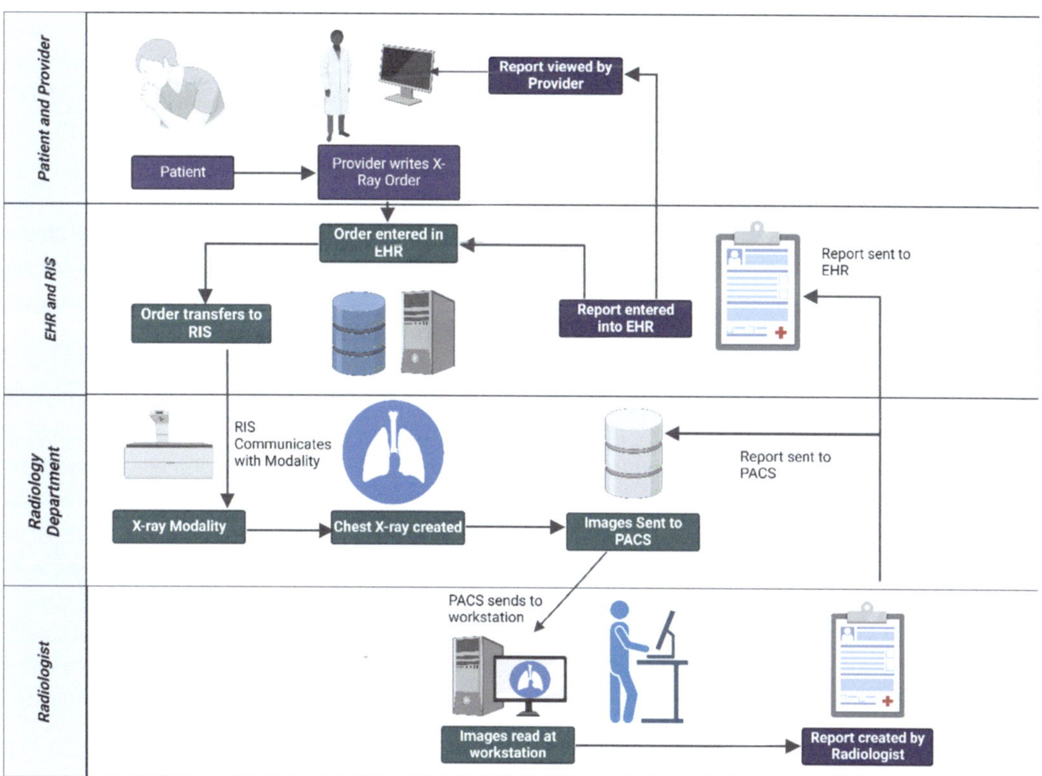

Fig. 10.2 Swim Lane diagram demonstrating flow of information from patient, provider, RIS, EHR, PACS, and Radiologist

prets the exam at a workstation using voice recognition software and signs the report. The signature closes the report, which is sent back to the RIS into EHR using *HL7* [8]. Once signed, a healthcare provider can view the radiology report in the EHR in a matter of minutes.

10.8 The Radiology Reading Room: Past and Future

Radiology reading rooms were once known as large working spaces with multiple films hung on several "alternators" which would rumble and chug-along using bicycle chains driving multiple panels of films in a revolving fashion. These rooms were at times loud, attracting many clinical visitors with the constant chatter of clinical discussions. This space was also used to review interesting cases to teach medical students and residents. Entire medical teams would come to conduct "radiology rounds" to evaluate their patients' daily progression and learn basic radiology. Fast forward to the future. As radiology became one of the first medical specialties to "computerize" it also became "our canary in the digital coal mine" [45]. The advent of the computerized *workstation, teleradiology*, and *remote workstations* brought a whole host of advantages [12], but also removed the restrictions of needing a physical space within the hospital to view films. A radiology workstation could now be placed anywhere, and a radiologist could now interpret radiology studies from across the country, and even across the world! While some mourn the loss of the communal space of the radiology reading room, teleradiology has become commonplace in daily operations with several added benefits. For example, teleradiology has helped to ease the radiologist labor shortage and [1] burnout with the advent of a hybrid remote and on-site work models [33]. Additionally, with the worldwide COVID-19 pandemic lockdown, teleradiology became an effective tool to overcome the physical barriers associated with the disease outbreak. A positive effect of the COVID-19 pandemic was the ability to leverage imaging informatics to rapidly adapt and scale teleradiology services.

10.9 Radiology Workflow and Technology

Radiologists use a wide variety of hardware and software applications in their daily workflow. A radiology workstation is composed of a desktop computer with multiple sets of monitors and powerful graphics cards able to display medical-grade images (Fig. 10.3). The standards for interpretation, transmission, and display of medical-grade images are overseen by the American College of Radiology (ACR), the American Association of Physicists in Medicine (AAPM), and the Society for Imaging Informatics in Medicine (SIIM) [31]. Additional recommendations for monitoring "luminance" and "ergonomic factors" are also provided by these societies, and their recommendations are critical for accurate and timely interpretation of images. As a result, desktop support is a critical component of a radiology department.

Proper interpretation of medical images is highly dependent on the clinical information provided by EHR; therefore, the interoperability of various systems is paramount to the operational workflow. This can be achieved using a RIS EHR module to provide the relevant clinical information through linked interoperable applications.

Voice recognition software has advanced significantly during the last few decades and is now commonplace to most radiology workflow operations.

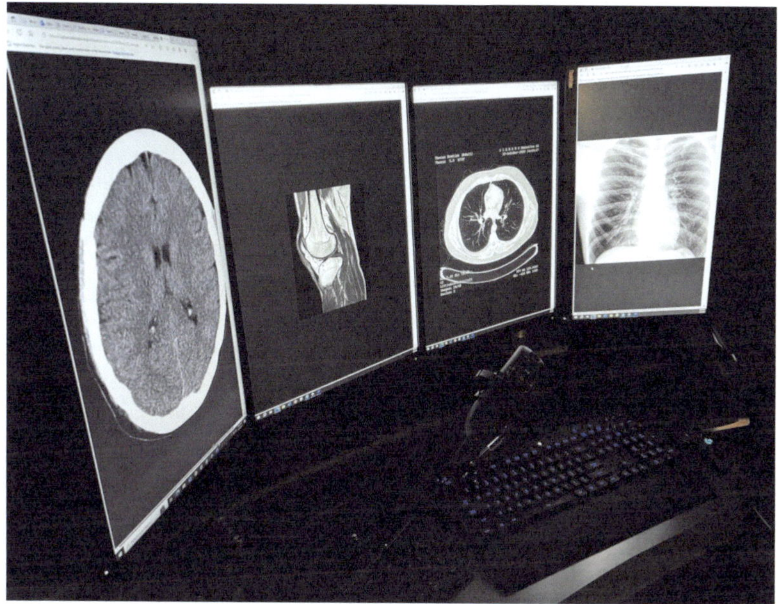

Fig. 10.3 Four-monitor workstation with lighted keyboard and dictation microphone. (Images on monitors courtesy of Wikipedia [25])

The voice recognition software package is specially formulated for radiology terminology and contains several tools which include spelling, template report creation, resident workflows, and critical result communication. Voice recognition software is integrated with the EHR RIS module and sends the completed report to the EHR. The addition of voice recognition software to the radiology workflow has been shown to significantly improve radiology report completion turnaround times [34].

10.10 Radiology Appropriate Use Criteria

Modern radiology is a complex specialty with numerous ways of tailoring imaging studies for patient needs. The options available to providers allow patients to receive bespoke imaging studies that precisely answer the clinically relevant question for each patient. However, all these options also present a problem: how does a healthcare provider order the correct study? This is a challenging problem within healthcare with high stakes. Modalities such as CT can harm patients through radiation. Other modalities such as MRI and PET are exceedingly expensive and not always available in all areas. Sometimes intravenous contrast is necessary to make a diagnosis, but other times it can obscure the diagnosis. Appropriately tailoring an imaging study for a patient can be difficult but is crucial to providing the best care.

Fortunately, the *American College of Radiology (ACR)* has created a solution for this problem: the *ACR Appropriateness Criteria*. The Appropriateness Criteria are a set of evidence-based guidelines that help healthcare providers choose the correct imaging study for the most common scenarios. These are created and maintained by panels of expert radiologists in each subspecialty within radiology. For example, an expert panel of musculoskeletal radiologists maintains several guidelines for common clinical scenarios, one of which is chronic shoulder pain. Within the chronic shoulder pain guidelines, the panel considers several variations of the scenario: pain with suspected rotator cuff injury, pain with suspected labral injury, pain in a patient who has had surgical rotator cuff repair, and others [29]. For each variation, the expert panel lists several potential imaging studies that could be performed along with their relative radiation levels. The panel provides one of three categories of recommendations for each study: "Usually Appropriate" (benefits outweigh the harms), "May be Appropriate" (the risk to benefit ratio is equivocal), and "Usually Not Appropriate" (harms outweigh the benefits).

In addition to the recommendations, the expert panels provide details on their research literature search along with an evidence table summarizing the research findings that support the panels' recommendations. For many clinical scenarios, the expert panels include a patient-friendly summary explaining their recommendations. These recommendations and evidence from the literature are reviewed and revised each year.

10.11 Artificial Intelligence in Radiology

Artificial intelligence (AI) refers to a type of algorithm that can learn how to perform tasks without explicitly being told the exact rules needed to perform those tasks. One example of AI is an algorithm that can name a household object when provided with just an image of that object. Although this task is straightforward for humans to perform, explicitly describing a full set of rules to create a non-AI algorithm to perform the same task is so complex that it is virtually impossible. However, in recent years, AI algorithms have been able to reach and even exceed human-level performance at this task [13].

In radiology, AI algorithms are still establishing a foothold, but several common applications have arisen. Some emerging applications involve high stakes tasks such as identifying hemorrhagic strokes (bleeding within the brain) and ischemic strokes (blockages in arteries supplying the brain with blood), which can help prioritize imaging studies for radiologists when there are multiple studies waiting to be read and notify the entire treatment team [28, 38]. Other applications involve detecting subtle but important findings such as lung nodules and fractures [28, 50].

AI algorithms are able to learn the rules to perform these kinds of tasks through training data. Training data consists of a large number of example inputs and their corresponding outputs after the task is successfully performed. Often, this training data is acquired manually and carefully reviewed to ensure high quality. Acquiring and curating this data can be the most time-consuming and expensive parts of developing an AI algorithm.

AI algorithms learn from training data by using techniques like random forests, decision trees, logistic regression, and neural networks. In recent years, neural networks have become the dominant technique used to create AI algorithms in part due to rapid improvements in the hardware needed to implement neural networks as well as their surprisingly strong performance [23]. These neural networks attempt to model the function of interconnected biological neurons in the human brain. Although the parallel between these two types of neurons is imperfect, neural networks in machine learning have served as the core architecture underlying many modern AI algorithms that have achieved human-level performance at tasks including handwritten digit recognition [18], image generation [49], and text generation [32]. In 2024, nearly all AI algorithms that perform relatively complex tasks on images and language are underpinned by neural networks.

10.12 Radiology AI Use Case

The FDA (Federal Drug Administration) regulates the use of medical devices through premarket clearance (510 k), De Novo Classification, or premarket approval [6]. These criteria are based on the overall risk of the product. The use of Artificial Intelligence and Machine Learning in healthcare is classified as Software as a Medical Device (SaMD) by the FDA. As of this publication, the FDA has approved more than 1000 clinical AI applications with radiology accounting for more than 70% [27]. The detection of pulmonary nodules is important in the early detection of lung cancer [21], and an AI pulmonary detection tool incorporated in the reading workflow could automate and improve the detection of pulmonary nodules [14]. Important factors to consider when selecting an AI application for healthcare include: the quality of the training data, bias, ethical implications, validation and testing, and integration with other systems [37].

Table 10.3 Professional societies

Professional organizations	Description
Radiological Society of North America (RSNA)	rsna.org Free student and in-training memberships Access to several leading radiology journals, including *Radiology* and *Radiology: Artificial Intelligence* AI Certificate program National Imaging Informatics Course (in conjunction with SIIM)
Society for Imaging Informatics in Medicine (SIIM)	siim.org Free student and in-training memberships. Access to the *Journal of Imaging Informatics in Medicine* (*JIIM*) Educational courses and CIIP training programs National Imaging Informatics Course
American Medical Informatics Association (AMIA)	amia.org Discounted student and in-training memberships Access to the *Journal of the American Medical Informatics Association* (*JAMIA*) Biomedical Imaging Informatics Work Group (BMII-WG)
Healthcare Information and Management Systems Society (HIMSS)	himss.org A membership organization for information technology workers in healthcare.

10.13 Imaging Informatics: Organizations and Professional Development

There are many routes to a career in imaging informatics: some professionals begin in a technical field, such as computer science or biomedical engineering, while others start out in clinical careers such as physicians, nurses, or imaging technologists. Either way, imaging informatics demands an understanding of information technologies and their applications to medical imaging. Imaging informatics professionals need to be able to work closely with clinical and IT colleagues and must know the properties of imaging techniques and workflow to best serve in their roles. The *Certified Imaging Informatics Professional* (CIIP) credential is one mark to demonstrate professional qualifications in this field.

The following professional organizations offer support and educational opportunities (Table 10.3):

Knowledge Check Questions

1. What is the transfer standard for medical images?
   (a) HL7
   (b) DICOM
   (c) LOINC
   (d) SCRIPT
2. What imaging modality does not use ionizing radiation?
   (a) Computed Tomography
   (b) Radiography
   (c) MRI
   (d) Fluoroscopy
3. Radiology is limited to a local network.
   (a) True
   (b) False
4. PACS consists of the following except:
   (a) Imaging modality
   (b) Network
   (c) Storage
   (d) Film
5. AI is not compatible with Imaging Informatics
   (a) True
   (b) False

Answers

1. b
2. c
3. b
4. d
5. b

References

1. Agrawal A. Emergency teleradiology-past, present, and, is there a future? Front Radiol. 2022;2:866643.
2. Agrawal JP, Erickson BJ, Kahn CE. Imaging informatics: 25 years of progress. Yearb Med Inform. 2016;1:S23–31.
3. Alzubaidi LZ, Humaidi A e. Review of deep learning: concepts, CNN architectures, challenges, applications, future directions. J Big Data. 2021;8:Article 53.
4. Andriole K. Picture archiving and communication systems: past, present, and future. J Med Imaging. 2023;10(6):061405.
5. Arora D, Mehta Y. Use of picture archiving and communication system for imaging of radiological films in cardiac surgical intensive care unit. J Anaesthesiol Clin Pharmacol. 2014;30:447–8.
6. Artificial Intelligence and Machine Learning in Software as a Medical Device. 2025, January 06. Retrieved from fda.com: https://www.fda.gov/medical-devices/software-medical-device-samd/artificial-intelligence-and-machine-learning-software-medical-device
7. Arvanitis T. Informatics opportunities and challenges in medical imaging: a journey. Stud Health Technol Inform. 2022;300:19–29.
8. Beek A What HL7 messages should a PACS Administrator learn? 2023, May 28. Retrieved from PACS Boot Camp: https://pacsbootcamp.com/what-hl7-messages-should-a-pacs-administrator-learn/#:~:text=A%20physician%20may%20place%20an,into%20the%20corresponding%20imaging%20modality
9. *Cloud PACS vs Onsite PACS*. 2024, July 31. Retrieved from Radsource: https://radsource.us/cloud-pacs-vs-onsite-pacs/
10. Computed Tomography (CT) Scans and Cancer. 2019, August 14. Retrieved from National Cancer Institue: https://www.cancer.gov/about-cancer/diagnosis-staging/ct-scans-fact-sheet#:~:text=CT%20imaging%20involves%20the%20use,low%20levels%20of%20ionizing%20radiation
11. DICOM. 2024. Retrieved from Digital Helathcare Research Archive: https://digital.ahrq.gov/dicom
12. Hanna T, Steenburg S, Rosenkrantz A, Pyatt R, Friedberg E. Emerging challenges and opportunities in the evolution of teleradiology. AJR. 2020;215(6):1411–6.
13. He K, Zhang X, Ren S, Sun J. Delving deep into rectifiers: surpassing human-level performance on ImageNet classification. 2015, February 06. Retrieved from arXiv: https://arxiv.org/abs/1502.01852
14. Hendrix W, Hendrix N, Scholten E, Mourits M, Trap-de-Jong J, Schalekamp S, et al. Deep learning for the detection of benign and malignant pulmonary nodules in non-screening chest CT scans. Nature. 2023;3(1):156.
15. Hersh W. Health informatics: practical guide. 8th ed. Orlando: Lulu; 2022.
16. Huang H. Short history of PACS. Part I: USA. Eur J Radiol. 2011;78:163–76.
17. Introduction to HL7 Standards. 2024. Retrieved from HL7 International: https://www.hl7.org/implement/standards/index.cfm?ref=nav
18. Islam K, Mujtaba G, Raj R, Nweke H. Handwritten digits recognition with artificial neural network. In: 2017 international conference on engineering technology and Technopreneurship (ICE2T). IEEE: Piscataway; 2017. p. 248–51.
19. Jacques S. Introduction to clinical engineering. Academic Press; 2020.
20. Khaleel H, Rahmat R, Zamrin D. Components and implementation of a picture. Rep Med Imaging. 2019:1–8.
21. Kondrashova R, Klimes F, Kaireit T, May K, Barkhausen J, Stiebeler S, et al. Comparison of AI software tools for automated detection, quantification and categorization of pulmonary nodules in the HANSE LCS trial. Sci Rep. 2024;14(1):27809.
22. Larobina M. Thirty years of the DICOM standard. Tomography. 2023;9:1829–38.
23. LeCun Y, Bengio Y, Hinton G. Deep learning. Nature. 2015;521:436–44.
24. Magnetic Resonance Imaging (MRI). 2023. Retrieved from National Institute of Biomedical Imaging and Bioengineering: https://www.nibib.nih.gov/science-education/science-topics/magnetic-resonance-imaging-mri
25. Medical Imaging. 2024. Retrieved from Wikipedia.
26. Miñano G. Radiating Hope Department Blog. 2018. Retrieved from Cincinati Childrens's: https://radiologyblog.cincinnatichildrens.org/when-film-was-king/
27. Murphy H. FDA has approved over 1,000 clinical AI applications, with most aimed at radiology. 2025, January 10. Retrieved from Health Imaging: https://healthimaging.com/topics/artificial-intelligence/fda-has-approved-over-1000-clinical-ai-applications-most-aimed-radiology#:~:text=Hannah%20Murphy%20%7C%20January%2010%2C%202025,the%20end%20of%20that%20year
28. Murray N, Unberath M, Hager G, Hui F. Artificial intelligence to diagnose ischemic stroke and identify large vessel occlusions: a systematic review. J Neurointerv Surg. 2020;12:156–64.
29. Nacey N, Fox M, Surasi D, Blankenbarker D, Chen D, Frick M, et al. ACR appropriateness criteria® chronic shoulder pain: 2022 update. JACR. 2023:S49–69.
30. Nett B. History X-Ray imaging. 2024. Retrieved from How Radiology Works: https://howradiologyworks.com/history-xray-imaging/

31. Norweck J, Seibert A, Andriole K, Clunie D, Curran B, Flynn M, et al. ACR–AAPM–SIIM technical standard for electronic practice of medical imaging. J Digit Imaging. 2013:38–52.
32. OPEN AI et al. GTP-4 technical report. 2023, March 15. Retrieved from arXiv: https://arxiv.org/abs/2303.08774v6
33. Petscavage-Thomas J, Hardy S, Chetlen A. Mitigation tactics discovered during COVID-19 with long-term report turnaround time and burnout reduction benefits. Acad Radiol. 2022;29:1786.
34. Prevedello L, Ledbetter S, Farkas C, Khorasani R. Implementation of speech recognition in a community-based radiology practice: effect on report turnaround times. J Am Coll Radiol. 2014;11:402–6.
35. Radiology Information System: How to Approach RIS Adoption. 2022, Jan 24. Retrieved from Altexsoft: https://www.altexsoft.com/blog/radiology-information-system/
36. Ridley E. Goodbye, PACS. Hello, MIMPS? FDA updates rules for radiology software. 2021, April 2021. Retrieved from Auntminnie.com: https://www.auntminnie.com/imaging-informatics/advanced-visualization/image-processing/article/15628226/goodbye-pacs-hello-mimps-fda-updates-rules-for-radiology-software
37. Sambir A. What to consider before implementing AI into your Healthcare Organization. 2023, November 10. Retrieved from Forbes: https://www.forbes.com/councils/forbesbusinesscouncil/2023/11/10/what-to-consider-before-implementing-ai-into-your-healthcare-organization/
38. Seyam M, Weikert T, Sauter A, Brehm A, Psychogios M, Blackham KA. Utilization of artificial Intelligence-based intracranial hemorrhage detection on emergent noncontrast CT images in clinical workflow. Radiol Artif Intell. 2022;4(2):e210168.
39. Shrestha. Guide to replacement PACS, version 2012. Appl Radiol. 2012.
40. Teleradiology. 2023. Retrieved from American College of Radiology: https://www.acr.org/Advocacy-and-Economics/Legislative-Issues/Teleradiology
41. Tubiana M. Wilhelm Conrad Röntgen and the discovery of X-rays. Bull Acad Natl Med. 1996;180:97–108.
42. Understanding Radiation Risk from Imaging Tests. Retrieved from American Cancer Society. 2024. https://www.cancer.org/cancer/diagnosis-staging/tests/imaging-tests/understanding-radiation-risk-from-imaging-tests.html
43. Vardeu M, Larentis O, Vechio I, Gorini I, Martini M, Bragazzi N, et al. History of use and abuse of X-ray: the early 20th century. Acta Biomed. 2020:113–7.
44. Varma D. Managing DICOM images: tips and tricks for the radiologist. Indian J Radiol Imaging. 2012;22:4–13.
45. Watcher R. The digital doctor: Hope, hype, and harm at the Dawn of medicine's computer age. McGraw Hill; 2017.
46. What is Imaging Informatics? 2022, November 11. Retrieved from SIIM: https://siim.org/communication/what-is-imaging-informatics/
47. What is medical ultrasound? 2023, December. Retrieved from National Institute of Biomedical Imaging and Engineering: https://www.nibib.nih.gov/science-education/science-topics/ultrasound
48. What is PACS? 2022, 01 24. Retrieved from intelerad: https://www.intelerad.com/en/2022/01/24/what-is-pacs/
49. Wolterink JM, Mukhopadhyay A, Leiner T, Vogl TJ, Bucher AM, Išgum I. Generative adversarial networks: a primer for radiologists. Radiographics. 2021;41:840–57.
50. Zech JS, Yi P. Artificial Intelligence (AI) for fracture diagnosis: an overview of current products and considerations for clinical adoption. AJR. 2022:869–78.

11 Clinical Decision Support System (CDSS)

Saptarshi Purkayastha and Thejomayi Malempati

Foundational Domains
This chapter addresses the following AMIA foundational domains: F4—Health Information Science and Technology, F5—Human Factors, and Socio-technical Systems.

Learning Objectives
1. Define Clinical Decision Support Systems (CDSS) and describe their key components and functionalities.
2. Differentiate between knowledge-based and non-knowledge-based CDSS.
3. Understand the historical development and evolution of CDSS.
4. Analyze the integration of CDSS within clinical workflows, including diagnostic support, treatment protocols, and real-time decision-making.
5. Evaluate the challenges and opportunities of CDSS implementation, including data integration, user adoption, and system maintenance.
6. Discuss the role of artificial intelligence (AI) in the future of CDSS, including applications in personalized medicine and population health management.

S. Purkayastha (✉)
Luddy School of Informatics, Computing, and Engineering, IUPUI, Indianapolis, IN, USA
e-mail: saptpurk@iu.edu

T. Malempati
EHR Associate Application Analyst, Prime Healthcare, Harlingen, TX, USA

11.1 Introduction

Clinical decision support systems (CDSS) serve as sophisticated computerized tools aimed at influencing clinician decision-making processes concerning individual patients in real-time scenarios. Following the heightened awareness surrounding the prevention of medical errors catalyzed by seminal reports such as the Institute of Medicine's "To Err Is Human" [1], there has been a significant emphasis on integrating computer-based physician order entry (CPOE) systems in conjunction with CDSS as pivotal components in enhancing patient safety within healthcare systems [2]. When used effectively, CDSS can revolutionize the traditional paradigms of medical education and practice. This chapter endeavors to offer an encompassing overview of CDSS, outline current empirical findings regarding their practical utility and impact, and furnish practical guidelines for their integration into commercial systems, extending beyond mere research and development domains.

C. Eldredge et al. (eds.), *Introductory Textbook in Health Informatics*, Health Informatics,
https://doi.org/10.1007/978-3-032-16657-9_11

11.1.1 Evolution and Historical Development

The earliest clinical decision support systems emerged in the 1970s from artificial intelligence research on building expert systems capable of replicating clinician reasoning [3]. Two pioneering examples were MYCIN for the diagnosis of bacterial infections using a rules-based approach and Internist-I for internal medicine differential diagnosis using probability networks [4]. However, these early systems performed poorly outside controlled environments.

In the 1980s, CDSS evolved to focus more on supporting clinician's decision-making rather than aiming to automate it completely [5]. Systems like QMR for diagnostics provided a ranked list of suggestions rather than a single solution. In the 1990s, guideline-based CDSS like ONCOCIN, which encoded expert protocols in logic frameworks, were developed [6]. This generation saw a transition from standalone systems to integration with EHRs.

The twenty-first century has witnessed exponential growth in healthcare data and analytics. Modern CDSS are increasingly embedded in clinical workflows and leverage advanced techniques like machine learning and predictive modeling rather than just expert knowledge [7]. However, lack of interoperability, knowledge base maintenance, and demonstration of tangible benefits continue to limit adoption [8].

11.2 Definition and Core Components

A Clinical Decision Support System (CDSS) is an information system designed to assist healthcare professionals in making clinical decisions for individual patients [7]. It integrates patient-specific data with medical knowledge and rules to provide recommendations or alerts to healthcare providers during the decision-making process [9]. The primary goal of CDSS is to improve the quality, safety, and efficiency of patient care by providing relevant and timely information to clinicians [10].

For example, suppose a physician is prescribing medication for a patient with multiple chronic conditions. The CDSS could analyze the patient's medical history, current medications, allergies, and other relevant data to provide real-time alerts about potential drug interactions or contraindications. This helps the physician make more informed decisions and avoid potential adverse events, ultimately improving patient safety and healthcare outcomes.

11.2.1 Types of Clinical Decision Support Systems

Depending on their underlying reasoning mechanisms for decision making, types of decision-making tasks they perform, and how they interact with end users and deliver recommendations, CDSS can be classified into two main types: knowledge-based systems and nonknowledge-based systems [11].

11.2.1.1 Knowledge-Based Systems

Knowledge-based systems are systems that utilize compiled medical information or "knowledge," typically in the form of IF-THEN rules that are derived from medical literature, subject matter experts, or evidence derived from clinical experience [11–13]. An example might be a system that alerts clinicians when a new imaging order is a duplicate of one that was ordered within the previous 48 h. The purpose of this type of alert is to prevent redundant testing [4].

Knowledge-based systems consist of following core components:

Knowledge Base: Contains the compiled clinical knowledge required to generate patient-specific advice, e.g., clinical guidelines, diagnostic algorithms, prediction models, rules, probabilistic associations, etc.

Inference Engine: Software containing reasoning logic to process the knowledge base and patient data to generate case-specific recommendations.

User Interface: Allows users to interact with the CDSS and displays the CDSS output using alerts, reminders, order sets, etc.

These components allow the CDSS to perform functions like providing diagnostic suggestions, preventing adverse events, optimizing treatment selection, and promoting adherence to clinical pathways. The knowledge base represents clinical intelligence, the inference engine provides the analysis, and the user interface enables communication with end-users.

Furthermore, the integration of these components allows the CDSS to adapt to diverse clinical contexts and cater to the specific needs of healthcare providers and patients. The knowledge base serves as a reservoir of evidence-based information, continuously updated with the latest research findings and clinical best practices. By leveraging this wealth of knowledge, the CDSS can offer timely and accurate recommendations aligned with current standards of care, thus promoting clinical excellence and patient safety.

The inference engine plays a pivotal role in transforming raw data into actionable insights by applying sophisticated algorithms and decision-making logic. Through data analysis and pattern recognition, the inference engine can identify trends, correlations, and potential risk factors, aiding clinicians in making informed decisions. Whether it is predicting disease progression, assessing treatment efficacy, or flagging medication interactions, the inference engine enhances clinical reasoning and augments healthcare professionals' diagnostic and therapeutic capabilities.

Moreover, the user interface serves as the primary point of interaction between healthcare providers and the CDSS, facilitating seamless integration into clinical workflows. A well-designed user interface ensures ease of use, accessibility, and relevance of information, thereby maximizing user acceptance and adoption. By presenting recommendations clearly and intuitively, the user interface empowers clinicians to leverage the CDSS effectively in their daily practice, leading to improved clinical outcomes and patient care.

In summary, the core components of a CDSS form a dynamic and synergistic system that enhances clinical decision-making processes and improves patient outcomes. By combining a comprehensive knowledge base, advanced inference engine, and user-friendly interface, CDSS empowers healthcare professionals with valuable insights, decision support, and guidance at the point of care. As technology and healthcare landscapes continue to evolve, CDSS will play an increasingly vital role in shaping the future of medicine, driving innovation, and delivering personalized, evidence-based care to patients worldwide.

11.2.1.2 Nonknowledge-Based Systems

Nonknowledge-based systems, on the other hand, are systems that simulate human thinking and learn from examples, analyzing patterns in patient data, and derive associations between signs and symptoms and diagnoses [14]. Nonknowledge-based systems apply machine learning (ML) algorithms such as artificial neural networks (ANN), genetic algorithms, or deep learning to learn various patterns and relationships from clinical data rather than predefined IF-THEN rules [15].

ANN-based systems simulate human thinking and learn from examples, analyzing patterns in patient data to derive associations between signs/symptoms and diagnoses [14]. Lastly, Genetic Algorithms (GA) are systems that use an evolutionary approach where they are iteratively recombining and mutating components of random solutions to find and suggest the best solution [17, 18]. Modern nonknowledge-based systems are adopting AI-driven models that are trained on using large volume of complex clinical data for more reliable and accurate decision making at various clinical settings [19].

Nonknowledge-based CDSS systems are usually composed of a data processing component where large-scale clinical data are gathered and processed for ML-based model training, the AI/ML engine that hosts the algorithms [15], the model training and validation pipeline that allows thorough training and evaluation of ML algorithms for reliable and accurate prediction, the inference engine that receives new patient data as inputs and applies them to the previously trained ML model and generates output, and the user interface to present the outputs to the end users [19].

As outlined by Middleton et al. [16], these two types of systems vary in their approaches and methodologies, with knowledge-based systems relying on established rules and guidelines while nonknowledge-based systems employ machine learning techniques as described above. Despite their effectiveness, concerns regarding transparency and interpretability exist, particularly with nonknowledge-based systems [19].

11.3 CDSS in Clinical Workflow

The successful integration of CDSS within clinical workflows is crucial for providing decision support at relevant points during care delivery [9]. Research has identified several keyways in which CDSS can enhance routine care processes:

(a) *Alerts and Reminders*
CDSS can automatically generate alerts and reminders regarding needed care, potential problems, or gaps in care by applying rules and logic to patient data [13]. Common examples include drug-allergy checking, drug interaction alerts, preventive care reminders, and duplicate test warnings [8]. Studies have shown that well-designed alerts can significantly reduce medication errors and improve patient safety [2].

(b) *Diagnostic Support*
CDSS can analyze patient findings such as symptoms, lab tests, and imaging results to generate a ranked list of likely diagnoses [7]. This supports clinicians during the diagnostic workup and helps reduce cognitive biases [14]. Diagnostic CDSS relies on technologies like probabilistic inference, machine learning, and natural language processing to provide suggestions [7].

(c) *Treatment Guidelines and Protocols*
Evidence-based clinical practice guidelines and standardized treatment protocols can be encoded into CDSS workflows [9]. This allows patient-specific recommendations regarding appropriate diagnostic tests, medications, or other interventions based on relevant guidelines [13]. CDSS can also track protocol adherence and outcomes, as demonstrated in multiple systematic reviews [14].

In summary, CDSS aligned with clinical workflows can provide concise, context-sensitive support to clinicians during care delivery to enhance decision quality and compliance with evidence-based practices. However, the utility and usability of such CDSS hinges on thoughtful integration into care team workflows and clinical environments. Poorly designed CDSS can be disruptive and get ignored or overridden.

(d) *Real-Time Decision Support*
Recent advances in CDSS technology, as outlined by Shortliffe and Sepúlveda [7], have enabled real-time analysis of patient data as it becomes available, offering actionable insights to clinicians during patient encounters. Studies have shown that real-time alerts and recommendations can significantly improve clinical decision-making and patient outcomes [3].

(e) *Patient-Specific Risk Assessment*
Modern CDSS implementations can conduct sophisticated patient-specific risk assessments by analyzing clinical data, demographic information, and medical history [16]. This capability enables proactive interventions and personalized care planning, which has been shown to improve outcomes in various clinical settings [5].

(f) *Automated Documentation and Reporting*
Integration with CDSS can streamline documentation processes through automated capture of decision-support interventions and clinical reasoning [10]. This automation has been demonstrated to improve both the quality and efficiency of clinical documentation [6].

(g) *Continuing Education and Training*
As highlighted by Berner [5], CDSS serves as a valuable educational tool by providing access to evidence-based guidelines and best practices. Through interactive modules and knowledge reinforcement, these systems support ongoing professional development [19].

(h) *Quality Improvement Initiatives*
Leveraging data collected by CDSS, healthcare organizations can conduct retrospective analyses to identify trends, patterns, and areas for improvement. Insights gleaned from CDSS usage data can inform quality improvement initiatives, protocol revisions, and clinical pathway optimizations to enhance care delivery and patient outcomes over time.

(i) *Remote Monitoring and Telehealth Support*
In the era of telehealth and remote patient monitoring, CDSS can play a crucial role in supporting virtual care delivery. By providing clinicians with decision support tools tailored for remote settings, CDSS can ensure consistent, evidence-based care delivery across various care modalities, improving access and continuity of care for patients.

Incorporating additional functionalities into CDSS enhances their value proposition and aligns them more closely with evolving healthcare delivery models and patient care needs. By leveraging CDSS to support real-time decision-making, risk assessment, documentation, education, quality improvement, and remote care, healthcare organizations can maximize the benefits of these systems and drive continuous improvements in care delivery.

11.4 CDSS Interoperability and Integration

The effectiveness of CDSS depends heavily on successful integration with existing health IT systems and clinical workflows [8]. Kuperman et al. [8] identify several critical factors for successful implementation, which are listed below.

(a) *Data Standards and Exchange*
Standardized data formats and exchange protocols are fundamental for seamless integration [9]. HL7, FHIR, SNOMED-CT, and related standards enable structured data representation and exchange, addressing interoperability challenges identified in multiple studies [6, 10].

(b) *CPOE and CDSS*
The integration of CDSS with Computerized Provider Order Entry (CPOE) systems has shown significant benefits in preventing medication errors and improving patient safety [2]. Studies have demonstrated up to a 55% reduction in serious medication errors through such integration [8].

Integration of clinical decision support capabilities into the CPOE system enhances its functionality by providing real-time support to clinicians during the order placement process. One key aspect of this integration is the implementation of drug-allergy checking, which alerts clinicians if a prescribed medication may cause an allergic reaction in the patient based on their known allergies stored in the EHR. By flagging potential allergies, the system helps prevent adverse drug events and allergic reactions, safeguarding patient well-being.

(c) *Alignment with Clinical Workflows*
Successful CDSS implementation requires careful attention to user workflows and con-

texts [13]. Poor integration can lead to alert fatigue and system avoidance, as documented in several implementation studies [17].

(d) *Knowledge Management*
Maintaining current clinical knowledge within CDSS requires robust governance and update processes [16]. Regular updates to reflect the latest evidence and practices are essential for maintaining system effectiveness [5].

With thoughtful interoperability, integration, and knowledge management, CDSS can become seamlessly embedded into the healthcare IT ecosystem and clinical practice to positively impact the quality, safety, and efficiency of care delivery.

11.5 Opportunities and Challenges

11.5.1 Opportunities and Applications

CDSS not only addresses clinical challenges but also presents opportunities to transform healthcare delivery by promoting evidence-based practice, engaging patients in their care, facilitating interdisciplinary collaboration, and supporting population health management initiatives. A strategic approach to CDSS implementation, coupled with ongoing evaluation and adaptation, can maximize these opportunities and ultimately improve patient outcomes and healthcare efficiency.

Table 11.1 presents a range of CDSS opportunities along with illustrative examples and relevant peer-reviewed references for further exploration.

Table 11.1 CDSS opportunities and applications

Opportunity	Example	Reference
Evidence-based medicine to support learning health systems	CDS tools may integrate relevant health research with patient-specific data to support evidence-based practice and improve care quality	Shiffman and Wright [22], AHRQ [23]
Quality improvement	An evidence-based CDS embedded in the EHR reduced inappropriate antibiotic prescribing for respiratory infections in primary care	McGinn et al. [24]
Personalized medicine	Multi-criteria CDS incorporates individual patient factors and preferences to support patient-centered decisions	Dolan [25]
Patient engagement	Patient decision support with patient-facing CDS that provides timely, tailored information that can strengthen engagement and shared decision-making	Liu et al. [26]
Supporting population health	Community-academic partnerships leverage data and structured input (e.g., concept mapping) to identify local priorities and guide interventions	Keller et al. [27]
Facilitating interdisciplinary collaboration	Interprofessional collaboration (IPC) supported by shared information and workflows can improve patient-reported outcomes	Kaiser et al. [28]

11.5.2 Challenges with the Use of CDSS

Despite the promise of CDSS in the clinical environment, several challenges to the use of these systems still exist, even in the age of artificial intelligence. One of the most pressing challenges is information "silos" due to the lack of data standards and interoperability. When CDSS cannot access complete and pertinent clinical information, the quality and reliability of its recommendations may degrade. Further, ethical and data privacy considerations remain prominent issues. Significant concerns about algorithmic decision bias and lack of transparency with the use of AI algorithms are the subject of an ongoing debate.

Questions of who is liable if the systems do not provide a quality recommendation or if the recommendation leads to an adverse event remain as regulations and governance regarding AI in medicine are still evolving [21]. Other issues involve costs to develop, adopt, and maintain these systems. Economic analyses have demonstrated both challenges and opportunities in CDSS implementation, and organizations should weigh the initial and ongoing investment costs with research on potential benefits [8]. Finally, proper implementation, training, and user support is required by a knowledgeable workforce, which considers important issues such as stakeholder input, usability, provider burnout, and alert fatigue.

11.6 Case Studies

11.6.1 Hospital CPOE-CDSS Implementation

Background

Medication errors and adverse drug events (ADEs) are significant challenges in healthcare, contributing to patient harm and increased healthcare costs. To address these issues, a 500-bed community hospital decided to implement a commercial computerized physician order entry (CPOE) system integrated with a medication-related clinical decision support system (CDSS). The goal was to improve patient safety by reducing medication errors and ADEs [2].

Implementation

The hospital carefully selected a CPOE system that could be seamlessly integrated with a CDSS. The CDSS was configured to include three key functionalities: drug allergy checking, drug-drug interaction alerts, and renal dose-checking rules. These features aimed to alert clinicians to potential medication-related problems during the ordering process.

To ensure a smooth transition and high user adoption, the project team conducted concurrent user training during the phased implementation period. This approach allowed clinicians to become familiar with the system gradually, while still having access to support and guidance from the project team.

One of the main concerns among clinicians was the potential for "alert fatigue," where an excessive number of alerts could lead to clinicians ignoring or overriding important warnings. To address this issue, the project team worked closely with clinicians to manage their expectations and fine-tune the CDSS rules to strike a balance between providing necessary alerts and minimizing irrelevant ones [17]. The team also actively sought feedback from users to identify and address any workflow concerns.

Results

One year after the implementation, the hospital observed a significant 50% reduction in ADEs, demonstrating the effectiveness of integrating CDSS with CPOE. Clinicians reported finding the relevant alerts useful in catching potential medication errors and improving patient safety. The focused scope of the CDSS rules, combined with the proactive management of alert fatigue, resulted in minimal instances of alert overload.

The successful implementation of the CPOE-CDSS system in this community hospital showcases the potential benefits of integrating these technologies. By providing real-time, patient-specific alerts and recommendations, the CDSS empowered clinicians to make more informed decisions and catch potential medication-related problems early in the ordering process [14].

Lessons Learned

This case study highlights several key lessons for successful CPOE-CDSS implementation:

1. Careful selection and configuration of the CDSS rules are crucial to ensure relevant and actionable alerts.
2. Proactive management of user expectations and concerns, such as alert fatigue, is essential for user adoption and satisfaction.
3. Concurrent user training during a phased implementation can help users adapt to the new system more effectively.

4. Ongoing monitoring and evaluation of the system's impact on patient safety and workflow are necessary to maintain and improve its effectiveness over time.

11.6.2 Primary Care Hypertension CDSS

Background

Hypertension, or high blood pressure, is a prevalent chronic condition that significantly increases the risk of cardiovascular disease and stroke. Managing hypertension effectively requires regular monitoring, lifestyle modifications, and often, pharmacological treatment. However, in an urban primary care clinic serving a predominantly uninsured and underserved population, nearly half of the patients had poorly controlled blood pressure. The clinic recognized the need to improve its hypertension management to enhance patient outcomes and reduce the risk of complications [9].

Workflow Analysis and CDSS Implementation

To address this challenge, the clinic first conducted a thorough analysis of its existing workflows related to hypertension management. This analysis revealed several areas for improvement, including inconsistent follow-up on overdue laboratory tests and a lack of standardized treatment recommendations based on the latest clinical guidelines.

Based on these findings, the clinic decided to implement a homegrown clinical decision support system (CDSS) module integrated with its electronic health record (EHR). The CDSS was designed to provide point-of-care reminders and individualized treatment recommendations to help clinicians better manage their hypertensive patients.

The CDSS module had two key features:

1. Point-of-care reminders: When a clinician opened a patient's EHR, the CDSS would alert them if the patient had any overdue laboratory tests related to hypertension management, such as blood work or urine analysis. These reminders helped ensure that clinicians had the most up-to-date information to make informed treatment decisions.
2. Individualized treatment recommendations: The CDSS incorporated clinical guideline logic to provide personalized treatment recommendations for each patient based on their specific characteristics, such as age, comorbidities, and current medications. These recommendations helped clinicians select the most appropriate pharmacological treatments and lifestyle modifications for each patient.

Results

Six months after implementing the hypertension CDSS module, the clinic observed a significant improvement in blood pressure control among its hypertensive patients. The percentage of patients with controlled blood pressure increased from 52% to 62%, demonstrating the positive impact of the targeted CDSS intervention.

Lessons Learned

1. Conducting a thorough workflow analysis is crucial to identify areas for improvement and ensure that the CDSS is designed to address specific needs.
2. Integrating the CDSS with the EHR allows for seamless delivery of point-of-care reminders and individualized treatment recommendations.
3. Incorporating clinical guideline logic ensures that the CDSS provides evidence-based recommendations tailored to each patient's unique characteristics.
4. Generating population health reports enables proactive outreach and focused care for patients with poorly controlled hypertension.

11.7 Conclusion

In summary, clinical decision support systems have evolved from humble beginnings in research labs to increasingly sophisticated tools integrated into mainstream clinical workflows [4]. When thoughtfully designed and implemented, CDSS can provide clinicians with patient-specific, evidence-based guidance at the right time and place to significantly enhance clinical practice.

However, realizing this potential necessitates overcoming adoption barriers and demonstrating tangible benefits. As healthcare continues transitioning to value-based care under constraints of cost and quality, CDSS can potentially serve as pivotal enablers. In the future, rapid growth in clinical data and analytics, along with evolving technologies like AI, promises to transform the scope and utility of clinical decision support.

Knowledge Check Questions

1. What are the key components of a CDSS to support clinical decision-making?
   (a) A knowledge base, inference engine, and user interface, which together store clinical rules, apply reasoning, and present recommendations to clinicians.
   (b) A database, printer, and communication module that help clinicians share documents.
   (c) A scheduling tool, billing module, and alert generator that organize clinical workflow.
   (d) A data warehouse and reporting tool that summarize hospital performance metrics.
   (e) All of the above.

2. Compare and contrast knowledge-based and non-knowledge-based CDSS. Provide examples of each type.
3. What role does CDSS play in improving patient safety? Select the best answer below.
   (a) CDSS improves safety by replacing all clinician decision-making.
   (b) CDSS improves safety by reducing staff and increasing cost of care.
   (c) CDSS improves safety by increasing documentation burden and alert fatigue.
   (d) CDSS improves safety by providing evidence-based alerts that can inform clinical decisions.
   (e) (a) and (b).
4. Which of the following are the best examples of how CDSS can prevent medication errors. Select all that apply.
   (a) CDSS can warn clinicians of drug–drug interactions during prescription ordering.
   (b) CDSS reminds clinicians to order more supplies for the pharmacy.
   (c) CDSS stores pharmacy inventory numbers for later review.
   (d) CDSS alerts clinicians to potential patient allergies.
5. List three important challenges associated with integrating CDSS into existing Electronic Health Records (EHR) systems.

Answers

1. (a)
2. Knowledge-based CDSS use handcrafted rules like IF-THEN statements. Examples are MYCIN and ONCOCIN. In contrast, non-knowledge-based CDSS rely on machine learning and pattern recognition such as AI-driven neural-networks.
3. (d)
4. (a) and (d)
5. Examples include addressing data interoperability issues, workflow disruption, alert fatigue, data privacy, data security, and high implementation costs.

References

1. Kohn LT, Corrigan JM, Donaldson MS. To err is human: building a safer health system. Washington, DC: National Academy Press; 2000.
2. Bates DW, Kuperman GJ, Wang S, Gandhi T, Kittler A, Volk L, et al. Ten commandments for effective clinical decision support: making the practice of evidence-based medicine a reality. J Am Med Inform Assoc. 2003;10(6):523–30.
3. Hunt DL, Haynes RB, Hanna SE, Smith K. Effects of computer-based clinical decision support systems on physician performance and patient outcomes: a systematic review. JAMA. 1998;280(15):1339–46.
4. Miller RA. Computer-assisted diagnostic decision support: history, challenges, and possible

paths forward. Adv Health Sci Educ Theory Pract. 2009;14(Suppl 1):89–106.
5. Berner ES. Clinical decision support systems: state of the art. AHRQ Publication No. 09-0069-EF. Rockville: Agency for Healthcare Research and Quality; 2009.
6. Wright A, Sittig DF. A framework and model for evaluating clinical decision support architectures. J Biomed Inform. 2008;41(6):982–90.
7. Shortliffe EH, Sepúlveda MJ. Clinical decision support in the era of artificial intelligence. JAMA. 2018;320(21):2199–200.
8. Kuperman GJ, Bobb A, Payne TH, Avery AJ, Gandhi TK, Burns G, et al. Medication-related clinical decision support in computerized provider order entry systems: a review. J Am Med Inform Assoc. 2007;14(1):29–40.
9. Osheroff JA, Teich JM, Middleton B, Steen EB, Wright A, Detmer DE. A roadmap for national action on clinical decision support. J Am Med Inform Assoc. 2007;14(2):141–5.
10. Wright A, Sittig DF, Ash JS, Feblowitz J, Meltzer S, McMullen C, et al. Development and evaluation of a comprehensive clinical decision support taxonomy: comparison of front-end tools in commercial and internally developed electronic health record systems. J Am Med Inform Assoc. 2011;18(3):232–42.
11. Sutton RT, Pincock D, Baumgart DC, Sadowski DC, Fedorak RN, Kroeker KI. An overview of clinical decision support systems: benefits, risks, and strategies for success. NPJ Digit Med. 2020;3:17. https://doi.org/10.1038/s41746-020-0221-y. PMID: 32047862; PMCID: PMC7005290.
12. Yang J, Xiao L, Li K. Modelling clinical experience data as an evidence for patient-oriented decision support. BMC Med Inform Decis Mak. 2020;20(Suppl 3):138. https://doi.org/10.1186/s12911-020-1121-4. PMID: 32646414; PMCID: PMC7346327.
13. Kawamoto K, Houlihan CA, Balas EA, Lobach DF. Improving clinical practice using clinical decision support systems: a systematic review of trials to identify features critical to success. BMJ. 2005;330(7494):765.
14. Bright TJ, Wong A, Dhurjati R, Bristow E, Bastian L, Coeytaux RR, et al. Effect of clinical decision-support systems: a systematic review. Ann Intern Med. 2012;157(1):29–43.
15. Taranath NL, Prabhu BPA, Dani R, Tiwari D, Darshan LM. Non-knowledge based decision support system. In: Shakya S, Balas VE, Haoxiang W, editors. Proceedings of third international conference on sustainable expert systems, Lecture notes in networks and systems, vol. 587. Singapore: Springer; 2023. https://doi.org/10.1007/978-981-19-7874-6_29.
16. Middleton B, Sittig DF, Wright A. Clinical decision support: a 25 year retrospective and a 25 year vision. Yearb Med Inform. 2016;Suppl 1:S103–16.
17. Sittig DF, Wright A, Osheroff JA, Middleton B, Teich JM, Ash JS, et al. Grand challenges in clinical decision support. J Biomed Inform. 2008;41(2):387–92.
18. Madhalaimuthu S, Radhakrishnan S. Clinical outcome prediction in pediatric respiratory infections using hybrid feature selection and a genetic algorithm-optimized machine learning. Sci Rep. 2025;15(1):36542. https://doi.org/10.1038/s41598-025-18258-6. PMID: 41120436; PMCID: PMC12540805.
19. Alkan M, Zakariyya I, Leighton S, Sivangi KB, Anagnostopoulos C, Deligianni F. Artificial intelligence-driven clinical decision support systems. arXiv [Internet]. 2025. Available from: https://arxiv.org/html/2501.09628v1.
20. Payne TH. Computer decision support systems. Chest. 2000;118(2 Suppl):47S–52S.
21. Labkoff S, Oladimeji B, Kannry J, Solomonides A, Leftwich R, Koski E, et al. Toward a responsible future: recommendations for AI-enabled clinical decision support. J Am Med Inform Assoc. 2024;31(11):2730–9.
22. Shiffman RN, Wright A. Evidence-based clinical decision support. Yearb Med Inform. 2013;22(1):120–7. https://doi.org/10.1055/s-0038-1638843.
23. AHRQ. About Learning Health Systems. 2019. https://www.ahrq.gov/learning-health-systems/about.html.
24. McGinn TG, McCullagh L, Kannry J, Knaus M, Sofianou A, Wisnivesky JP, Mann DM. Efficacy of an evidence-based clinical decision support in primary care practices: a randomized clinical trial. JAMA Intern Med. 2013;173(17):1584–91. https://doi.org/10.1001/jamainternmed.2013.8980.
25. Dolan JG. Multi-criteria clinical decision support. Patient. 2010;3(4):229–48. https://doi.org/10.2165/11539470-000000000-00000.
26. Liu LG, Ancker JS, Masterson Creber RM. Improving patient engagement through patient decision support. Am J Prev Med. 2021;60(3):438–41. https://www.ajpmonline.org/article/S0749-3797(20)30389-5/fulltext.
27. Keller AO, St. Arnold Bell L, Haglund K. Engaging a community–academic partnership to implement community-driven solutions. Prev Chronic Dis. 2025;22:240334. https://doi.org/10.5888/pcd22.240334.
28. Kaiser L, Conrad S, Neugebauer EAM, Pietsch B, Pieper D. Interprofessional collaboration and patient-reported outcomes in inpatient care: a systematic review. Syst Rev. 2022;11:169. https://doi.org/10.1186/s13643-022-02027-x.

Virtual Care 12

Velma L. Payne and Brittany Partridge

Abbreviations

3D	Three-Dimensional
CMS	Centers for Medicare and Medicaid Services
ED	Emergency Department
ER	Emergency Room
HIPAA	Health Insurance Portability and Accountability Act
HMD	Head-Mounted Display
LLMs	Large Language Models
NICU	Neonatal Intensive Care Unit
RPM	Remote Patient Monitoring
VLAN	Virtual Local Area Network
VR	Virtual Reality

Foundational Domains

This chapter addresses the following AMIA Foundational Domains: F1—Health, F4—Health Information Science and Technology.

Learning Objectives

1. Describe components of a prominent virtual care conceptual framework.
2. Discuss current solutions and associated workflows comprising the virtual care landscape.
3. Summarize best practices when embarking on a virtual care project.

12.1 Introduction

Virtual care has transformed healthcare delivery through the use of technology enabling patients to have a visit with healthcare providers remotely without going into a clinic, hospital, or other healthcare setting. Virtual care can include synchronous or asynchronous patient and provider interaction using any form of communication technology [3]. Virtual care provides many benefits such as improving patient engagement and patient satisfaction by enabling patients to "partner" in their care through the use of videoconferencing software, interconnected records, remote health monitoring, and wearable devices that gather patient data [3].

This chapter will provide an overview of aspects of virtual healthcare delivery including discussion of terminology, conceptual framework, current state and landscape, associated technologies, best practices and recommendations, and a look at the future of this type of healthcare service delivery.

V. L. Payne (✉)
The University of Arizona, Center for Biomedical Informatics and Biostatistics, Tucson, AZ, USA
e-mail: paynevl@arizona.edu

B. Partridge
UC San Diego Health, San Diego, CA, USA

C. Eldredge et al. (eds.), *Introductory Textbook in Health Informatics*, Health Informatics,
https://doi.org/10.1007/978-3-032-16657-9_12

12.2 Virtual Care Terminology

A term used for remote healthcare delivery is *digital or virtual care*. Virtual care is often used interchangeably with the term telemedicine. The goal of *telemedicine* is to replicate the one-on-one experience of in-person care using digital technology without changing fundamental aspects of care [17]. Virtual care is delivery of a broader scope of remote healthcare services including clinical and non-clinical support for a variety of conditions delivered online or via apps to manage and maintain care [2, 17]. Essentially, telemedicine digitizes in-person care, and virtual care redesigns care delivery, putting the patient at the center, by leveraging technology to enable proactive and continuous care management [2]. Virtual care incorporates use of technologies such as video conferencing and integrated web-based technology to connect patients and providers in remote locations, facilitates real-time video consultation, patient-provider communication, data sharing, follow-up visits, rehabilitation and therapy services, outpatient care, emergency services, and health professional online training and education [13].

12.3 Virtual Care Conceptual Model

A conceptual model depicting aspects of virtual care including information, people, process, policy, and infrastructure is depicted in Fig. 12.1. People associated with virtual care include clinicians, families, and patients. The information aspect of virtual care includes healthcare data and artificial intelligence. Virtual care processes include care models and clinical workflow. Policy aspects of virtual care include regulations, legislation, standards, and funding models. The final component is technical architecture and infrastructure which includes software, network, devices, and cybersecurity. Virtual care models may include additional components or items within these categories, depending on the organi-

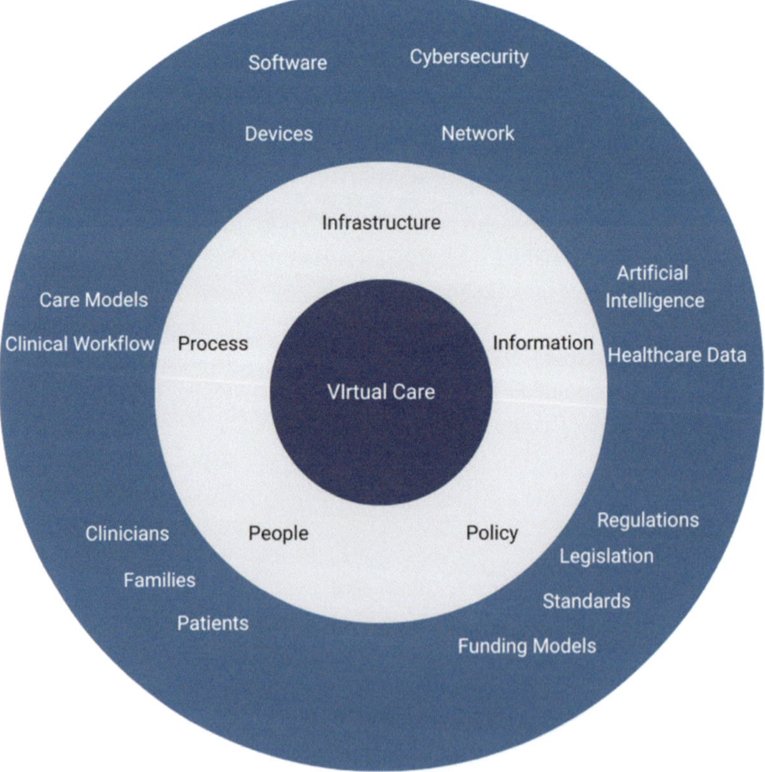

Fig. 12.1 Virtual care conceptual model. (Figure created by authors; adapted from Perimal-Lewis et al. [18])

zation needs, and the solution adopted by individual organizations. We will use this conceptual model as a foundation for our discussion of virtual care healthcare delivery.

12.4 Virtual Care Landscape

The current landscape of virtual care is composed of many diverse workflows. In this section, we will walk through many of the examples of what is currently in existence in the healthcare environment, keeping in mind that it is a sector that is continuously evolving, changing, and improving.

12.4.1 Inpatient Settings

Virtual care in inpatient environments has a wide variety of approaches and use cases. Some examples include the following:

Remote Rounding Think of a specialist physician covering multiple inpatient hospitals and clinics. Their patient and the patient's nurse might need a quick check-in from the physician while they are offsite, perhaps because there is a change in patient status that could use the physician's eyes. Rather than having to wait for their clinic appointment to be over or for the physician to physically drive to the new location, a virtual round using either a mobile cart or an in-room camera allows the interaction to take place more quickly, saving time and improving access to care.

Team Collaboration Perhaps the patient treatment team is a wide array of physician specialists and teaching teams with complex schedules that make it challenging to arrive in the same physical location at the same time. Telemedicine can allow them to discuss the case with one physician in the patient's room and the rest attending from their specific departments to foster better care and collaboration.

Acute Specialty Consults

1. *TeleStroke*: Think of a patient that enters a rural hospital Emergency Department (ED) that does not have an in-house Neurology team. The patient is experiencing stroke symptoms. With the use of a TeleStroke Cart, an advanced trained Neurologist is able to remotely evaluate the patient and advise the clinical staff on next steps in clinical care such as tissue plasminogen activator (tPA) administration, a clot buster procedure that is essential to administer quickly after a stroke.
2. *Remote Mental Health Consultations*: With the shortage of mental health providers there are often access challenges with mental healthcare. Patients may show up in the emergency room with acute mental health needs. Having a mental health telehealth program allows Psychiatrists to cover multiple hospitals and provide real-time care and consultations with emergency room staff and ED Physicians.

Family and Patient Engagement

1. *Discharge Education*: Using telehealth technology, a bedside nurse is able to team up with a virtual nurse to complete discharge education. The virtual nurse is able to spend targeted time answering patient questions and bringing family in remotely to attend the teaching. During a study performed on the virtual discharge model of care it was found "patient satisfaction communication scores improved significantly, and patients maintained a low 7-day readmission rate" [19].
2. *Family Meetings*: Family meetings are often scheduled to make sure that family caretakers and decision makers are included in a patient's healthcare decisions, allowing them to ask questions and hear about difficult topics directly from the physician. Family members and caregivers may have work commitments, live out of state, or be limited by a hospital's visitor policies. Using virtual care technology may aid in aligning the schedules of all the appropriate care team members. In a study

conducted during the COVID-19 pandemic, Kuntz et al. [12] said "Family meetings likely happened sooner and with far more participants than would have been possible without the use of the technology". The team of this study created an e-family meeting procedure framework that helped everyone involved including healthcare providers and family members to follow best practices.

12.4.2 Ambulatory (Outpatient) Settings

12.4.2.1 Ambulatory Video Visit

Currently, the most pervasive type of telehealth generally exists in two models. The first is a scheduled appointment with a patient's physician or specialist where each party joins an audio-visual meeting at the scheduled time and conducts the appointment on screen. The second is the patient joins a queue, most often used in urgent care type models and is seen by the next available care team member to be assessed for minor illnesses, also conducted fully over audio/visual software for real-time, face-to-face interactions.

12.4.2.2 eVisit

eVisit is defined by the Centers for Medicare and Medicaid Services (CMS) as "non-face-to-face patient-initiated communications through an online patient portal" [4]. eVisits are utilized specifically to respond to patient-initiated health concerns often through triage-type forms inside of a patient portal. These forms contain branching logic and can guide a patient through including all pertinent information for a physician to provide medical advice. eVisits can be billed for reimbursement if they meet all appropriate criteria and allow patients to get their concerns addressed without the need to complete a full appointment, thus increasing access. The findings of Bhargava et al. [1], which looked at over 20,000 eVisits, suggest most eVisits quickly and effectively address patient needs without necessitating follow-up visits.

12.4.2.3 Virtual Second Opinion Consults

Allow patients who live far from cutting-edge research and academic medical centers to access virtual second opinion consultations from specialists for specific targeted conditions. Second opinion consults are often cash pay services that allow a patient to upload their medical records and imaging studies into a portal (or have the consulting program request the appropriate records). Patients are then matched with the most appropriate specialist for their condition. Next, the specialist reviews all the information, scans, labs, and notes and provides a written second opinion to the patient (and their initial physician if the patient so chooses).

12.4.3 Clinical Surveillance

12.4.3.1 Remote Patient Monitoring

Remote Patient Monitoring (RPM) is a type of virtual care that uses data collected from patients through a variety of pathways and devices while the patient is outside of a traditional hospital setting (usually at home). This data allows healthcare teams to monitor patients' vital signs and health in near real time to make changes to their care plans or bring them in for a higher level of care as needed. Data is collected through wearables, connected vital devices like scales and O2 (oxygen) monitors as well as patient-entered data into applications and portals [8].

12.4.3.2 TeleSitters or eSitters

In inpatient settings, TeleSitters or eSitters use audiovisual technology to view patients from a remote "control center". Technicians or nurses monitor these patients who are at an elevated fall risk or have an altered mental state and might need extra communication. The staff can provide reminders to the patients to stay in bed, not to pull on their lines, tubes, and drains, and provide reassurance and orientation. They can also alert nurses if escalations are needed. It is a cost-effective way to improve safety for patients who do not need the acuity of a 1:1 sitter.

12.4.3.3 Virtual Nursing

Also known as Telenursing or Tele-ICU Nursing, depending on levels of care or hospital vernacular. Virtual care nurses are not meant to replace bedside nurses, instead the idea is that they will augment the current floor staff. The virtual nurses focus on non-physical tasks such as admissions, care plans, education, and discharge planning to alleviate some of the administrative burden from the floor nurses. Virtual nurses are often nurses with many years of experience and they can also mentor, precept, and support floor nurses during their shifts [6].

12.5 Virtual Care Requirements and Best Practices

When beginning a new virtual care project or looking to roll out telemedicine in your clinical practice or a hospital, the task can be overwhelming. The sheer volume of vendors that exist in the market along with understanding how they fit in the current architecture can be a daunting task. While there are many ways to roll out a new technology project, starting with the basics and scaling from there often increases the success of the project.

12.5.1 Define the Problem Statement—Get Specific

Ask yourself the following questions:

1. What problem are we trying to solve?
   An example might be patients are unable to make it across town through traffic for their weekly in-person group nutrition counseling. Often at this point both end users and technologists want to jump right into picking vendors and developing a solution, but it is really important that you get clear on the need and use case prior to that step.
2. What is the patient and clinician population that will be using this technology?
   It is important to define the users (stakeholders) and their needs prior to beginning the project. Once the users are defined, set time to interview each group to obtain requirements information as well as uncover specific challenges and needs that might not be evident. Then list the care team's roles and ask pertinent questions such as: What clinic do they work for? Do they have administrative support? Do the patients live in areas that have connectivity? Do they have access to a smartphone or computer? What are their primary languages? Are they signed up for the system's patient portal?
   You can use these demographics to inform a requirements document to use to assure you are selecting the correct vendor and the build documents contain the appropriate access changes and build points. Once these requirements are defined, you will want to bring these to the vendor meetings with you. Beyond the patient and clinical requirements, there are some baseline technology requirements and teams to include that are important to keep in mind.

12.5.2 Technology

Please see below for more description on the technology requirements that should be considered in virtual care.

12.5.2.1 Connectivity

- *Internet Bandwidth*: While you cannot control the patient's home network you do have control over the clinic, hospital, and provider attestation that their home networks (if they are practicing there) stand up to telemedicine requirements. Telemedicine requires a reliable and high-speed internet connection (ideally above 50 Mbps) to ensure smooth audio and visual transmission. Think about potential network congestions at peak times and consider putting all your telemedicine equipment on their own virtual local area network (VLAN).

- *Latency*: Aim for a latency (delay before a transfer of data begins) below 150 ms to minimize lag and delays in performance. Real-time consultation and assessment require a smooth video feed.
- *Back-Up Options*: If the primary Internet provider goes down, or an access point fails what are your back-up plans. Is there a secondary provider? Can you use a wired connection? Are you able to switch to mobile?

12.5.2.2 Hardware

- *Clinician Devices*: Often virtual care software platforms perform slightly differently on different devices. It is important to know what devices you will support your clinicians using for their workflow to make sure clinician devices meet the technical requirements for the software solution. It is also important to determine if these devices will be managed by the institution or whether clinicians can use personal devices.
- *Patient Devices*: To support patients in completing virtual care workflows, you will want to publish what the minimum standards are for devices. This can help inform knowledge base creation, the technical sector process of adding to a central repository of knowledge for quick reference by front-line support staff and the help desk. This information can also inform patient-facing tipsheets.
- *Updates and Maintenance*: Ensure there is communication with vendors as software continues to update to ensure you are not caught with hardware that cannot run the new software. Have enough runway (lead time) to update to newer hardware prior to the software updates.

12.5.2.3 Software

- *Telemedicine (Audio Visual) Software*: There are many software vendors that support telemedicine options. It is important that you create a requirements list of all the workflows your clinicians need; they will inform conversations about technical feasibility. Some things to think about include the following:
  - Is it available on both mobile and desktop? Clinicians and patients use a variety of devices throughout their daily lives and clinical workflows including tablets, mobile phones, laptops, and desktop computers. When analyzing software options, it is important to determine if the software has the same set of features across devices and to be able to speak to the differences. This information will allow the technical team to select the best option for current workflows and be able to support patients across an array of devices.
  - Does it integrate with the health system's primary electronic health record? In the healthcare systems clinicians spend a significant proportion of their workflow in the main Electronic Health Record (EHR), each time they have to go outside of that system it causes a disruption in their flow and creates the potential for missed information. Ensuring that selected software has the ability to integrate with the current EHR, allows the technical teams to support clinicians and patients with an effective clinical workflow that ensures data accuracy.
  - Does it integrate with other software needed during a video visit (e.g., interpreters, sharing of imaging studies, pulling in family members, etc.)?
- *Supporting Workflow Software*: What other software do you need to enable a clinician to fully complete their telemedicine session? For example: Do the stroke neurologists have the ability to remotely view the scans and images they need to diagnose and treat remotely?

12.5.2.4 Security

Ensure that you connect with the information security team before starting any new software project. They will be able to best inform you of the specific needs your environment has. Some items a security team might ask about are:

- *User Authentication*: How will end users attempting to gain access to the system be verified?
- *Data Security and Privacy*: What type of encryption is in place? Does the system meet Health Insurance Portability and Accountability Act (HIPAA) standards?
- *Disaster Recovery Plan*: How will your team handle cyber-attacks, natural disasters, or power outages to your system? What are the downtime procedures? How will you educate end-users to keep the impacts on clinical care at a minimal level?
- *Security Review*: Formal process where the security team works with the vendor to ensure they meet all the information security standards of your healthcare system.

12.5.2.5 Support

- Who is going to support this software/hardware? Do you have a help desk? Once a new technical workflow is implemented, users will continue to need a place to go with questions and issue reports. The organization will need to identify a technical team that owns the solution going forward post implementation. When the help-desk receives a call from the users and creates a ticket they need to know where to route it to have the issue resolved. Sometimes it is a group of teams that will support different pieces of the workflow. For example, you may have "User Security and Access" receive the ticket if the user cannot log into the software, you might have the "Network" team on point if the ticket says the cameras are offline and the "Virtual Care Team" would receive the ticket if the launch button from the EHR to the video visit is suddenly missing. It is important to have a clear matrix for the help-desk on where to route these tickets so there is no delay in issue resolution.
- Have you created the knowledge base articles and resources to help them in supporting the end-users (patient/clinician). What does your field support team need to know about this solution?
- How is the support team contacted if there is an issue?

12.5.2.6 Operations

While you will work with your operational stakeholders when implementing a technical solution, some areas to consider are:

- *Budget*: Who is paying for the initial implementation? Who is covering the cost of the hardware? Who is paying for any ongoing subscription costs?
- *Needs Assessment*: Who can you work with on the operational side to determine the current state of this workflow? Who can answer questions on future state vision, to ensure technical solutions meet their need?
- *Policy, Legal, and Compliance*: With almost all virtual care solutions, it is important to contact policy, legal, and compliance departments within your institution early to ensure that all regulations, policies, consent processes, and billing requirements are being met and planned for.

12.5.2.7 Training

- *Clinician Training*: What modality of training is best for this solution: classroom, videos, tipsheets, etc.? How will this information be disseminated: clinician newsletters, governance meetings, internal websites?
- *Patient Training*: What type of education does a patient need to complete their virtual care workflow? When can this information be shared? Are there multiple ways a patient can access and learn about this technology?

12.6 Looking to the Future

As with any technological solution it is difficult to fully predict what the future holds and how the ever-changing landscape of healthcare legislation, security and reimbursement will affect the emerging technical advances of virtual care. However, even with all the unknowns there are a few innovations with the potential to have a major impact on virtual care.

12.6.1 Wearable Devices

The first area of interest is the continued evolution of wearable devices and remote monitoring solutions. While these tools exist in the market today, manufacturers are making continuous improvements around their portability, connectivity, and power technology. The rapid evolution in device technology has allowed these tools to be more readily available to a broader group of patients. This has allowed for higher adoption rates, leading to earlier detection of health challenges and better management of disease states. Some leading-edge examples include the following:

- "Very soft, thin, flexible skin like" wireless sensors: These can be used on fragile patients such as Neonatal Intensive Care Unit (NICU) babies [5].
- Electrochemical sensing fibers: These sensors are for use in clothing as wearable health monitoring devices [20].
- Continuous molecular health monitoring through biomarkers: Recent developments have focused on electrochemical and optical biosensors, together with advances in the non-invasive monitoring of biomarkers including metabolites, bacteria, and hormones [11].

12.6.2 Virtual and Augmented Reality

Another area of technological advancement that may impact virtual care is virtual and augmented reality. *Virtual Reality* (VR) is defined as "computer-generated, three-dimensional virtual environment that users can interact with, typically accessed via a computer that is capable of projecting 3-Dimensional (3D) information via a display, which can be isolated screens or a wearable display, e.g., a Head-Mounted Display (HMD), along with user identification sensors" [9]. Augmented reality provides increased knowledge and awareness of users about their environment and the subjects they interact with through the enhancement of one or more of the senses [16]. Some examples of their future impact on virtual care are as follows:

- *Immersive Telemedicine Visits*: Clinicians have reported the ability to build trust more rapidly with patients while jointly viewing scans in VR and conducting therapy visits with VR avatars [15]. "VR has also been promoted over non-VR alternatives for benefits such as more comfortable treatment, higher engagement, greater satisfaction, more consistent practice, greater skill transfer, and facilitation of nonverbal communication that improves therapist-client contact" [14].
- *Visual Augmentation*: Wearable feedback in a heads up display or handheld device. Some examples include vein visualization devices to locate veins more easily for intravenous (IV) insertions, or surgical navigation systems that provide 3D visualization of a patient's anatomy during surgery.
- *Remote Mentoring from Clinician to Clinician*: This type of mentoring is the real-time remote guidance of healthcare procedures or skills where the mentoring clinician can see through the eyes of the performing clinician [7].

12.6.3 Artificial Intelligence

While there are other emerging technologies that will have an impact on virtual care, the last one this chapter will cover is *Artificial Intelligence* (AI). Some examples include the following:

12.6.3.1 Generative AI

Generative AI is defined as models, such as Large Language Models (LLMs), that generate new content, including images, text, and even music based on its training data set. In the healthcare space, there are some specific Generative AI models that have been extensively trained on industry-specific data known as *Industry Tailored LLMs*. In the medical space, they might be trained on medical texts and case studies to provide more accurate healthcare answers. One example of such a model is Google's Med-PaLM 2.

Two areas where Generative AI might be used to further virtual care are as follows:

- *Chat Bots*: Trained on medical industry-tailored LLMs, chatbots can help patients answer questions about their healthcare and help them engage the healthcare system at the appropriate level of care. For example, after a discussion with the chat bot a patient might be directed to schedule an appointment at the local urgent care, directed to drive to the nearest Emergency Room (ER) or escalated to a virtual call with a triage nurse.
- *Clinical Documentation*: Artificial intelligence models may be added into telehealth visits to aid clinicians in their documentation. This model can use the audio from a telehealth visit to compile a clinical process note for the physician's review based on the information gathered during the visit. As the model has been extensively trained across many clinical notes, it will be able to structure the note in the best format(s) to meet billing requirements, prepare prior authorization documents, or create a patient-friendly discharge summary.

12.6.3.2 Computer Vision

"Computer vision is a field of artificial intelligence that enables computers and systems to derive meaningful information from digital images, videos, and other visual inputs—and take actions or make recommendations based on that information. If AI enables computers to think, computer vision enables them to see, observe and understand" [10]. Areas where this type of technology could augment virtual care are as follows:

- *Fall Risk Detection*: Using vision-based surveillance, AI can augment eSitters in a hospital setting and alert them to patients that might be at imminent risk for a fall event.
- *Augmenting Telemedicine Visits*: Through computer vision overlay on telemedicine visits, the clinicians' assessment can be enhanced through models analyzing facial expressions and body language to provide insight into pain levels and mental health status. Models might also supplement with longitudinal analysis of wound healing or supporting neurological assessments through eye tracking of the patient. These advances are in no way meant to replace the clinician but to help them filter through the vast amounts of information coming through the screen and support them in targeting the best intervention.
- *Access to Rehabilitation Support*: Computer vision might help increase access to patients in more remote areas through the augmentation of physical therapy sessions. After an initial in-person assessment with a physical therapist, interim sessions might be supported by a computer model that corrects positioning and gives real-time feedback on exercises to get the most out of in-home practices.

All these emerging technologies are exciting and will likely have a substantial impact on virtual care. There are also many technological evolutions to be seen over the coming years that we are unable to predict. However, as technologists continue to push for newer and more advanced technology it is very important that the safety and data security of the patient is kept at the forefront of the research.

Knowledge Check Questions

1. Which of the following are aspects of virtual care?
   (a) Remote delivery of a broad scope of healthcare services for a variety of conditions
   (b) Delivery of services including clinical care and non-clinical support
   (c) Delivery of care and/or support using online or mobile applications
   (d) All of the answers are applicable
2. The 7 areas to keep in mind when deploying a new virtual care solution are Training,

Support, Operations, Hardware, Software, Security, and Connectivity.
   (a) True
   (b) False
3. An example of a LLM that is specifically trained for healthcare is:
   (a) Disney's WALL-E
   (b) Meta's LLAMA 2
   (c) Google's Med-paLM 2
   (d) OpenAI's GPT

Answers

1. (d)
2. (a)
3. (c)

References

1. Bhargava R, Gayre G, Huang J, et al. Patient e-visit use and outcomes for common symptoms in an integrated health care delivery system. JAMA Netw Open. 2021;4:e212174. https://doi.org/10.1001/jamanetworkopen.2021.2174.
2. Bradley T. Virtual care is transforming the future of healthcare. 2022. https://www.forbes.com/sites/tonybradley/2022/11/07/virtual-care-is-transforming-the-future-of-healthcare/?sh=fbf6a36659e5. Accessed 31 Dec 2023.
3. Burton L, Rush KL, Smith MA, et al. Empowering patients through virtual care delivery: qualitative study with micropractice clinic patients and health care providers. JMIR Form Res. 2022;6(4):e32528.
4. Centers for Medicare and Medicaid Services. E-visits. https://www.medicare.gov/coverage/e--visits#:~:text=E%2Dvisits%20allow%20you%20to,Clinical%20nurse%20specialists. Accessed 12 Nov 2023.
5. Chung HU, Kim BH, Lee JY, et al. Binodal, wireless epidermal electronic systems with in-sensor analytics for neonatal intensive care. Science. 2019;363:6430. https://doi.org/10.1126/science.aau0780.
6. Cloyd B, Thompson J. Virtual care nursing. Nurse Lead. 2020;18:147–50. https://doi.org/10.1016/j.mnl.2019.12.006.
7. Dinh A, Yin AL, Estrin D. Augmented reality in real-time telemedicine and telementoring: scoping review. JMIR Mhealth Uhealth. 2023;11:e45464. https://doi.org/10.2196/45464.
8. El-Rashidy N, El-Sappagh S, Islam S. Mobile health in remote patient monitoring for chronic diseases: principles, trends, and challenges. Diagnostics. 2021;11:607. https://doi.org/10.3390/diagnostics11040607.
9. Hamad A, Jia B. How virtual reality technology has changed our lives: an overview of the current and potential applications and limitations. Int J Environ Res Public Health. 2022;19:11278. https://doi.org/10.3390/ijerph191811278.
10. IBM. What is computer vision. 2023. https://www.ibm.com/topics/computer-vision. Accessed 10 Feb 2023.
11. Kim J, Campbell AS, de Ávila BE-F, et al. Wearable biosensors for healthcare monitoring. Nat Biotechnol. 2019;37:389–406. https://doi.org/10.1038/s41587-019-0045-y.
12. Kuntz JG, Kavalieratos D, Esper GJ. Feasibility and acceptability of inpatient palliative care e-family meetings during COVID-19 pandemic. J Pain Symptom Manag. 2020;60:e28–32. https://doi.org/10.1016/j.jpainsymman.
13. Li C, Borycki EM, Kushniruk AW. Connecting the world of healthcare virtually: a scoping review on virtual care delivery. Healthcare. 2021;9(10):1325–51. https://doi.org/10.3390/healthcare9101325.
14. Mantovani E, Zucchella C, Bottiroli S, et al. Telemedicine and virtual reality for cognitive rehabilitation: a roadmap for the COVID-19 pandemic. Front Neurol. 2020;11:926. https://doi.org/10.3389/fneur.2020.00926.
15. Morris ME. Enhancing relationships through technology: directions in parenting, caregiving, romantic partnerships, and clinical practice. Dialogues Clin Neurosci. 2020;22(2):151–60. https://doi.org/10.31887/DCNS.2020.22.2/mmorris.
16. Navab N, Martin-Gomez A, Seibold M, et al. Medical augmented reality: definition, principle components, domain modeling, and design-development-validation process. J Imaging. 2022;9:4. https://doi.org/10.3390/jimaging9010004.
17. Omada Health and Digital Medicine Society. The state of virtual care. 2022. https://resourcecenter.omadahealth.com/thought-leadership-resource/the-state-of-virtual-care-how-buyers-perceive-virtual-care-in-2022. Accessed 14 Jan 2024.
18. Perimal-Lewis L, Williams PAH, Mudd G, et al. Virtual care: the future for telehealth. In: Maeder AJ, Higa C, van den Berg MEL, Gough C, editors. Telehealth innovations in remote healthcare services delivery, vol. 277. Amsterdam: IOS Press Ebooks; 2021. p. 106–13. https://doi.org/10.3233/SHTI210033.
19. Perpetua Z, Seitz S, Schunk J. Virtual discharge. J Nurs Care Qual. 2023;38:234–42. https://doi.org/10.1097/NCQ.0000000000000689.
20. Tian H, Ma J, Li Y. Electrochemical sensing fibers for wearable health monitoring devices. Biosens Bioelectron. 2024;246:115890. https://doi.org/10.1016/j.bios.2023.115890.

Telehealth: Overview, Policy, and Reimbursement

13

Velma L. Payne

Abbreviations

AAMC	Association of American Medical Colleges
CAA	Consolidated Appropriations Act
CCHP	Center for Connected Health Policy
CDC	Centers for Disease Control and Prevention
CMS	Centers for Medicare and Medicaid Services
COVID-19	Coronavirus Disease 2019
CPT	Common Procedural Terminology
CTBS	Communication Technology Based Service
DEA	Drug Enforcement Agency
DoD	Department of Defense
FFS	Fee for Service
FQHC	Federally Qualified Health Centers
HCPCS	Healthcare Common Procedure Coding System
HHS	Health and Human Services
MAC	Medicare Administrative Contractors
NCTRC	National Consortium of Telehealth Resources Centers
OCR	Office for Civil Rights
PHE	Public Health Emergency
POS	Place of service
REH	Rural Emergency Hospitals
RHC	Rural Health Centers
RTM	Remote Therapeutic Monitoring
WHO	World Health Organization

V. L. Payne (✉)
The University of Arizona, Center of Biomedical Informatics and Biostatistics, Tucson, AZ, USA
e-mail: paynevl@arizona.edu

Foundational Domains
This chapter addresses the following AMIA Foundational Domains: F1—Health, F4—Health Information Science and Technology, F8—Professionalism.

Learning Objectives
1. Describe terminology, technology, and services associated with telehealth
2. Discuss telehealth regulation modifications related to the COVID-19 Public Health Emergency
3. Summarize the timeline for telehealth waivers established during COVID-19
4. Explain telehealth reimbursement payers, codes, and applicable services

13.1 Introduction

Traditional healthcare delivery models have consisted of in-person face-to-face conversation and information exchange between patient and provider within clinical settings such as a physician office,

C. Eldredge et al. (eds.), *Introductory Textbook in Health Informatics*, Health Informatics,
https://doi.org/10.1007/978-3-032-16657-9_13

hospitals, and outpatient clinics. Technological advances enable significant changes to how and when healthcare is delivered [38]. Even though healthcare has been slow to implement technology and adopt procedures for remote care delivery, there has been progress in implementing telecommunication technology facilitating distance care and digital interaction between patients and providers [40].

This chapter will provide an overview of telehealth including: an introduction of terminology, technology enabling telehealth services, telehealth policies, federal and state telehealth regulations, Coronavirus Disease 2019 (COVID-19) waivers associated with privacy and security, location, provider eligibility, provider licensure requirements, controlled substance regulations, financial and service reimbursement policies constraining telehealth use, and patient and provider experiences using telehealth.

13.2 Telehealth Terminology, Technology, and Services

There are numerous terms, and a lack of standard definitions used to describe delivery of healthcare services when the patient and clinician are in separate locations. Telehealth is healthcare service delivery involving patients and healthcare professionals who are in separate locations when care is delivered. The United States Department of Health and Human Services (HHS) defines telehealth as "the use of electronic information and telecommunication technology to support long-distance clinical healthcare, patient and professional education, public health, and health administration" [17]. The definition the Center for Medicare and Medicaid Services (CMS) uses is "use of telecommunications and information technology to provide access to health assessment, diagnosis, intervention, consultation, supervision, and information across distance" [7]. Telehealth enables clinicians to care for patients without an in-person office visit, commonly with the patient attending from home and the clinician in a medical facility [18, 41]. Telehealth enables patients to receive a variety of services including *general services* such as prescription management, lab result review, follow-up appointments; *specialized care* including urgent care and physical, occupational, and mental health therapist appointments; and *remote monitoring services* for chronic condition management. Telehealth includes live patient-provider communication using technology such as video chat, computers, mobile devices, telephone, email, secure messaging and file exchange, and remote monitoring devices to transmit data to clinicians [18].

13.3 Telehealth Utilization

Telecommunications technology supporting delivery of telehealth services has been available and used in healthcare for some time. However, telehealth utilization rates changed significantly when the COVID-19 pandemic commenced in 2020.

13.3.1 COVID-19 Pandemic Timeline

In December 2019, individuals in Wuhan, China began to experience pneumonia-like symptoms that were nonresponsive to treatment [6]. By early January 2020, China public health officials identified the agent causing the outbreak as coronavirus, which was later referred to as "2019 Novel Coronavirus" by the World Health Organization (WHO). By January 19, 2020, there were 282 laboratory-confirmed cases of the novel coronavirus reported in China, Thailand, Japan, and the Republic of Korea. Soon thereafter the Centers for Disease Control and Prevention (CDC) reported the first laboratory-confirmed case of the coronavirus in the United States in Washington state and activated an emergency center to monitor the outbreak. Soon thereafter as a result of the coronavirus, determined to be person-to-person spread, travel advisories to avoid unnecessary travel to certain countries was established, which eventually led to mandatory lockdowns in various countries, and federal quarantine orders in the United States. By the end of January 2020, the US HHS Secretary declared the 2019 Novel Coronavirus outbreak a public health emergency [6]. As of May 2024, the WHO reports over 775 million coronavirus cases and over 7 million deaths reported worldwide, with

Table 13.1 Factors impacting telehealth utilization [35, 48, 52]

Inconsistent and inadequate health system reimbursement
Inconsistent coverage policies across insurers
Restrictions at the US state-level
Patient and provider location restrictions
High startup and per-service cost
Privacy regulations requiring secure telecommunication technology
Interstate provider licensing restrictions
Prescription policies
Healthcare workflow reconfiguration
Clinician buy-in
Patient lack of awareness and interest
Telehealth not suitable for certain patients or situations

103 million cases and 1.2 million deaths in the United States [53, 54].

13.3.2 Telehealth Usage Prior to the COVID-19 Pandemic

Prior to COVID-19, although steadily increasing, telehealth use in the United States was minimal [48, 52]. Research shows that during this time 82% of Americans had not used telehealth and 18% of those using telemedicine resided in rural areas [1]. Factors impacting low utilization include those listed in Table 13.1.

13.3.3 Telehealth Usage During the COVID-19 Pandemic

The COVID-19 pandemic rapidly transformed the US healthcare system with primary drivers of change being use of telemedicine and the sudden shift in telehealth adoption [39]. Telehealth adoption rose significantly in response to the coronavirus due to shelter in place and social distancing mandates and restrictions on in-person care delivery. Widespread healthcare policy changes from governments and insurers including relaxed restrictions on telehealth policies by the US federal government Medicare program allowing beneficiaries from any location to access services remotely and HHS issuing waivers on enforcement of HIPAA for telemedicine were also contributors that increased telehealth usage [15, 31].

An example of the impact of COVID-19 on healthcare is New York University Langone Health, where between March 2 and April 14, 2020, telemedicine urgent care visits increased by 683% (from 102.4 to 801.6 visits daily), coinciding with a decline of over 80% in-person visits [39]. COVID-19-related telemedicine urgent care visits comprised 56.2% of all virtual visits, with 17.6% nonurgent visits being COVID-19 related. Within a 6-week period, there were 144,940 video visits involving 115,789 unique patients and 2656 unique providers [39]. Another study conducted by Omada Health and Digital Medicine Society [44] revealed that during COVID-19 there was a 38-fold increase in telemedicine utilization from pre-COVID-19 baseline.

It is anticipated that telemedicine healthcare will continue to be an integral part of medical care, especially with changes to reimbursement for telehealth and modifications to telehealth federal and state policies.

13.4 Telehealth Policy and Regulation

Regulations regarding insurance coverage and reimbursement for telehealth services vary by payer/insurer, geographic location, and federal/state policies. The US federal government regulates Medicare and self-insured plans. Medicaid and fully insured private plans comply with federal and state requirements, with state regulations varying on a state-by-state basis. This section will discuss critical telehealth regulations, modifications, and the longevity of regulations and waivers implemented during COVID-19.

13.4.1 Privacy and Security Regulations

It is important that all health information remains confidential and private to protect the rights of patients, providers, and organizations delivering healthcare services, regardless of the mode of delivery. The protection of health information is essential when using telecommunication technology for provision of telehealth services.

Telemedicine platforms used to connect patients and providers during telehealth sessions are required to comply with the HIPAA federal privacy protection regulations including the Privacy Rule for protection of individually identifiable information, and the Security Rule for protection of confidentiality, integrity, and availability of electronic protected health information [19, 20].

On March 17, 2020, HHS issued the "Notification of Enforcement Discretion for Telehealth Remote Communications During the COVID-19 Nationwide Public Health Emergency (PHE)" stating enforcement discretion would be exercised by not imposing penalties for noncompliance with HIPAA regulatory requirements against covered healthcare providers who were acting in good faith when using telecommunication technology to provide healthcare services during the COVID-19 Public Health Emergency [15, 16, 31, 52]. Three years later, due to the PHE expiring, the US Office for Civil Rights (OCR) announced the notification of enforcement discretion issued under HIPAA during the COVID-19 PHE would expire on May 11, 2023. The OCR granted a 90-day transition period through August 9, 2023, to allow covered healthcare providers to comply with HIPAA rules for telehealth; enforcement of HIPAA penalties resumed after this extension period. Currently, all telehealth services covered by health plans provided by eligible providers must comply with HIPAA rules, use technology vendors that comply with HIPAA rules, and enter into HIPAA business associate agreements when using remote video communication technologies for telehealth [20].

13.4.2 Telehealth Location Regulations

There are location-based requirements and restrictions associated with delivery of healthcare services using telecommunications technology. This section discusses specific terms and regulations associated with the location of provider delivering services and patient receiving services.

An *Originating Site* is the location of the patient at the time healthcare services are provided via telecommunications systems during a telehealth encounter, or where store-and-forward (asynchronous) services are provided [9]. For Medicare reimbursement, the originating site must meet certain requirements. Prior to the COVID-19 PHE, eligible originating sites included physician offices, hospitals, critical access hospitals, rural emergency hospitals, federally qualified health centers, rural health clinics, renal dialysis facilities, hospital or critical access hospital-based renal dialysis centers, skilled nursing facilities, community mental health centers, mobile stroke units, homes of Medicare beneficiaries with end-stage renal disease receiving home dialysis, and homes of patients receiving treatment for opioid abuse and co-occurring mental health disorders. During 2023, these requirements were waived rendering the patient home eligible for telehealth-delivered services. Due to the Consolidated Appropriations Act (CAA) of 2023, this policy was temporarily in place until December 31, 2024.

A *Distant Site* is the location of the provider at the time telehealth services are rendered; restrictions may apply due to licensure policies [9]. The rate of Medicare reimbursement will be dependent on the provider's distant site location, taking into account cost-of-living adjustments. The Medicare Act which bans foreign payments may also impose restrictions for physicians who are permanently or temporarily located outside of the United States when providing telehealth services. A temporary policy related to provider location was implemented after the PHE declaration stating during COVID-19 providers were permitted to use their work address even if telehealth services were provided from the physician's home so as to maintain confidentiality of providers' residence address.

13.4.3 Provider Regulations

Eligible Providers are providers who are authorized to deliver and be reimbursed for telehealth services through Medicare [9]. In order to practice and be reimbursed by Medicare for telehealth services, providers must be approved as an eligible provider. Prior to COVID-19 eligible providers included physicians, nurse practitioners, physician assistants, nurse-midwives, clinical nurse specialists, certified registered nurse anesthetists, clinical psychologists, clinical social workers, registered dietitians, and nutrition professionals. During the COVID-19 PHE, all eligible Medicare providers, Rural Health Centers (RHC), and Federally Qualified Health Centers (FQHC) were eligible for reimbursement for telehealth services including hospital outpatient therapies, counseling, and educational services beyond mental and behavioral health services. This extended policy was in effect until December 31, 2024.

13.4.4 Licensure Regulations

In order to practice medicine within a US state, healthcare professionals are required to meet state licensing requirements where the *provider* is located *and* be licensed or legally permitted to practice in the state where the *patient* is located [21]. The US licensure process, intended to protect the general public and ensure patient safety, involves healthcare professionals providing verification of educational qualifications and satisfactory performance on qualifying examinations, participating in background checks, maintaining/renewing licenses, completing continuing education, and self-reporting disciplinary actions [21]. Since licensing requirements may differ across US states, there may be additional requirements to practice in multiple states. Licensing requirements also differ by specialty type, which adds additional requirements.

It should be noted that US federal laws permit interstate practice of healthcare for specific situations and patient populations including the Uniform Emergency Volunteer Health Practitioners Act that applies during a declared state emergency and the Sports Medicine Licensure Clarity Act permitting sports medicine professionals to provide services to athletes when not in their home state. In addition, providers employed by the US Department of Veterans Affairs, US Department of Defense (DoD), and Indian Health Service are permitted to provide interstate healthcare services to Veterans, DoD employees, and American Indian and Alaska Natives, respectively [21].

Multi-State Licensure Compacts are licensing standards that apply when care is delivered in-person or virtually through telehealth, brought forth due to the increase in telehealth utilization during the COVID-19 PHE. Broadening cross-state licensure to include telehealth services by recognizing licenses in other states, known as *multi-state licensure compacts*, are agreements between states to streamline the licensing application process using one application, while preserving state oversight and quality [21, 22, 32]. During COVID-19 many US states expanded licensure policies to permit out-of-state providers (e.g., physicians, nurses, psychologists, audiologists, speech therapists) in good standing to provide telehealth services in another state after completing *Telehealth Registration* requirements. Telehealth registration enables out-of-state providers to provide telehealth services without obtaining a state license in the state where services are rendered. Each state is permitted to implement variation in telehealth registration; however, typically providers must have a current, valid, unrestricted license in a US state, not be subject to any past disciplinary proceedings in any state where they hold a professional license, maintain and provide evidence of professional liability insurance, not open an office or provide in-person treatment in the state where telehealth services are rendered, and annually register and pay a fee with the appropriate state licensing authority in their home state. These changes resulted in a number of US states establishing a telehealth advisory oversight committees to monitor access and patient safety of healthcare delivered through telehealth.

13.4.5 Controlled Substance Regulations

The US Federal Drug Enforcement Agency (DEA) maintains oversight of controlled substances under the Controlled Substances Act which indicates an in-person evaluation must be performed before a provider can prescribe a controlled substance [23, 52]. This stipulation limited use of telemedicine for individuals who have controlled substance problems. In March 2020 during the COVID-19 PHE, exceptions were implemented permitting DEA-regulated providers to use telemedicine to issue prescriptions for controlled substances to patients without an in-person evaluation in accordance with state laws regulating telemedicine and controlled substances. On May 10, 2023, the "First Temporary Rule" was jointly issued by DEA and HHA extending exceptions through November 11, 2023. A "Second Temporary Rule" was enacted to extend controlled substance DEA regulation for new practitioner-patient relationships through December 31, 2024 [42].

13.5 Telehealth Regulation: COVID-19 Public Health Emergency

The COVID-19 pandemic required assessing policies and procedures related to the practice of medicine, delivery of healthcare services, and provision of telehealth services. With the COVID-19 PHE declaration, US Congress made significant changes to Medicare telehealth restrictions including where services could originate and be provided, service reimbursement, approved technology/platforms, interstate practices, and privacy regulations [48]. Soon thereafter state and private payers collectively implemented temporary flexibilities to policies, regulations, and requirements on an emergency waiver basis [52].

Figure 13.1 reflects the progression of the COVID-19 outbreak in the US, declaration of the PHE, and policy waivers that have occurred. A declaration of the COVID-19 PHE occurred on January 31, 2020, through the Public Health Service Act (§ 319). The PHE was renewed several times through May 11, 2023, at which time the COVID-19 PHE expired [13, 15, 16]. The Consolidated Appropriations Act of 2023 extended some telehealth PHE waivers through November 30, 2023. There was a second extension of a few telehealth flexibilities through December 31, 2024. Some telehealth flexibilities have been made permanent, although most were implemented temporarily [24, 51].

Listed below are temporary Medicare telehealth waivers implemented for the COVID-19 PHE through December 31, 2024 [24, 51].

- FQHCs and RHCs are approved distant site providers for non-behavioral/mental telehealth services
- Medicare patients can receive telehealth services in their home
- No geographic originating site restrictions exist for non-behavioral/mental telehealth services
- Some non-behavioral/mental telehealth services may be delivered using audio-only communication platforms
- An in-person visit within 6 months of an initial behavioral/mental telehealth service, and annually thereafter, is not required
- All eligible Medicare providers may provide telehealth services

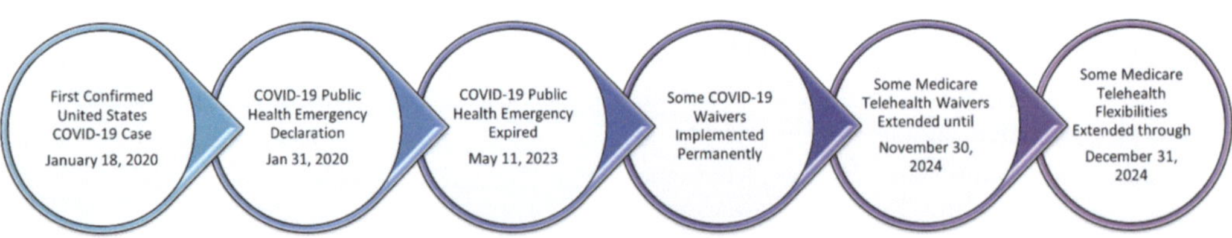

Fig. 13.1 COVID-19 and PHE Waiver Timeline. (Original figure created by authors)

The list below reflects Medicare telehealth flexibilities implemented during the COVID-19 PHE that have been approved as permanent changes [8, 10, 24, 49–51]

- FQHCs and RHCs are approved distant site providers for behavioral and mental telehealth services
- Medicare patients can receive telehealth services for behavioral and mental healthcare at home
- No geographic originating site restrictions exist for behavioral and mental telehealth services
- Behavioral and mental telehealth services may be delivered using audio-only communication platforms
- Rural Emergency Hospitals (REH) are eligible originating sites for telehealth

Additional information on regulatory and financial aspects of telehealth can be found on the HHS telehealth website (telehealthTelehealth.hhs.gov) and the CMS website (cms.gov). The National Consortium of Telehealth Resources Centers (NCTRC) provides no-cost up-to-date information and resource guides on telehealth (https://telehealthresourcecenter.org).

13.6 Financial Aspects of Telehealth

13.6.1 Telehealth Billing and Reimbursement

There are three types of reimbursable telehealth services including asynchronous (also called store-and-forward), synchronous, and remote patient monitoring; each type has specific billing and reimbursement rules. There are three primary entities involved in reimbursement of telehealth services including:

Medicare Program (Federal)
The CMS Physician Fee Schedule, updated annually, specifies Medicare payment policies, payment rates, telehealth services, and billing codes [8, 10]. CMS also provides information for safety net providers who provide healthcare services to the uninsured, Medicaid, and other vulnerable patients, and Medicare Administrative Contractors (MAC) or private healthcare insurers with geographic authority to process Medicare Part A, Part B, and durable medical equipment claims [25].

Medicaid Programs (State)
All US state Medicaid programs reimburse healthcare providers/organizations for synchronous services where the patient interacts with a provider directly. Reimbursement for other telehealth services varies and is determined by individual state Medicaid programs. Some, but not all US states, have expanded Medicaid coverage for telehealth to include reimbursement for services offered asynchronously, over the telephone, electronically, virtually, and when the originating site is the patient's home. The HHS State Medicaid Telehealth Coverage website provides information on state Medicaid telehealth reimbursement policies [26]. For each US state, this resource designates if Medicaid reimbursement is provided for live video, store-and-forward, remote patient monitoring, or audio only; if private payer laws exist; payment parity availability; types of interstate compacts; and consent requirements for professional requirements. The Center for Connected Health Policy (CCHP) website provides information on Medicaid state telehealth laws, reimbursement policies, private payer laws, and professional requirements for each US state, the District of Columbia, Puerto Rico, and the US Virgin Islands [2–4].

Private Payers
The majority of US states have a private payer program that requires *parity*, with parity policies varying from state to state [5]. There are two types of telehealth parity requirements including:

- *Service Parity* (also referred to as *Coverage*) requires the same services to be covered by payers when delivered via telehealth as would be covered if delivered in person. This type of

parity does not guarantee the same rate of payment for telehealth and in-person care.
- *Payment Parity* requires reimbursement at the same payment rate for telehealth services as in-person care/services. This type of parity is less common among US states.

The HHS Billing for Telehealth website [27] provides information on billing and reimbursement for telehealth services including the following:

- Medicare Payment Policies [30]
- Medicaid and Medicare Billing for Asynchronous Telehealth [30]
- Billing and coding Medicare Fee-for-Service Claims [28]
- Billing Medicare as a Safety-Net Provider [25]
- State Medicaid Telehealth Coverage [26]
- Private Insurance coverage for Telehealth [29]

13.6.2 Billing and Reimbursement Coding/Codes

Reimbursement for telehealth services is based on various billing codes including Common Procedural Terminology (CPT) Codes and Healthcare Common Procedure Coding System (HCPCS). Request for reimbursement are made using specific forms including the CMS-1500 form for reimbursement to individual practitioners, and the UB-04 form for reimbursement to facilities.

CPT Codes
Common procedural terminology codes used by Medicare, Medicaid, and other payers serve as a uniform language for coding medical services and procedures based on the following categories:

- *Category I* code descriptors corresponding to a procedure or service are organized into subcategories based on anatomy, procedure, or service type
- *Category II* codes are optional supplemental performance measurement tracking codes
- *Category III* are temporary codes for developing technologies, procedures, and services used for data collection, assessment, and payment of procedures/services not meeting Category I criteria

The number of CPT codes increased substantially in 2020 to accommodate COVID-19-related procedures and services. However, some codes are temporary and will not be listed on the permanent list; updates to the code list occur frequently.

Code Modification/Modifiers
Code modifiers, used to identify how the service was delivered, provide additional information to payers. Modifiers are not applicable for every CPT code category. Examples of CPT code modifiers for Medicare Fee for Service (FFS), FQHC, RHC, and other program services are listed below.

- *G0*: Telehealth services for diagnosis, evaluation, and treatment of symptoms of acute stroke
- *FR*: Supervising practitioner of physicians-in-training present during audio or video communication
- *FQ*: Telehealth service using real-time audio-only communication technology
- *93*: Synchronous telemedicine services via interactive audio-only telecommunications systems
- *95*: Synchronous telemedicine services via interactive audio and video telecommunications system

Place of Service Codes
Place of service (POS) codes are based on provider and patient location during the telehealth encounter. Specific reporting requirements are required for payment parity, where applicable. Reimbursement of services based on location are dependent on policies in place before the COVID-19 PHE, during the PHE extension period, and/or if the policy was deemed permanent. Specific policies may also apply for mental health services. Examples of location codes are:

- *02*: Telehealth services not in the patient's home provided/received via telecommunication technology
- *10*: Telehealth services in the patient's home provided/received via telecommunication technology
- *11*: Telehealth services in a location other than a hospital, skilled nursing facility, military treatment facility, community health center, public health clinic, intermediate care facility where the health professional routinely provides services
- *19*: Off-campus hospital location providing services not requiring hospitalization
- *22*: Hospital main campus location providing services not requiring hospitalization

Revenue Codes
Revenue codes are used to indicate the type of service provided by a facility, or the amount charged for hospital services provided to a patient, specifically if the service was performed in an emergency room, operating room, or another department.

Service Codes
Service codes designate what telehealth service was performed based on specific categories including:

- *Evaluation & Management*: Codes used primarily for outpatient office visits, although also used for inpatient, observation, and other care sites including prolonged care in non-outpatient settings
- *Communication Technology-Based Service (CTBS)*: Codes describing technology-based services not labeled telehealth by CMS. During the PHE, reimbursement was allowed for services for new patients; however, post-PHE reimbursement will only be permitted for established patients
- *Remote Evaluation & Virtual Check-In*: Codes for remote evaluation of asynchronous/store-and-forward image interpretation for patient follow-up and brief communication technology-based services (e.g., virtual check-ins) within specific conditions
- *Care Management*: Codes relating to services not involving direct face-to-face patient discussion important in caring for simple or complex medical conditions
- *Remote Physiological or Patient Monitoring*: Subset of care management codes for patients requiring chronic, post-discharge, or senior care, RPM services for high-risk patients with an established relationship with a clinical practice that began prior to the COVID-19 PHE
- *Remote Therapeutic Monitoring (RTM)*: Codes associated with monitoring progression of therapies performed by the patient based on a plan (e.g., respiratory/musculoskeletal therapies)
- *eVisit/eConsult/Interprofessional Consultation*: Codes associated with provider-to-provider-based activities such as specialist referrals and specialized disease consultations

13.7 Telehealth Experiences

13.7.1 Patient Experiences

Patients using telehealth prior to the March 2020 COVID-19 pandemic had positive impressions of remote visits, with convenience, time savings, decreased travel time, perceived improved outcomes and quality of care, faster service, shorter wait times, improved communication, and cost savings as factors contributing to their satisfaction [1, 34, 37, 45–47]. A systematic review conducted by Orlando et al. [45] revealed patients living in rural and remote areas attending an outpatient visit using videoconferencing were generally satisfied with telehealth due to improved access to healthcare, quality of patient-provider communication, patients feeling listened to, patient involvement in information sharing and decision-making, quality of care, thoroughness of the clinical assessment, ease in discussing personal matters difficult to discuss in person, and time and cost savings for travel. Patient concerns and dissatisfaction include lack of a physical examination, data security concerns, increased risk of breach of health information confidentiality, difficulty using equipment, and reduced audio-visual quality [14, 45]. When examining patient experiences with telehealth for follow-up care, Donelan et al. [12] found 62.6% of patients reported no difference in overall visit quality between in-person and virtual video visits. In terms of personal connection between patient and provider, 32.7% of patients reported better personal connection in in-person office visits than virtual visits; although 59.1% of patients indicated there was no difference between visit types [12].

13.7.2 Provider Experiences

Prior to the COVID-19 pandemic, provider use of telehealth was minimal, with the lack of use being largely due to inexperience with the technology [48], concern about suboptimal personal connection during virtual visits, and feeling that visit quality is better with in-person visits [12]. A Berkshire Hathaway study [1] designed to understand clinicians' perspectives and practices on telehealth shows 72% of 444 clinicians are interested in telehealth to expand patient access and reach; however, lack of reimbursement, program cost, and clinician resistance are barriers to implementation. Barriers to telehealth cited by clinicians in a study conducted by Klink et al. [36] include clinicians feeling telehealth was an inefficient use of their time, concerns regarding the quality of care, potential liability issues, lack of training, equipment costs, and inadequate reimbursement.

Educating clinicians on telehealth practices, technology, and ways to enhance virtual visits to ensure personal connectivity are areas to improve clinician experiences. The National Consortium of Telehealth Resource Centers provides free assistance and resources to help healthcare organizations and professionals understand telehealth technologies and ways to enhance telehealth services [43].

13.8 Telehealth and Informatics

The implementation of telehealth services has been challenging due to the lack of technologies and personnel with adequate technology-oriented skills required to realize the full benefit of telehealth. Telehealth can democratize healthcare, address healthcare disparities, promote a patient-centric approach to healthcare, and enhance patient engagement. Although telehealth alone is not enough.

The integration of telehealth and informatics has the potential to enhance healthcare delivery and health outcomes. Telehealth uses technology to remotely provide healthcare services; whereas informatics utilizes technology to store, manage, and provide access to patient information. Telehealth technology enables remote/virtual medical visits, remote patient monitoring by tracking vital signs real-time, access to medical specialists, and improved communication between patients and healthcare providers. Health informatics involves use of technology to store, retrieve, and transfer patient information, improve decision-making, standardize care, and predict potential health issues allowing early intervention. Amalgamating telehealth and health informatics allows for continuous observation and recording of patient health information through hospital-grade wearables equipped with secure data integration; ongoing data collection processes using biometric devices to ensure patient health status is constantly updated and aiding in timely medical responses. Benefits of the integration of telehealth and informatics include enhancing patient safety through facilitating the continuum of services across providers and care settings, and timeliness of care and communication.

In order to offer such sophisticated leading-edge healthcare, trained personnel with knowledge and skills in technology, telehealth, and informatics are needed. It is essential that academic informatics programs include curriculum to build learners' knowledge, skill, and competency in emerging technologies such as telehealth, virtual care, remote patient monitoring, etc. Health informatics students need to acquire the knowledge and skills required to implement and evaluate telehealth technology and services and train healthcare personnel and patients on proper use of the technology. Such education will prepare students for careers in implementing cutting-edge medical technologies to meet the needs of patients and healthcare professionals and enhance healthcare.

13.9 Resource List

Below are some resources available to learn more about telehealth:

- Health and Human Services Telehealth Website Resources for Providers and Patients [33]
- State Telehealth Laws and Reimbursement Policies [2]
- Billing for Telehealth Encounters. An Introductory Guide on Fee-For-Service [4]
- Telehealth for Providers: What You Need to Know [11]
- National Consortium of Telehealth Resource Centers [43]

Knowledge Check Questions

1. Once the COVID-19 Public Health Emergency ended, all regulatory waivers and flexibilities established during the pandemic related to privacy and security, location of service, controlled substance prescribing, and healthcare professional licensing requirements were implemented permanently.
   (a) True
   (b) False
2. The requirement that the same payment rate be issued for telehealth services as is issued for in-person care services is known as:
   (a) Payment parity
   (b) Service parity
3. Regulation modifications implemented during COVID-19 to support telehealth include which of the following:
   (a) Originating and Distant Location
   (b) Eligible Providers
   (c) Controlled Substances
   (d) All of the Above
   (e) None of the Above
4. Which type of code is associated with the type of service provided by a facility such as hospital services?
   (a) Place of service codes
   (b) Revenue codes
   (c) Service codes
5. Benefits of the integration of Telehealth and Health Informatics include which of the following?
   (a) Storage, retrieval, and transfer of patient information that improves decision-making
   (b) Facilitates continuous observation and recording of patient health information through hospital-grade wearables equipped with secure data integration
   (c) Enables ongoing data collection processes using biometric devices to ensure patient health status is constantly updated
   (d) Enables timeliness of care and communication
   (e) All of the Above

Answers

1. (b)
2. (a)
3. (d)
4. (b)
5. (e)

References

1. Berkshire Hathaway. Providers push for telehealth while patient uptake lags. 2017. https://www.businesswire.com/news/home/20171218005231/en/Providers-Push-Telehealth-Patient-Uptake-Lags. Accessed 12 Nov 2023.
2. Center for Connected Health Policy. State telehealth laws and reimbursement policies. Spring 2023 summary chart of key telehealth policy areas. 2023. https://www.cchpca.org/2023/05/Spring2023_SummaryChart.pdf. Accessed 23 Jan 2024.
3. Center for Connected Health Policy. Policy finder. 2023. https://www.cchpca.org/all-telehealth-policies. Accessed 23 Jan 2024.
4. Center for Connected Health Policy. Billing for telehealth encounters. An introductory guide on fee-for-service. 2023. https://www.cchpca.org/2023/07/2023BillingGuideFINAL.pdf. Accessed 16 Jan 2024.
5. Center for Connected Health Policy. Private payer parity. 2023. https://www.cchpca.org/topic/parity. Accessed 23 Jan 2024.
6. Centers for Disease Control and Prevention. CDC Museum COVID-19 Timeline. n.d. https://www.cdc.gov/museum/timeline/covid19.html. Accessed 25 Jan 2024.
7. Centers for Medicare and Medicaid Services. Telemedicine. 2020. https://www.medicaid.gov/medicaid/benefits/telemedicine/index.html. Accessed 2 May 2023.
8. Centers for Medicare and Medicaid Services. CY 2022 telehealth update medicare physician fee schedule. 2022. https://www.cms.gov/files/document/mm12549-cy2022-telehealth-update-medicare-physician-fee-schedule.pdf. Accessed 15 Nov 2023.
9. Centers for Medicare and Medicaid Services. Medicine learning network fact sheet: telehealth services. MLN90175. 2023. https://www.cms.gov/files/document/mln901705-telehealth-services.pdf. Accessed 15 Nov 2023.
10. Centers for Medicare and Medicaid Services. CY 2023 telehealth update medicare physician fee schedule. 2023. https://www.cms.gov/medicare/payment/fee-schedules/physician. Accessed 15 Nov 2023.
11. Coverage to Care. Telehealth for providers: what you need to know. 2023. https://www.cms.gov/files/document/telehealth-toolkit-providers.pdf. Accessed 28 Nov 2023.
12. Donelan K, Barreto EA, Sossong S, et al. Patient and clinician experiences with telehealth for patient follow-up care. Am J Manag Care. 2019;25:40–4.
13. Executive Office of the U.S. President. Statement of administration policy. H.R. 382 bill to terminate the public health emergency declared with respect to COVID-19. 2023. https://www.whitehouse.gov/wp-content/uploads/2023/01/SAP-H.R.-382-H.J.-Res.-7.pdf. Accessed 23 Jan 2024.
14. Haluza D, Naszay M, Stockinger A, et al. Prevailing opinions on connected health in Austria: results from an online survey. Int J Environ Res Public Health. 2016;13(8):813–26. https://doi.org/10.3390/ijerph13080813.
15. Health and Human Services. Notification of enforcement discretion for telehealth remote communications during the COVID-19 nationwide public health emergency. 2020. https://www.govinfo.gov/content/pkg/FR-2020-04-21/pdf/2020-08416.pdf. Accessed 23 Jan 2024.
16. Health and Human Services. Notification of enforcement discretion for telehealth remote communications during the COVID-19 nationwide public health emergency. 2021. https://www.hhs.gov/hipaa/for-professionals/special-topics/emergency-preparedness/notification-enforcement-discretion-telehealth/index.html. Accessed 23 Jan 2024.
17. Health and Human Services. Telemedicine and telehealth. 2023. https://www.healthit.gov/topic/health-it-health-care-settings/public-health/telemedicine-and-telehealth. Accessed 2 Jan 2024.
18. Health and Human Services. HHS fact sheet: telehealth flexibilities and resources and the COVID-10 public health emergency. 2023. https://www.hhs.gov/about/news/2023/05/10/hhs-fact-sheet-telehealth-flexibilities-resources-covid-19-public-health-emergency.html#:~:text=Telehealth%20includes%20services%20provided%20through,an%20in%2Dperson%20office%20visit. Accessed 2 Jan 2024.
19. Health and Human Services. HIPAA rules for telehealth technology. 2023. https://telehealth.hhs.gov/providers/telehealth-policy/hipaa-for-telehealth-technology. Accessed 23 Jan 2024.
20. Health and Human Services. Prescribing controlled substances via telehealth. 2023. https://telehealth.hhs.gov/providers/telehealth-policy/prescribing-controlled-substances-via-telehealth. Accessed 23 Jan 2024.
21. Health and Human Services. Getting started with licensure. 2023. https://telehealth.hhs.gov/licensure/getting-started-licensure. Accessed 2 Jan 2024.
22. Health and Human Services. Health Information Privacy. 2023. https://www.hhs.gov/hipaa/index.html. Accessed 23 Jan 2024.
23. Health and Human Services. State medicaid telehealth coverage. 2023. https://telehealth.hhs.gov/providers/billing-and-reimbursement/state-medicaid-telehealth-coverage. Accessed 23 Jan 2024.
24. Health and Human Services. Billing for telehealth. 2023. https://telehealth.hhs.gov/providers/billing-and-reimbursement?section=1,2,4#billing-medicare-for-fee-for-service-telehealth. Accessed 12 Nov 2023.
25. Health and Human Services. State medicaid telehealth coverage. 2023. https://telehealth.hhs.gov/providers/billing-and-reimbursement/state-medicaid-telehealth-coverage. Accessed 4 Jan 2024.
26. Health and Human Services. Private insurance coverage for telehealth. 2023. https://telehealth.hhs.gov/providers/billing-and-reimbursement/private-insurance-coverage-for-telehealth. Accessed 4 Jan 2024.

27. Health and Human Services. Billing and coding medicare fee-for-service claims. 2023. https://telehealth.hhs.gov/providers/billing-and-reimbursement/billing-and-coding-medicare-fee-for-service-claims. Accessed 4 Jan 2024.
28. Health and Human Services. Billing medicare as a safety-net provider. 2023. https://telehealth.hhs.gov/providers/billing-and-reimbursement/billing-medicare-as-a-safety-net-provider. Accessed 4 Jan 2024.
29. Health and Human Services. Medicare payment policies. 2023. https://telehealth.hhs.gov/providers/billing-and-reimbursement/medicare-payment-policies. Accessed 12 Nov 2023.
30. Health and Human Services. Medicaid and medicare billing for asynchronous telehealth. 2024. https://telehealth.hhs.gov/providers/billing-and-reimbursement/medicaid-and-medicare-billing-for-asynchronous-telehealth. Accessed 23 Jan 2024.
31. Health and Human Services. FAQs on telehealth and HIPAA during the COVID-19 nationwide public health emergency. n.d. https://www.hhs.gov/sites/default/files/telehealth-faqs-508.pdf Accessed 23 Jan 2024.
32. Health and Human Services. Licensure compacts. n.d. https://telehealth.hhs.gov/licensure/licensure-compacts. Accessed 23 Jan 2024.
33. Health and Human Services. Telehealth hub for patients and providers. n.d. https://telehealth.hhs.gov. Accessed 23 Jan 2024.
34. Hsu H, Greenwald PW, Clark S, et al. Telemedicine evaluations for low-acuity patients presenting to the emergency department: implications for safety and patient satisfaction. Telemed JE Health. 2020;26(8):1010–5. https://doi.org/10.1089/tmj.2019.0193.
35. Hyder MA, Razzak J. Telemedicine in the United States: an introduction for students and residents. J Med Internet Res. 2020;22(11):e20839.
36. Klink K, Coffman M, Moore M, et al. Family physicians and telehealth: findings from a national survey project report. Robert Graham Center; 2015. https://www.graham-center.org/content/dam/rgc/documents/publications-reports/reports/RGC%202015%20Telehealth%20Report.pdf. Accessed 2 Dec 2023.
37. Kruse CS, Krowski N, Rodriguez B, et al. Telehealth and patient satisfaction: a systematic review and narrative analysis. BMJ Open. 2017;7(8):e016242.
38. Majerowicz A, Tracy S. Telemedicine: bridging gaps in healthcare delivery. J AHIMA. 2010;81(5):52–3.
39. Mann DM, Chen J, Chunara R, et al. COVID-19 transforms health care through telemedicine: evidence from the field. J Am Med Inform Assoc. 2020;27(7):1132–5.
40. Marx EW, Padmanabhan P. Healthcare digital transformation: how consumerism, technology and pandemic are accelerating the future. New York: Productivity Press; 2020.
41. Mayo Clinic Press. Telehealth: technology meets health care. 2022. https://www.mayoclinic.org/healthy-lifestyle/consumer-health/in-depth/telehealth/art-20044878. Accessed 2 Jan 2024.
42. National Archives and Records Administration. Second temporary extension of COVID-19 telemedicine flexibilities for prescription of controlled medications. 2023. https://www.federalregister.gov/documents/2023/10/10/2023-22406/second-temporary-extension-of-covid-19-telemedicine-flexibilities-for-prescription-of-controlled. Accessed 23 Jan 2024.
43. National Consortium of Telehealth Resource Centers. n.d. https://telehealthresourcecenter.org. Accessed 8 Sept 2023.
44. Omada Health and Digital Medicine Society. The state of virtual care. 2022. https://resourcecenter.omadahealth.com/thought-leadership-resource/the-state-of-virtual-care how-buyers-perceive-virtual-care-in-2022. Accessed 14 Jan 2024.
45. Orlando JF, Beard M, Kumar S. Systematic review of patient and caregivers' satisfaction with telehealth video conferencing as a mode of service delivery in managing patients' health. PLoS One. 2019;14(8):e0221848.
46. Pflugeisen BM, Mou J. Patient satisfaction with virtual obstetric care. Matern Child Health J. 2017;21(7):1544–51.
47. Polinski JM, Barker T, Gagliano N, et al. Patients' satisfaction with and preference for telehealth visits. J Gen Intern Med. 2016;31(3):269–75.
48. Shaver J. The state of telehealth before and after the COVID-19 pandemic. Prim Care Clin Office Pract. 2022;49:517–30. https://doi.org/10.1016/j.pop.2022.04.002.
49. U.S. Congress. Consolidated appropriations act, 2021. 2021. https://www.congress.gov/116/plaws/publ260/PLAW-116publ260.pdf. Accessed 2 Dec 2023.
50. U.S. Congress. Consolidated appropriations act, 2022. 2022. https://www.govinfo.gov/content/pkg/BILLS-117hr2471enr/pdf/BILLS-117hr2471enr.pdf. Accessed 2 Dec 2023.
51. U.S. Congress. Consolidated appropriations act, 2023. 2023. https://www.congress.gov/117/bills/hr2617/BILLS-117hr2617enr.pdf#page=1440. Accessed 2 Dec 2023.
52. Weigel G, Ramaswamy A, Sobel L, et al. Opportunities and barriers for telemedicine in the U.S. during the COVID-19 emergency and beyond. 2020. https://www.kff.org/womens-health-policy/issue-brief/opportunities-and-barriers-for-telemedicine-in-the-u-s-during-the-covid-19-emergency-and-beyond Accessed 3 Feb 2024.
53. World Health Organization. Number of covid-19 cases reported to WHO cumulative total. 2024. https://data.who.int/dashboards/covid19/cases. Accessed 25 May 2024.
54. World Health Organization. Number of covid-19 deaths reported to WHO cumulative total. 2024. https://data.who.int/dashboards/covid19/deaths?n=o. Accessed 25 May 2024.

Clinical Research Informatics

14

James E. Andrews

Foundational Domains

This chapter addresses the following AMIA Foundational Domains: F1—Health, F4-Health Information Science and Technology, F8—Professionalism, F9—Interprofessional Collaborative Practice.

Learning Objectives

1. Describe the basic features of clinical research informatics as a subdiscipline of health informatics.
2. Explain how health informatics approaches support clinical research design, conduct of clinical research, and the sharing of discoveries.
3. Summarize the key functions of clinical research systems and the processes they support, such as protocol management, patient identification and accrual, and reporting and analyses.
4. Examine different clinical data registries and other data and information resources utilized by clinical researchers.
5. State and briefly discuss the importance of standards to clinical research informatics.

J. E. Andrews (✉)
University of South Florida, School of Information, Tampa, FL, USA
e-mail: jimandrews@usf.edu

14.1 Introduction

Clinical research is critical to understanding and improving health and medicine. This branch of medical science involves discovery, safety and effectiveness of drugs and medications, various interventions, medical devices, and other products that are meant for use and treatment of humans in the overall diagnosis and management of disease [1]. The amount and diversity of information and data generated through clinical research activities, and the concomitant activities needed in their documentation, communication, and exchange, requires specialized attention by those working in the subdiscipline of Clinical Research Informatics.

Clinical Research Informatics (CRI) can be broadly defined as "the sub-domain of biomedical informatics concerned with the development, application, and evaluation of theories, methods and systems to optimize the design and conduct of clinical research and the analysis, interpretation, and dissemination of the information generated" [1]. AMIA supports the CRI Working Group (WG) whose website offers additional perspectives on the scope of professional and research activities that define this rapidly growing area [2]. The foci of CRI per the CRI-WG reflect the processes and needs of clinical research, such as: development and implementation of the technology needed to support a clinical research ecosystem; improvement and

C. Eldredge et al. (eds.), *Introductory Textbook in Health Informatics*, Health Informatics,
https://doi.org/10.1007/978-3-032-16657-9_14

optimization of various systems and data resources supporting research, management of workflow across all data and information resources and services; and standardization that enables sharing and interoperability [2]. The CRI-WG is also charged with promotion and advancement of CRI's emergence as a subdiscipline focused on supporting the research enterprise with tools adopted from the broader biomedical informatics tool chest. CRI utilizes these with the goal of making research safer, more effective and efficient, and interoperable in support of advancing science and improving health and quality of life.

In this chapter, we very briefly discuss foundational aspects of CRI to give readers a sense of the scope and purpose of this informatics domain. This includes the clinical research environment followed by where informatics tools and methods are brought to bear to help manage and enable clinical research processes. While not exhaustive, it is presented to promote a basic level of understanding of this subdiscipline of informatics that can be used as a starting point for further investigation.

14.2 Clinical Research Basics

Clinical research has innate features that differentiate this area of medical science from other contexts (namely, clinical medicine, public health, etc.) The National Institutes of Health (NIH) offers a definition of clinical research that is appropriately comprehensive: "clinical research is [...] patient-oriented research conducted with human subjects (or material of human origin that can be linked to an individual)" [3]. Research can involve many types of populations, have different aims or hypotheses, and utilize a variety of methods to explore "human disease, therapeutic interventions, clinical trials, development of new technologies, epidemiology, behavioral studies, and outcomes and health services research" [1]. In other words, clinical research encompasses the overall pursuit of new knowledge and processes to ultimately improve people's health.

Methodologies differ in the conduct of human subjects-based clinical research, and draw from a range of tools, processes, and research questions driving an inquiry. At one level, these could be observational or more passive, such as studying data longitudinally over time and stored in an existing patient information database or Electronic Health Record (EHR). At a different level, *Randomized Controlled Trials (RCTs)* are considered among the most rigorous for clinical research. RCTs can be used in many types of experimental contexts, but the robust nature of RCTs is particularly useful in determining the safety and efficacy of medical treatments and interventions for humans.

Rigor in RCTs comes first from the random assignment of subjects to study groups within an experiment. Randomization is key to ensuring an equal chance of assignment to a group, thus reducing issues such as selection bias. The goal is to provide equally comparable study groups. Most RCTs are divided into control and experimental intervention groups. As the name suggests, the control group is held constant with either no treatment or whatever the standard treatment may be. The experimental intervention group will receive the new treatment that is being tested, and results or outcomes are then compared with the control [4, 5].

The method of *Blinding* in research is often utilized to afford further rigor and reduction of bias. This refers to when the investigator, subject, or both, are prevented from knowing who is assigned to which group. Single-blind studies are when participants do not know their group assignment; double-blind studies are where both participants and subjects are unaware. The idea is to prevent bias in group assignment or other potential preconceptions that might influence a study. A double-blinded, randomized, placebo (no treatment), controlled trial can be seen as the most robust type of study (or gold standard) assuming it is feasible for a given experiment and study group [4].

RCTs can occur in phases, such as in the case of testing a new drug or other therapeutic intervention. Each phase, from I through IV, builds upon the knowledge gained through the outcomes and evaluation of the previous and using increasingly larger study populations to ensure safety, efficacy, and effectiveness of a treatment in humans. At each level of these studies there are strict regulatory guidelines and requirements, and other supporting systems and processes to support research [also see, 6].

There are some common steps or phases, regardless of study design, that most clinical research studies are likely to include. Payne [4] outlines these in terms of the broad steps in a study along with the concomitant information needs or data management requirements involved. The early, or preparatory phase, is where a study is conceived of and formalized in a protocol. Here, patient cohorts are identified and recruited. Next, the actual study is conducted, with data collection, interventions, and monitoring of the results. Finally, results are analyzed and disseminated or reported as required or needed to appropriately share findings and document the study. Throughout these phases there are information, data, and related informatics needs, requiring different resources and tools, that fall within the purview of CRI.

14.3 Essentials of Clinical Research Collection and Management

CRI emerged to develop solutions that facilitate work within the clinical research environment to develop enabling technology solutions to relevant research processes and aims, and to ensure results can ultimately be translated to support healthcare delivery. While it is outside the scope of this chapter to examine every area that falls within this broad charge of CRI, the below are a representation of some basic areas where CRI is focused to improve research. Readers are encouraged to explore the thorough treatment of these as found in *Clinical Research Informatics* [7] or other resources on the topic.

14.3.1 Study Protocols

A clinical research study is articulated in a plan that guides the investigation known as a *study protocol*. The study protocol outlines the research study's conceptual scientific structure, including a detailed description of the actions needed to complete the study, the measurements and tests to be conducted, and the procedures for analyzing and reporting the results [8]. These plans can be manifest in different formats, from a textual document to a fully instantiated computer-based protocol. Protocols enable study management, conduct, and reporting, which are among the foundational features of clinical research processes supported by CRI.

Computing tools have been integral in serving general management of the specific components of study protocols, from study documents and related artifacts, regulatory reporting, managing versions of protocols and documents, and so on. Niland et al. [8] outline how CRI is increasingly utilized to build highly integrated systems to support the full spectrum of the clinical study cycle. The phases (as noted earlier, and reflected generally in Fig. 14.1) range from conceptualization and design, to execution of the study, to analysis, with CRI offering potential solutions within each phase. For instance, in designing a study, there are methods to help conceptualize the best approach for a given study, help in the design of data capture forms (known as CRFs or *Case Report Forms*), and utilize standards for representation of data elements and their values. Once a study is underway, informatics can offer more efficient patient or cohort identification and recruitment [see 9], reporting of participant adverse events during the study, and supporting data management across each study arm. After the study is complete, CRI tools and methods support not only the statistical and technical analyses of the results, but also the critically important sharing of results for future use and analysis [8].

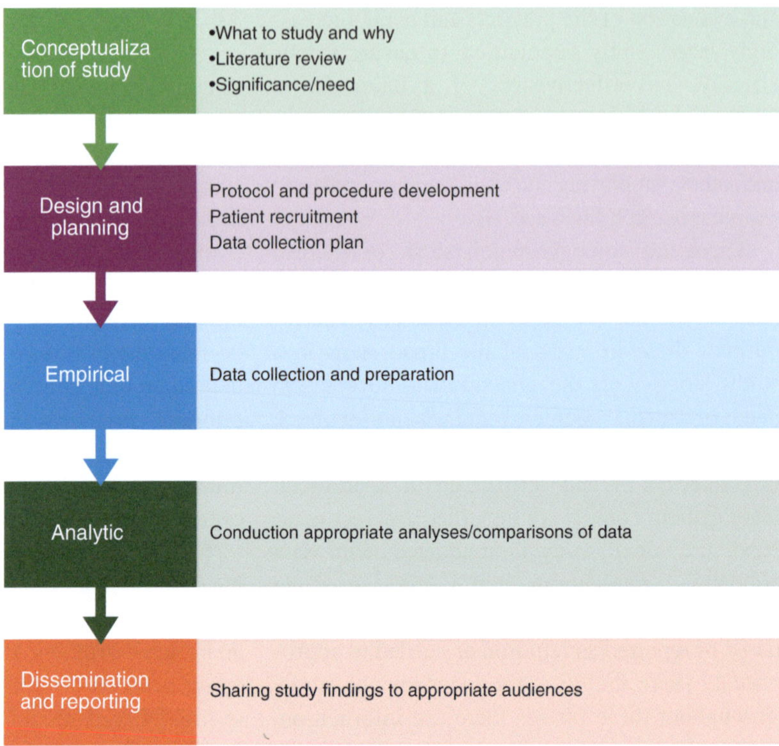

Fig. 14.1 General research phases. (Reference: https://obssr.od.nih.gov/sites/obssr/files/Design-Decisions-in-Research.pdf)

14.3.2 Clinical Research Management Systems

The intersecting functions and tasks of a research study pose challenging technological problems. Systems designed to support and integrate many of these functions are commonly referred to as *Clinical Research* (or Clinical Trial) *Management Systems (CRMS or CTMS)*, or *Clinical Research Information Systems (CRIS)*. These systems support a host of needs across clinical research activities (often beyond trials) and can help in reducing the rising costs of clinical research and enable more efficient data sharing and use [4, 6, 10]. A couple of the core components of these systems are discussed below.

14.3.2.1 Data Capture/Case Report Forms

One of the core activities in a CRMS is to ensure accurate, standardized, and timely data capture throughout the study. A primary tool for doing this in a computer-based system is through properly modeled electronic *Case Report Forms* (CRF). These forms are structured to collect specific data points relevant to the study for each subject participating in the protocol. A range of data items are collected, including elements of the subject's medical history, treatment interventions, lab results, and any adverse events experienced [8]. Although there are similarities between EHRs (see Chap. 10) and a CRMS given that they often share data across systems for certain purposes (e.g., patient history, communicating with care providers outside the study, etc.), the scope and purpose of each is clearly different. For data capture using CRFs, the main purpose is collection, management, regulatory compliance, and support for analysis and reporting within the scope of the clinical study and its goals [10].

14.3.2.2 Participant Selection and Recruitment

One of the greatest challenges to clinical research is the identification and recruitment of trial participants; that is, those who both meet eligibility requirements and are willing and able to sign on to a study. As noted in the above discussion of research study design, it is important to limit bias and include only participants who fall within certain parameters outlined by the protocol (age, sex, various measures related to a given disease, current or past treatments, allergic reactions, etc.). Naturally, this means only a limited number of participants will ultimately meet eligibility criteria, be accessible for participation in the study, or even be willing to participate.

CRI systems are created to assist in accurately identifying eligible participants and in providing necessary support to retain them throughout the life of the study. Integration with EHRs is one highly effective way to identify potential participants [10], as are registries, discussed later. CRMSs that enable searching patient records and databases based on specific criteria and characteristics of interest to the study can be quick and accurate. Once identified, further interviewing is necessary to ensure patients are fully informed on the study, its risks, and if there are other issues that might preclude their involvement (some new condition or situation yet to be reflected in the EHR). Beyond EHRs, there are other sources where patients might be matched with appropriate clinical research studies. There are increasing numbers of sites on the Web that allow patients (and physicians and researchers) to search for trials and to help determine matches for eligibility [see 9, 11]. Also, data warehouses have been used with informatics tools to identify cohorts for studies. These can perform functions similar to linking to an EHR but are focused more on patient data recording and less on the care continuum [9].

Despite the role of informatics technologies, research still faces serious challenges in attempting to recruit for, and successfully complete, a study. Some literature has noted less than 3% of eligible cancer patients might enroll in a clinical trial, and so many studies are not able to go forward due to lack of patient recruitment [12]. While individuals might have altruistic motivations to participate in a trial to help advance science and cutting-edge treatments, there are many reasons people may choose not to be part of a trial. Some of the reasons may stem from a misunderstanding of how clinical research studies are conducted, which can lead to fear of receiving lesser treatment, or being used as a "guinea pig" (despite the fact that very high levels of care are standardly offered in clinical trials). Informatics and health communication tools can be useful in ensuring that eligible participants understand the benefits and risks associated with participating in a study with fully informed consent. Recently, there have been a number of efforts to improve patient and stakeholder engagement and empowerment in the clinical research process, from design through completion and reporting [11]. Greater knowledge and understanding, and integrated participation in clinical study design and conduct, may lead to greater participation and retention of eligible individuals.

14.3.2.3 Protocol Management

An effective CRMS should enable overall management of the study as outlined in the approved protocol. As stated, the e-protocol is the blueprint of the clinical research and outlines the goals, measures, activities, and other features of the study; the CRMS must successfully support implementation and execution of these to support efficiency, transparency, and compliance with regulatory oversight.

Protocol management is supported by a CRMS by means of a variety of functions. For instance, an important one is the tracking of components of the protocols throughout their lifecycle, from original form through eventual amendments and revisions. Maintaining version control across these ensures only the most recent version of the protocol is available to study staff, preventing erroneous errors from use of earlier versions. Protocol management also supports core functions such as access control and permissions so that only authorized personnel have editing and approval authority and supports other collaborations across the team staff. Importantly, the CRMS protocol management functions are meant to integrate with other systems that support data capture and exchange, can work with data from EHRs (as noted earlier for patient matching), and generally streamline and support information sharing, recording, and use. Also, CRMS should have components that provide convenient scheduling of study visits, hopefully in concert with their primary care provider and organization [4, 10]. The systems should ideally support management of subjects throughout the study might include tracking enrollment.

14.3.2.4 Patient Monitoring and Safety

Patient safety is of central concern to clinical researchers, so the CRMS should provide tools to support monitoring and safety. For instance, identification of adverse events experienced by subjects is essential to their well-being and the safety of others. These can range from mild side effects caused by the treatment or intervention, to severe reactions or even death. A CRMS will have the ability to identify, record, and report adverse events experienced by participants. These can be entered directly into the system and subsequently reported as required by federal regulations (e.g., events graded at some base level or higher require reporting and sometimes suspension of the study); or, built-in automated alerts can trigger the system to notify investigators of potential problems from deviations in lab values, vital signs, patient-reported outcomes, etc. [10, 13]

In addition to adverse event recording and response, overall monitoring can ensure continued compliance with the approved, current protocol across various areas, such as patient enrollment and retention, different regimens, assessments, etc. The goal is to automate this in the CRMS to ensure quality of the study and compliance with appropriate regulations, guidelines, and protocols. Also, reporting and documentation can be facilitated to be more efficient with a well-designed CRMS. Moreover, facilitating communication with patients during and after the study can ensure that patients' concerns, progress, and any unforeseen impacts on them from the study are carefully monitored and addressed and to support patient engagement [10, 11].

Integrating tools from the CRMS that assist in patient safety and monitoring with other care-focused systems and appropriate investigator oversight can help achieve the goal of patient welfare and safety and ensure research quality and integrity. Those charged with the collection and management of clinical research data are generally required to be well-versed in clinical data management (CDM) practices and policies, including developing and enacting detailed data management plans to cover CDM from early phases in the study through the storage and archiving of the results [14].

14.4 Models to Enable Use of Clinical Research Data

Clinical and other biomedical research endeavors do not live in isolation; ideally, their processes and results should be stored and shared so as to build upon knowledge and speed up discovery. CRI seeks to utilize informatics tools and methods for storage and curation of these diverse resources so that they are retrievable for use in other research studies, by advanced systems examining findings and data across a range of studies, or for other research aims. Moreover, there is a need for transparency and accountability of clinical research that have motivated openly accessible resources such as trial registries. Additional forms of registries and repositories support other goals within the clinical research broader ecosystem. Below we briefly look at a few models that support the management, sharing, and use of clinical research and represent a range of these resources.

14.4.1 Registries

A registry is an open-access tool that allows for the reporting and organization of research studies, patient data, or other health-related elements from a range of study types and for different purposes. By and large, the motivation for registries comes from the need for transparency and accountability, which are critical to building trust about clinical research by the public and key stakeholders. Registries are used to further research and speed discovery and innovation by sharing results and data across studies; they can reduce redundancy, identify gaps, prevent publication bias [15], and generally lead to improved health [15–17]. The number and types of registries have proliferated internationally over the past few decades, and are generally sponsored and supported by different organizations or government agencies.

14.4.1.1 Clinical Trial Registries

Clinical trial registries are open-access, online repositories of protocol information from reported clinical trials [17]. Different elements can be collected, depending on the trial registry and the country. Most involve a number of metadata elements related to the study protocol. For instance, critical dates and contact information, sponsors of the study, and a series of elements to describe the health issue being studied, as well as the intervention's aims, sample size and participant criteria, and other information particular to the protocol [16]. Clinical trial registries usually provide information about ongoing and completed trials, and many provide at least summary results.

There are different ways to explore and access records of clinical trials registries internationally. Within the United States, the National Institutes of Health (NIH) has created a public online database, ClinicalTrials.gov, to provide access to metadata on clinical research studies and their results [18]. The site supports both required and voluntary submission of research study data from sponsors and researchers of both clinical trials and observational studies. Investigators submit data according to laws and regulations governing their research [18].

At the international level, the World Health Organization (WHO) developed the International Clinical Trials Registry Platform (ICTRP) [16]. This is a portal that allows searching a large number of clinical trials from a number of countries' registries, referred to as "primary registries". Primary registries included in the WHO network must meet specific criteria and requirements of the ICMJE [16, 17]. Investigators do not register their studies with the ICTRP but through the primary registries, which are searchable through the portal and also include searching of ClinicalTrials.gov.

14.4.1.2 Patient Registries

The Agency for Healthcare Research and Quality (AHRQ) defines patient registries as, "...an organized system that uses observational study methods to collect uniform data (clinical and other) to evaluate specified outcomes for a population defined by a particular disease, condition, or exposure, and that serves one or more stated scientific, clinical, or policy purposes" [19]. As Richesson et al. [20] note, patient registries have a long tradition in supporting observation of patients over time to study etiology of diseases, epidemiological monitoring of such illnesses as cancer, and in support of clinical research study design and conduct (e.g., cohort identification, recruitment, safety monitoring, etc.). Patient registries, then, are similar to clinical trials registries but have distinctly different aims. While trials databases are meant to provide information on studies that are ongoing or completed to support transparency and accountability (among other benefits, describe previously), patient registries are focused on the patients and their data (either individuals or cohorts) as the core unit of analysis [20] and serve the broader need of studying the health over time across populations [17].

The specific data managed within a given patient registry is determined by its purpose. A registry might primarily collect specific information relevant to its context or purpose (e.g., a rare disease registry), and clinical data from other systems might be plausible in augmenting this. However, most registries find it difficult to incorporate EHR or other clinical data into a registry due to such issues as the specificity of the data needed, which is often not easily retrievable in an EHR, or costly processing of data that is potentially relevant but is unstructured. Increasingly, registries are including data outside of clinical encounters and the EHR, such as patient-reported outcomes (PROs). These are data that are reported directly by patients outside the clinical encounter and that reflect useful information that can measure health status and functioning [6]. There are a number of tools being developed that seek more standard ways to collect this information, such as the PROMIS system [21].

Patient registries are continuing to grow as useful tools for supporting healthcare research. For instance, the value of patient registries in supporting RCTs is becoming more apparent. Richesson [20] outlines several evolving research contexts where registries are central to research design and quality, such as an expanded role in providing real-world evidence. In fact, there are increasing numbers of registry-based RCTs being conducted that are based solely on registry data that are far more cost-effective, have strong internal validity (due to randomization), and, high levels of data quality once rigorous assessments of these are done [20, 22]. Of course, registry development, maintenance, and proper use to support research can be supported by CRI and related informatics tools and methods.

Similar to clinical trial registries, there are lists of patient registries meant to support sharing and use, such as by the NIH (https://www.nih.gov/health-information/nih-clinical-research-trials-you/list-registries) and AHRQ's Registry of Patient Registries (https://www.nih.gov/health-information/nih-clinical-research-trials-you/list-registries) [6, 20].

14.4.1.3 Research Data Repositories and Resources

Other types of databases and repositories allow for sharing and use of clinical research data and information. Like registries, these can play a vital role in advancing medical science and generating new knowledge and are also equally varied in their scope and purpose. The following are just a few examples of such resources and services.

Advances in research involving genetic data have continued to evolve rapidly over the past few decades, as has the need to develop large-scale systems that allow sharing and additional use of various *-omics* research data (i.e., genomics, metabolomics, etc.) [23]. These sources include government-supported and developed biorepositories, sequencing data and tools, data and results from exploring genotype and phenotype, bioinformatics tools, and other resources. These artifacts of the postgenomic era are available to increase the rate of discovery, support translational medicine, and to deliver precision medicine that is individualized to patients' needs. Please see the chapters in this textbook on genomics and translational informatics for more information.

An excellent listing of prominent molecular biology databases regularly used to support clinical research is provided by Meyestre et al. [23, p. 311]. These, and hundreds of others outside of this list, house massive amounts of molecular and genetic data as well as highly specialized computational tools to allow their access and use. Among the many sources, a few examples are worth noting. For instance, *GenBank*, developed by the NIH, National Center for Biotechnology Information (NCBI) (https://www.ncbi.nlm.nih.gov/genbank/), is a large database of annotated DNA sequences and genetic data and part of a larger international effort. *dbGAP* is another tool developed by NCBI that is designed to enable storage and retrieval of various studies of the interactions of genotype and phenotype in humans (https://www.ncbi.nlm.nih.gov/gap/). Part of dbGAP's value is that it provides tools for the secondary analysis of quality datasets to match a study's research parameters.

Resources across academic health centers that are heavily engaged in clinical research have provided an array of clinical research data resources via the *Clinical and Translational Science Award (CTSA)*. Created by the National Center for Advancing Translational Sciences (NCATS), participating institutions (more than 60 of top medical institutions in the country) have formed a network to foster collaborations, store and share data from clinical studies and related research, and ultimately help improve the effectiveness and efficiency of translational science (i.e., moving from the research study to the application of its results in clinical care) [24]. A number of sub-networks and hubs have emerged from this broader CTSA network, thus expanding the goal of sharing knowledge and tools [4].

The Patient-Centered Outcomes Research Network (PCORnet) is a non-profit, very large collaborative network that also seeks to leverage and integrate data and resources from a number of clinical research networks. Members of PCORnet have access to large data repositories including EHRs and real-world evidence, claims data, and patient-reported information [25]. This network has been important to a wide spectrum of clinical and healthcare research, and has a particular emphasis on engagement with patients, advocacy groups, and other stakeholders.

The *i2b2* (Informatics for Integrating Biology and the Bedside) *TranSMART* foundation is another successful initiative to share resources across research enterprises [i2b2.org]. The ultimate goal is to enhance precision medicine "through the sharing, integration, standardization, and analysis of heterogeneous data from healthcare and research" [26] and is committed to open source and open data to ensure maximum sharing and use across communities.

14.4.2 Standards

The critical role of standards in healthcare and informatics is described in Chap. 24. As noted there and elsewhere in this text, health informatics plays a major role in encouraging and supporting the development and appropriate implementation of standards. Without attention to this, and without continually seeking new systems and approaches to successfully integrate standards across the health information ecosystem, the ability to capture, exchange, and reuse data and information is greatly impeded. As the reader can surmise, standards are no less important in support of CRI goals.

There are a variety of areas across the clinical research enterprise requiring standards development and use. Richesson et al. [27] discuss the full spectrum of standards use in clinical research, including development and maintenance organizations, support and promotion efforts, and research processes that are supported by specific standards. They note how an idealized and fully integrated healthcare and research system involves standards to support many functions we have already discussed, such as: core clinical research tasks (e.g., patient identification and accrual, specimen management); data collection and capture during visits; data quality support (e.g., collected by the right person and in compliance with protocol specifications); search and retrieval of core study data elements; efficient and accurate data analysis and reporting; and, adverse event identification and reporting in compliance with regulatory safety and reporting guidelines [27].

A major international effort related to promotion of clinical research standards involving work across industry, governmental agencies, academia, and the public, is the Clinical Data Interchange Standards Consortium (CDISC) (https://www.cdisc.org/). CDISC is a non-profit organization that either develops or advances standards to support data and information interoperability and reuse, and is supported by organizations from 90 countries and a vast number of research organizations [6, 8, 27]. For instance, Health Level 7 (HL7) is a standards development organization that supports a number of data exchange and communication and other administrative and clinical data functions. They collaborate with CDISC in support of their Regulated Clinical Research Information Management (RCRIM) model, which is an attempt to harmonize standards and support messages, document structure, semantics, and other functions largely related to drug and device studies and development [4].

In the last several years, a set of Fast Health Interoperability Resources (FHIR) was developed to help simplify the complex suite of HL7 standards and modeling. The goals of FHIR are to enable faster and more efficient clinical application development that use newer technologies, reducing barriers to spur innovation. This effort has led to FHIR's popularity and rapid adoption by developers, and there is much optimism about expanding FHIR-based applications in research [27; see also Chap. 23].

In addition to information exchange and messaging, other standardization tools are needed to support the clinical research ecosystem. For instance, controlled terminologies and related systems are important to the standardized representation of research data and information. Described in more detail elsewhere (e.g., Chap. 25). For instance, clinical terminologies that cover a broad range of health-related concepts include SNOMED

CT (https://www.snomed.org/) and ICD (https://icd.who.int/browse10/2019/en) and are used in a number of EHR and other clinical data systems. ICD 10 is a classification of diseases, conditions, signs, treatments, etc. that is presented hierarchically across several "chapters" based on systems and disease classes. SNOMED CT is more expansive in its coverage and is organized in polyhierarchical model (i.e., a concept can have multiple parents) with semantic relationships connecting concepts (e.g., *x* is-a *y* is-a *z*; or, *viral pneumonia* IS-A *infectious pneumonia* IS-A *pneumonia* IS-A *lung disease*) [28]. While SNOMED CT is more comprehensive in coverage than ICD 10, particularly since one can utilize its syntax rules that enable very precise concepts to be constructed through post-coordination, this ironically also can make it difficult to use or employ as a clinical terminology in research contexts [29].

Other standardized terminologies include LOINC (https://loinc.org/) (Logical Observation Identifiers Names and Codes), which is focused on laboratory and clinical measurements and observations. It is used in clinical contexts and within patient record systems but has obvious uses in clinical research where such data require standardization and consistent recording. Similarly, RxNorm (https://www.nlm.nih.gov/research/umls/rxnorm/index.html) employs standard names for drugs to enable linking to other systems focused on pharmaceuticals but that use different standard terminologies.

There is much overlap and redundancy across a number of standards in healthcare and that are employed to support clinical research. Most have their own governing bodies that oversee their maintenance and evolution, and some require membership to access and use while other standards are open source. The complexities involved in selection and utilization of certain standards for a given research study are non-trivial and might include, but certainly not limited to: availability and appropriateness to a study; coverage of concepts and data elements; difficulty of use by study personnel; cost to implement; regulatory obligations; and so on. Because of this, there are increased movements internationally to better harmonize standards so that they can effectively link and interoperate more efficiently and support data sharing and reuse. Various efforts to encourage such collaborations, as well as the many issues involved, are detailed by Richesson et al. [27].

14.5 Summary

Clinical Research Informatics integrates many of the foundations of health informatics, as covered in this text, and concentrates these to improve the more specific area of clinical research. Research across the medical sciences is complex and by nature information-intensive, involving interactions across a number of processes and stakeholders. Central to these is supporting safe and efficient research studies while producing new knowledge and cures. CRI develops and evaluates systems to support all phases of clinical research, from conceptualization to reporting and analysis. This includes the array of data registries and other information repositories that manage everything from patient-reported data, to trial information and results, to massive biorepositories or other molecular and biological databases and tools. Throughout all of this, the continued development, promotion, and integration of standards helps ensure that these data are of consistently high quality and are able to be shared and used across the systems and research community with the goal of improving care and expanding biomedical knowledge.

References

1. Fultz Hollis K, Andrews JE, Richesson R. Introduction to clinical research informatics. In: Richesson RL, Andrews JE, Fultz Hollis K, editors. Clinical research informatics. 3rd ed. London: Springer; 2023.
2. AMIA. Clinical Research Informatics Working Group. https://amia.org/community/working-groups/clinical-research-informatics. Accessed 1 Apr 2024.
3. NIH. The NIH Director's panel on clinical research report. https://grants.nih.gov/grants/NIH_Directors_Panel_Clinical_Research_Report_199712.pdf 12/97. Accessed 1 Apr 2024.
4. Payne PR, Embi PJ, Cimino JJ. Clinical research informatics. In: Shortliffe EH, Cimino JJ, editors.

Chiang MF, co-editor. Biomedical informatics: computer applications in health care and biomedicine. 5th ed. Cham: Springer; 2021.
5. Connaway L, Radford ML. Research methods in library and information science. 7th ed. Santa Barbara: Libraries Unlimited; 2021.
6. Fultz Hollis K, Winden T. Clinical research informatics. In: Hersh W, editor. Healthcare informatics: practical guide. 8th ed. Lulu.com; 2022.
7. Richesson RL, Andrews JE, Fultz Hollis K. Clinical research informatics. 3rd ed. London: Springer; 2023.
8. Niland J, Horn J, Hmwe S. Study protocol representation. In: Richesson RL, Andrews JE, Fultz Hollis K, editors. Clinical research informatics. 3rd ed. London: Springer; 2023.
9. Weng C, Embi PJ. Informatics approaches to patient recruitment. In: Richesson RL, Andrews JE, Fultz Hollis K, editors. Clinical research informatics. 3rd ed. London: Springer; 2023.
10. Nadkarni P. Clinical research information systems. In: Richesson RL, Andrews JE, Fultz Hollis K, editors. Clinical research informatics. 3rd ed. London: Springer; 2023.
11. Andrews JE, Eldredge C, Applequist J, Johnson JD. Evolving opportunities and challenges for patients in clinical research. In: Richesson RL, Andrews JE, Fultz Hollis K, editors. Clinical research informatics. 3rd ed. London: Springer; 2023.
12. Allison M. Can web 2.0 reboot clinical trials? Nat Biotechnol. 2009;27:895–902.
13. Richesson RL, Malloy JF, Paulus K, Cuthbertson D, Krischer JP. An automated standardized system for managing adverse events in clinical research networks. Drug Saf. 2008;31(10):807–22.
14. Walden A, Garza M, Rasmussen L. Best practices for research data management. In: Richesson RL, Andrews JE, Fultz Hollis K, editors. Clinical research informatics. 3rd ed. London: Springer; 2023.
15. Chan AW, Hróbjartsson A. Promoting public access to clinical trial protocols: challenges and recommendations. Trials. 2018;19(1):116.
16. WHO. International Clinical Trials Trials Registry Platform (ICTRP). https://www.who.int/clinical-trials-registry-platform. Accessed 15 Apr 2024.
17. Krleza-Jeric K, Mahmic-Kaknjo, El Emam K. Clinical trial registries, results databases, and research data repositories. In: Richesson RL, Andrews JE, Fultz Hollis K, editors. Clinical research informatics. 3rd ed. London: Springer; 2023.
18. NIH. ClinicalTrials.gov. https://clinicaltrials.gov/. Accessed 15 Apr 2024.
19. Agency for Healthcare Research and Quality. Research report: registries for evaluating patient outcomes: a user's guide. 4th ed. Rockville: Agency for Healthcare Research and Quality; 2020.
20. Richesson R, Vehik K. Patient registries: utility, validity and inference. Adv Exp Med Biol. 2010;686:87–104.
21. NIH. Patient Reported Outcome Measurement Information System (PROMIS). https://commonfund.nih.gov/promis/index. Accessed 15 Apr 2024.
22. Ecker BL, Brajcich BC, Ellis RJ, Ko CY, D'Angelica MI. Registry-based randomized clinical trials in surgery: working with ACS-NSQIP and the AHPBA to conduct pragmatic trials. J Surg Oncol. 2022;125(1):89–92.
23. Meystre SM, Gouripeddi R, Alekseyenko AV. Molecular, genetic, and other omics data. In: Richesson RL, Andrews JE, Fultz Hollis K, editors. Clinical research informatics. 3rd ed. London: Springer; 2023.
24. NCATS. Clinical and Translational Science Award (CTSA). https://ncats.nih.gov/research/research-activities/ctsa. Accessed 15 Apr 2024.
25. PCORI. Patient-Centered Outcomes Research Network (PCORnet). https://pcornet.org/. Accessed 15 Apr 2024.
26. I2b2 tranSMART. Informatics for integrating biology and the bedside (i2b2). i2b2.org Accessed 15 Apr 2024.
27. Richesson RL, Lynch CO, Hammond WE. Developing and promoting standards for clinical research. In: Richesson RL, Andrews JE, Fultz Hollis K, editors. Clinical research informatics. 3rd ed. London: Springer; 2023.
28. Wikipedia. SNOMED CT. https://en.wikipedia.org/wiki/SNOMED_CT. Accessed 15 Apr 2024.
29. Richesson RL, Andrews JE, Krischer JP. Use of SNOMED CT to represent clinical research data: a semantic characterization of data items on case report forms in vasculitis research. J Am Med Inform Assoc. 2006;13(5):536–46.

Population Health

15

Kelli Nam and Sue S. Feldman

Foundational Domains
This chapter addresses the following AMIA Foundational Domains: F1—Health, F6—Social and Behavioral Aspects of Health.

Learning Objectives
After reading this chapter, the learner will be able to:

1. Define population health and compare it to the field of public health.
2. Explain how population health practice is applied to the field of health care.
3. Identify opportunities for improved health outcomes in the field of population health.
4. Identify challenges to improved health outcomes in the field of population health.

K. Nam (✉)
Department of Health Informatics, Nova Southeastern University, Davie, FL, USA
e-mail: kn507@nova.edu

S. S. Feldman
Graduate Programs in Health Informatics, University of Alabama at Birmingham, Birmingham, AL, USA
e-mail: sfeldman@uab.edu

15.1 Background on the Field of Population Health

The population health approach has no exact origins and no definitive history [1]. Throughout history, sovereigns have held an interest in the overall volume of their populations and its direct influence on their military and economic prowess [1]. In the sixteenth century, leaders became interested in reducing disease outbreak occurrences within towns [1, 2]. By the eighteenth century there was an attention shift toward diseases of civilization that could impact economic and urban growth including, but not limited to, gout and communicable conditions like tuberculosis and other respiratory infections [1, 3]. In the 1990s, the term *population health* was initially described as pertaining to the health outcomes of a certain set of individuals or a group [4, 5]. Within the last two decades, population health has been centered around a defined community such as the individuals within a city or county or state [4]. Additionally, the term has evolved to the point where population health professionals account for relational interactions: (a) between individuals, (b) between individuals and their contexts, and (c) between individuals and the accessible services they use, as well as how these different interactions result in the health of a population [6]. Population health, as a field of study, is a discipline that examines the health differences of people within a population and also

C. Eldredge et al. (eds.), *Introductory Textbook in Health Informatics*, Health Informatics,
https://doi.org/10.1007/978-3-032-16657-9_15

Table 15.1 Definitions

Term	Definition
Health disparity	A difference in health that is linked to disadvantages impacting population groups at social, economic, or environmental levels [10]
Health equity	An aim to achieve the highest attainment of health for all populations [11]
Health inequity	A type of health disparity influenced by social determinants such as cultural and normative values and structural determinants such as policies that negatively impact the health of population groups [11]
Health inequality monitoring	Used to assess and quantify existing health inequalities within defined populations to identify areas for improvement [12]
Population health	A discipline that includes the examination of the differences among and between the health outcomes of groups of people [7]
Public health	Focuses on the population's health as a whole and is the science and art of preventing disease, prolonging life, and promoting health through organized efforts and informed choices of society, organizations, public and private communities, and individuals [4, 9]
Social determinants of health (SDOH)	Factors such as one's employment status, housing, gender, race, and income level as well as other factors that influence health, such as literacy, attitudes, beliefs, and behaviors as related to health [11, 13–15]. The societal hierarchies and inequities that exist between these factors for groups of people influence their health risks and health care access [14]
Stakeholder	An individual or organization with an interest in or that will be affected by the results of an initiative or project [16]

studies health outcome differences between populations [7]. Epidemiologists are professionals who measure relationships between population groups and their environments and are thus essential in describing the health status of populations that inform population health [8]. It is important to note that the term population health and public health are not synonymous. Unlike population health which focuses on the health outcomes of a certain set of individuals or groups and is narrower in scope than public health, public health is concerned with the health promotion and protection of all people [4, 5, 9] (Table 15.1).

15.2 Models and Strategies

Population health professionals initially based their conceptual framework on studying why some population groups tend to be healthier than others [4, 5]. Attempts were also made to develop conceptual models to understand these health differences such as with the development of bioactuarial models in the 1970s that were models used to predict population-level health characteristics such as lung cancer morbidity and mortality among American men from 1950 to 1977 [17]. Population health strategies have evolved to focus on health equity improvements, policy changes, and factors/determinants that can have an effect on the health outcomes of a population [4, 5]. In more recent times, population health methods include the "consideration of the social, economic, environmental, and health care system factors" that influence the health outcome differences between groups of people [7]. As mentioned earlier, *social determinants of health (SDOH)* are factors which encompass a person's living conditions such as one's employment status and housing, in addition to their community (available recreation, play, etc.) [11, 13, 14]. Other social determinants of health include factors such as literacy, attitudes, beliefs, and behaviors as related to health [15]. Societal hierarchies and inequities that exist between these factors for groups of people influence their health risks and health care access [14]. An individual's behaviors are linked to SDOH and are consequences of the individual's social environment and the structural conditions around them [18].

It is important to note that different industries implement population health methods, models, and applications differently and they also define the term population health differently. Health insurers consider population health as any effort to enhance the health of their members [19]. The trade organization America's Health Insurance Plans (AHIP) defines population health to include clinical research, public and private partnerships between health insurance providers, government agencies, and non-profit organizations, as well as the exploration of SDOH [20]. The American Hospital Association (AHA) considers population health as that which aims to improve the health outcomes of a defined group of people and requires initiatives to: (a) increase the prevalence of preventive health behaviors and evidence-based preventive health services, (b) improve patient safety and care quality, and (c) advance care coordination across the health care continuum [19, 21]. Harm reduction practitioners have accounted for factoring in population health perspectives to address America's opioid epidemic [22]. For example, applying a broad approach to identify: (a) upstream and midstream opioid misuse prevention factors and (b) access to evidence-based intervention downstream factors for the health of individuals and populations [22]. In this context, population health includes proactive partnerships among individuals, families, and multiple industry sectors including health care providers, emergency management personnel, judicial personnel, police, the pharmaceutical industry, and governmental agencies [22]. These partnerships establish coalitions to examine communal knowledge and attitudes to identify root causes, care gaps, disparities, and opioid misuse prevalence to formulate evidence-based treatments and policies toward community recovery support [22].

15.3 Health Disparities

Health disparities result from differences in health linked to disadvantages such as social, economic, or environmental level disadvantages for population groups [10]. Health advocates can establish whether health disparities exist in communities by comparing relative differences in health outcomes for population groups [23]. A *health inequity* is a type of health disparity influenced by (a) social determinants such as cultural and normative values and (b) structural determinants such as policies that shape an individual's residential segregation, access to education, and social position [11].

15.3.1 Opportunities

15.3.1.1 Contextualizing Health Improvement

Opportunities exist in the field of population health for shifting the attention away from solely intervention(s) and moving toward an overall focus on generating lasting health outcomes within existing population groups while keeping in mind health system improvements scaled up to the public health level [24]. It is worthy to note that it is more time-consuming and costly to develop a new intervention than it is to implement an improvement adaptation that accounts for contextual relevance and cultural compatibility with a population group [25]. When inciting changes to benefit population health, it is imperative for these approaches to be evidence-based. Evidence-based changes describe methods that have already been assessed to be effective [25]. Appropriate population health management techniques are also needed to foster system-wide changes and include proactive management of at-risk population(s) using layers of individual, cultural, and organizational considerations across disciplines [26–28].

15.3.1.2 Social Media

The role of social media should not be underestimated by population health professionals. Social media can be a valuable tool to distribute customized preventive health recommendations to various population groups [29]. In addition, during emergency preparedness and response scenarios, social media can be leveraged to identify projections of population health indices based on the analysis of: (a) social media content data types such as hashtag keywords, text strings, and numeric data, (b) linguistic styles within textual data, and (c) graph-based representations of influential health factors within textual data [29, 30].

15.3.1.3 Health Equity

As mentioned earlier, *health equity* is an aim to achieve the highest attainment of health for all populations [11]. To increase population health equity between communities, an opportunity exists for health advocacy professionals to evaluate the severity of barriers to health care access in communities by implementing Community Health Needs Assessments (CHNAs) [23]. CHNA is a tool that can be utilized to measure stakeholders' needs to efficiently coordinate public health, health care, and community organization activities that address identified needs [23]. Population health projects can be regularly measured with specified measurement framework(s) that define what to measure, to ensure accountability, and to incorporate reliability, validity, and scientific approaches [23].

15.4 Clinical Education

In clinical and medical education contexts, instead of teaching medical professionals about SDOH as facts to be known, the focus on training future clinicians to challenge and change the factors that contribute to systemic health care inequities could result in increased patient health [14]. Hospitals and academic medical centers could collaborate and partner with epidemiologists and local community-based organizations to conduct CHNAs, design, implement, and evaluate geographical area-wide, community-engaged, disease prevention and health improvement projects [31].

15.5 Healthy People Initiative

Healthy People is a long-standing public health initiative with new priorities established every decade. Healthy People State and Territorial Coordinators often work on population health initiatives as part of greater Healthy People initiatives, thus partnering with these coordinators alongside the stakeholders mentioned above would increase interprofessional collaborations in the discipline of population health. Each US state or territory has these coordinators who work as liaisons with the Office of Disease Prevention and Health Promotion (ODPHP) [32]. The coordinators and the ODPHP work together to establish improvement plans that address the current decade of *Healthy People 2030* leading health indicators, which are the areas for improvements affecting communities that require

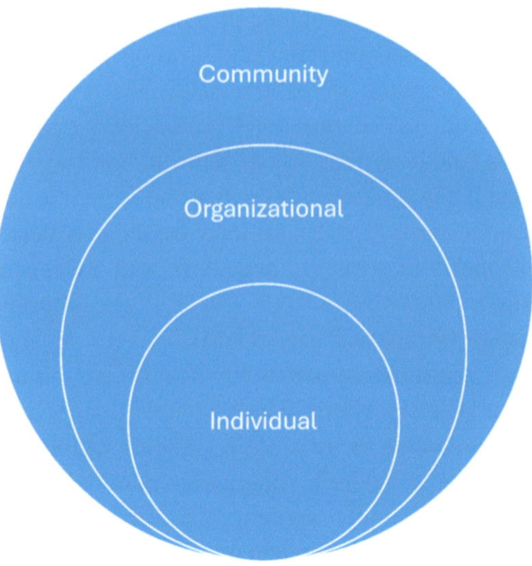

Fig. 15.1 Contextualize health initiatives at the individual, organizational, and community level

multi-sectoral actions toward human health advancement within the next decade [32, 33]. Population health professionals work to identify and address how cultures and social structures feed into destructive systems of economic, racial, and social inequities [34, 35]. In 2023, the World Health Organization launched the *Health Inequality Data Repository* that includes over 2,000 indicators, 22 dimensions of inequality, and populations across the globe [12]. Population health advocates may seize opportunities to engage with such resources to contribute to health inequality monitoring strategies [12]. As mentioned earlier, *health inequality monitoring* is used to assess and quantify existing health inequalities within defined populations to identify areas for health outcome improvements [12]. These improvements include contextualizing health initiatives at the individual, organizational, and community levels toward increased access to care for all community individuals and sustained behavioral change [11] (Fig. 15.1).

15.6 Public Health Policy Development

Population health and public health have an existing synergistic relationship with the potential to benefit human health [4]. The scope of public health is broader compared to population health and can include diverse health aspects, spanning from the environment (Environmental Health) to work spaces (Worksite Health), to living places (Community Health), and the management of infectious disease outbreaks [4, 36]. Multi-sectoral policies influence the health of populations [37]. Thus, during the development of population health policies, it would be prudent to: (a) enhance stakeholder engagement in policy development, (b) partner with stakeholders at historical institution structures across jurisdictions to remove barriers, and (c) mobilize social health advocacy actors named policy entrepreneurs who can articulate specific issues and who are aware of how policy agendas relate to new or existing policy solutions [37]. Policymakers, alongside stakeholders could integrate evidence-based behavioral services into primary, specialty, and community settings [38–40]. Since population health touches upon a myriad of sectors and disciplines, this underscores the need for diverse advocacy professionals and groups to work with policy entrepreneurs [37]. Policy stakeholders, researchers, and policy advocacy organizations (including public health organizations) could also collaborate on establishing a systems approach (discussed further in Chap. 8 on human factors) when implementing health policies [41]. Ongoing, systematic examination of policy implementation by engaged stakeholders is equally crucial since each public sector is governed by ranges of policies at national, state, and local levels for diverse communities [41].

15.6.1 Challenges

What is not measured cannot be fixed [42]. Unfortunately, population health measurement efforts "in the United States are poorly developed and uncoordinated" [23]. Populations with health disparities are negatively impacted based on factors such as socioeconomic disadvantage, race, ethnicity, sexuality, gender, individuals with disabilities, and populations living in or originating from underserved rural areas (i.e., SDOH) [43–45]. Cultural and structural racism has also fueled inequities across social and health policy decision-making in health care [34]. Communities of color have fewer opportunities and greater barriers to quality health services due to policies around land use, employment, housing, and access to care [46]. An individual's zip code has more significance in shaping their overall health than their genetic code [46, 47]. Even worse, SDOH tend to be systemic, intergenerational, cyclical, and population-based; effectively addressing them will require multi-policy and multi-sector initiatives for improvements in population health, likely over generations [10]. Despite this, system-wide integration and improvement approaches remain underutilized to scale up equitable health models among population groups [24]. Population health interventions tend to be at the policy, systems, and environmental levels geared toward reaching majority populations which are predominantly white and middle class and not as frequently based on research for health disparity populations [11]. Additionally, there has often been a lack of evidence-based approaches in community health improvement projects as well as limited collaborations between the health care system and communities [31].

15.7 Case Study

Background*:

Dr. Barbara Campbell is an epidemiologist that monitors the health of population groups. She examines the health of a small rural community, Maplevalley, with her team of epidemiologists. Maplevalley is located in a rural area where access to health care services is limited. Dr. Campbell's team conducts a community health needs assessment using surveys, assesses the community for potential health risks, and identifies trends and issues in the survey data that disproportionately affect rural elderly residents' access to care. She performs further statistical analyses to quantify areas for improvement for the elderly population in Maplevalley. Her team collaborates with population health professionals to account for social determinants of health such as senior residents' living conditions, structural environment, local policy influences, mobility status, relative proximity to a health care facility, access to transportation, and their health attitudes, beliefs, and behaviors to contextualize health improvements at the individual, organizational, and community levels. Her team also collaborates with community stakeholders such as elderly residents, the local health department, local hospitals, emergency services, policy professionals, clinics, community centers, family members, caregivers, and community health workers to establish a community health monitoring system that provides data important for informing the design of evidence-based health treatment access and prevention programs for seniors ages 65 and older. The health monitoring system helps her team and interprofessional stakeholders to track the local elderly population's health disparities and other emerging health issues within the Maplevalley community. The data from the system are used for the development of tailored health programs to improve Maplevalley's population health outcomes. *This case study includes example scenarios for educational purposes and is not indicative of real-life occurrences.

Discussion Question:

How is the work of Dr. Barbara Campbell and her team of epidemiologists important to inform population health improvement efforts?

15.7.1 Professional Organizations

15.7.1.1 AHA Community Health Improvement (ACHI)

ACHI is a national association for population health professionals and community benefit professionals that offers professional development resources, networking opportunities, and educational tools to achieve community health goals [48].

15.7.1.2 United Against Inequities in Disease (UAID)

An organization led by students for students and the communities in which they serve [49]. UAID focuses its efforts on local communities and collaborates with local partners to leverage the power of research and an interdisciplinary approach to reduce health inequities in communities, empower public health advocates, and affect sustainable change [49].

15.7.1.3 The National Association of Community Health Centers (NACHC)

Promotes high-quality, efficient, comprehensive health care that is accessible, culturally and linguistically competent, community-directed, and patient-centered for all [50].

Knowledge Check Questions

1. How has the definition of population health changed over time?
2. Describe one way in which public health and population health differ.
3. Provide an example of a social determinant of health that can influence population health.
4. Different industries uniquely utilize population health methods. Provide an example of one of the ways a specific industry uses population health methods.
5. Describe how the field of population health can address health inequalities.
6. Describe one challenge to the field of population health.

Answers

1. Population health was initially described as pertaining to the health outcomes of a certain group of people. Over time, this definition expanded to account for relational interactions between individuals, their contexts, and the accessible services they use to result in the health of a population.
2. Population health examines differences in health outcomes for groups of people. Public health is different and has a broader scope encompassing health promotion for all people.

3. The health literacy levels of individuals within a population is a social determinant of health that can influence the population's health.
4. The American Hospital Association (AHA) uses population health methods to advance care coordination across the healthcare continuum.
5. Population health examines differences between the health outcomes of groups of people. Health inequality monitoring is used to assess why different groups of people experience different health outcomes to identify areas for equity and improvements.
6. A challenge to the field of population health is that population health measurement efforts tend to be poorly developed and uncoordinated. Thus, evidence-based approaches are needed to improve assessments, collaborations, and health promotion efforts toward improved population health.

References

1. Szreter S. The population health approach in historical perspective. Am J Public Health. 2003;93:421–31. https://doi.org/10.2105/ajph.93.3.421.
2. Bates DG, Cipolla CM. Public health and the medical profession in the renaissance. Am Hist Rev. 1977;82:138. https://doi.org/10.2307/1857269.
3. Bynum WF. Darwin and the doctors: evolution, diathesis, and germs in 19th-century Britain. Gesnerus. 1983;40:43–53.
4. Baba Z, Belinske S, Post D. Public health, population health, and planning:: ideas to improve communities. Dela J Public Health. 2018;4:14–8. https://doi.org/10.32481/djph.2018.03.004.
5. Kindig D, Stoddart G. What is population health? Am J Public Health. 2003;93:380–3. https://doi.org/10.2105/ajph.93.3.380.
6. Roux AVD. On the Distinction – or Lack of Distinction – Between Population Health and Public Health. Am J Public Health. 2016;106:619–20. https://doi.org/10.2105/AJPH.2016.303097.
7. Wright KD, Alston AD, Piatt L. Definition and history of population health. In: Gary FA, Lotas MJ, editors. A population health approach to health disparities for nurses: care of vulnerable populations. Springer; 2022. https://doi.org/10.1891/9780826185044.0002.
8. Gulis G, Fujino Y. Epidemiology, population health, and health impact assessment. J Epidemiol. 2015;25:179–80. https://doi.org/10.2188/jea.JE20140212.
9. Winslow CE. The untilled fields of public health. Science. 1920;51:23–33. https://doi.org/10.1126/science.51.1306.23.
10. Hill-Briggs F, Ephraim PL, Vrany EA, Davidson KW, Pekmezaris R, Salas-Lopez D, Alfano CM, Gary-Webb TL. Social determinants of health, race, and diabetes population health improvement: black/african americans as a population exemplar. Curr Diab Rep. 2022;22:117–28. https://doi.org/10.1007/s11892-022-01454-3.
11. Trinh-Shevrin C, Islam NS, Nadkarni S, Park R, Kwon SC. Defining an integrative approach for health promotion and disease prevention: a population health equity framework. J Health Care Poor Underserved. 2015;26:146–63. https://doi.org/10.1353/hpu.2015.0067.
12. Kirkby K, Bergen N, Baptista A, Schlotheuber A, Hosseinpoor AR. Data resource profile: world health organization health inequality data repository. Int J Epidemiol. 2023;52:e253–62. https://doi.org/10.1093/ije/dyad078.
13. Marmot M, Friel S, Bell R, Houweling TAJ, Taylor S, Commission on Social Determinants of Health. Closing the gap in a generation: health equity through action on the social determinants of health. Lancet. 2008;372:1661–9. https://doi.org/10.1016/S0140-6736(08)61690-6.
14. Sharma M, Pinto AD, Kumagai AK. Teaching the social determinants of health: a path to equity or a road to nowhere? Acad Med. 2018;93:25–30. https://doi.org/10.1097/ACM.0000000000001689.
15. Braveman P, Egerter S, Williams DR. The social determinants of health: coming of age. Annu Rev Public Health. 2011;32:381–98. https://doi.org/10.1146/annurev-publhealth-031210-101218.
16. Centers for Disease Control and Prevention (CDC) Identifying and Determining Involvement of Stakeholders. https://www.cdc.gov/std/Program/pupestd/Identifying%20and%20Determining%20Stakeholders.pdf
17. Manton KG, Stallard E. Bioactuarial models of national mortality time series data. Health Care Financ Rev. 1982;3:89–106.
18. Trinh-Shevrin C. Applying a population health equity framework in the clinical setting-incorporating social and behavioral determinants of health into estimations of risk. JAMA Netw Open. 2020;3:e2021771. https://doi.org/10.1001/jamanetworkopen.2020.21771.
19. Sharfstein JM. The strange journey of population health. Milbank Q. 2014;92:640–3. https://doi.org/10.1111/1468-0009.12082.
20. America's Health Insurance Plans (AHIP). Population health: our position. 2017. https://www.ahip.org/issues/population-health
21. American Hospital Association (AHA). Managing population health: the role of the hospital. 2012. http://www.hpoe.org/resources/ahahret-guides/805
22. Salmond S, Allread V. A population health approach to america's opioid epidemic. Orthop

Nurs. 2019;38:95–108. https://doi.org/10.1097/NOR.0000000000000521.
23. Stoto MA. Population health measurement: applying performance measurement concepts in population health settings. EGEMS (Wash. DC). 2014;2:1132. https://doi.org/10.13063/2327-9214.1132.
24. Koorts H, Rutter H. A systems approach to scale-up for population health improvement. Health Res Policy Syst. 2021;19:27. https://doi.org/10.1186/s12961-021-00679-0.
25. Movsisyan A, Arnold L, Copeland L, Evans R, Littlecott H, Moore G, O'Cathain A, Pfadenhauer L, Segrott J, Rehfuess E. Adapting evidence-informed population health interventions for new contexts: a scoping review of current practice. Health Res Policy Syst. 2021;19:13. https://doi.org/10.1186/s12961-020-00668-9.
26. Steenkamer BM, Drewes HW, Heijink R, Baan CA, Struijs JN. Defining population health management: a scoping review of the literature. Popul Health Manag. 2017;20:74–85. https://doi.org/10.1089/pop.2015.0149.
27. Swarthout M, Bishop MA. Population health management: review of concepts and definitions. Am J Health Syst Pharm. 2017;74:1405–11. https://doi.org/10.2146/ajhp170025.
28. van Ede AFTM, Minderhout RN, Stein KV, Bruijnzeels MA. How to successfully implement population health management: a scoping review. BMC Health Serv Res. 2023;23:910. https://doi.org/10.1186/s12913-023-09915-5.
29. Nguyen H, Nguyen T, Nguyen DT. A graph-based approach for population health analysis using Geo-tagged tweets. Multimed Tools Appl. 2021;80:7187–204. https://doi.org/10.1007/s11042-020-10034-0.
30. Merchant RM, Lurie N. Social media and emergency preparedness in response to novel coronavirus. JAMA. 2020;323:2011–2. https://doi.org/10.1001/jama.2020.4469.
31. Kaplan SA, Gourevitch MN. Leveraging population health expertise to enhance community benefit. Front Public Health. 2020;8:88. https://doi.org/10.3389/fpubh.2020.00088.
32. United States Department of Health and Human Services (HHS) Healthy People in States and Territories. https://health.gov/healthypeople/tools-action/healthy-people-states-and-territories
33. Pronk NP, Kleinman DV, Richmond TS. Healthy people 2030: moving toward equitable health and well-being in the United States. EClinicalMedicine. 2021;33:100777. https://doi.org/10.1016/j.eclinm.2021.100777.
34. Cogburn CD. Culture, race, and health: implications for racial inequities and population health. Milbank Q. 2019;97:736–61. https://doi.org/10.1111/1468-0009.12411.
35. Griffith DM, Johnson J, Ellis KR, Schulz AJ. Cultural context and a critical approach to eliminating health disparities. Ethn Dis. 2010;20:71–6.
36. American Medical Informatics Association ® (AMIA ®) About AMIA. https://amia.org/about-amia
37. Béland D, Katapally TR. Shaping policy change in population health: policy entrepreneurs, ideas, and institutions. Int J Health Policy Manag. 2018;7:369–73. https://doi.org/10.15171/ijhpm.2017.143.
38. Crowley M, Green L, Scott T, Long E. Behavioral health policy for improving population health and wellbeing: opportunities for investment in evidence-based policymaking. Transl Behav Med. 2020;10:590–7. https://doi.org/10.1093/tbm/ibz173.
39. Katon W, Unützer J, Wells K, Jones L. Collaborative depression care: history, evolution and ways to enhance dissemination and sustainability. Gen Hosp Psychiatry. 2010;32:456–64. https://doi.org/10.1016/j.genhosppsych.2010.04.001.
40. Wagner EH, Austin BT, Von Korff M. Organizing care for patients with chronic illness. Milbank Q. 1996;74:511–44. https://doi.org/10.2307/3350391.
41. Oh A, Abazeed A, Chambers DA. Policy implementation science to advance population health: the potential for learning health policy systems. Front Public Health. 2021;9:681602. https://doi.org/10.3389/fpubh.2021.681602.
42. Gostin LO, Friedman EA. Health inequalities. Hast Cent Rep. 2020;50:6–8. https://doi.org/10.1002/hast.1108.
43. Benson RT, Koroshetz WJ. Health disparities: research that matters. Stroke. 2022;53:663–9. https://doi.org/10.1161/STROKEAHA.121.035087.
44. National Institutes of Health (NIH). Overview: populations with health disparities. 2023. https://www.nimhd.nih.gov/about/overview/
45. The Lancet Public Health. Disability-a neglected issue in public health. Lancet Public Health. 2021;6:e346. https://doi.org/10.1016/S2468-2667(21)00109-2.
46. Iton A, Ross RK, Tamber PS. Building community power to dismantle policy-based structural inequity in population health. Health Aff (Millwood). 2022;41:1763–71. https://doi.org/10.1377/hlthaff.2022.00540.
47. Callahan RF, Bhattacharya D. Public health leadership. Routledge; 2017.
48. AHA Community Health Improvement (ACHI) About ACHI. https://www.healthycommunities.org/about-ACHI
49. UAID The UAID Approach. https://www.uaid.org/approach
50. National Association of Community Health Centers (NACHC) Mission. https://www.nachc.org/about-nachc/mission/

16 Public Health Information Systems

Kelli Nam and Sue S. Feldman

Foundational Domains

This chapter addresses the following AMIA Foundational Domains: F4—Health Information Science and Technology.

Learning Objectives

After reading this chapter, the learner will be able to:

1. Define a public health information system.
2. Identify the role of the health informaticist relative to public health information systems.
3. Explain the applicability of public health information systems in the field of health care.
4. Identify opportunities for utilizing public health information systems.
5. Identify challenges to efficiently utilizing public health information systems.

K. Nam (✉)
Department of Health Informatics, Nova Southeastern University, Davie, FL, USA
e-mail: kn507@nova.edu

S. S. Feldman
Graduate Programs in Health Informatics, University of Alabama at Birmingham, Birmingham, AL, USA
e-mail: sfeldman@uab.edu

16.1 Background on Public Health Information Systems

Across civilizations, illnesses, remedies, and results have been recorded for public health posterity [1]. In ancient Greece, public health philosophies and principles have been in existence since the Hippocratic physiology of the four humors being in equilibrium (black bile, blood, phlegm, and yellow bile) whenever nutrition, exercise, rest, and excretion remain in perfect balance for human health [1, 2]. In the 1800s, industrialization and the large-scale migration of populations into cities with inadequate waste disposal systems sparked outbreaks of water-borne diseases including, but not limited to, cholera, dysentery, typhoid fever, and tuberculosis [3]. The infamous 1848–1854 cholera epidemic claiming over 53,000 lives in England and Wales was extensive in scale [3]. In 1854, John Snow, a physician by trade, conducted a pioneering epidemiological investigation into the epidemic; calculating cholera death rates among district of London homes, classifying outcomes in matrices, then providing groundbreaking epidemiological evidence that contaminated water from the River Thames was the origin of the cholera epidemic [3]. Through this event, John Snow established the basic methodology of modern public health investigations [3]. In the latter half of the nineteenth century, Florence Nightingale, a nurse by trade, advocated for the systematic collection and use of health statistics that could be acquired

C. Eldredge et al. (eds.), *Introductory Textbook in Health Informatics*, Health Informatics,
https://doi.org/10.1007/978-3-032-16657-9_16

from the records of patients treated in hospitals to inform social and public health reforms [4]. John Snow, making use of health data to inform a groundbreaking epidemiological investigation, and Florence Nightingale, making use of patient record data for health improvements are among the salient innovators and events that have helped to shape the field of public health, and public health investigations, into what they are today.

With an increase in the tracking and storage of public health data, safeguarding sensitive health information became imperative. The Health Insurance Portability and Accountability Act (HIPAA) was passed by Congress in 1996 to secure the confidentiality and security of protected health information [5]. *Protected health information (PHI)* is defined as any type of health information that can identify an individual and is in the possession of or can be transmitted by a covered entity or its business associates [6]. A covered entity is a health plan, health care provider, or health care clearinghouse that is a part of collecting, storing, using, or transferring protected health information [7]. A business associate performs services or activities on behalf of, or to, a covered entity [7].

Over time, United States federal laws began to incentivize the adoption of health information technology systems, primarily electronic health records (EHRs) [8]. In 2004, the federal government's first step toward creating a nationwide health information exchange occurred with Executive Order 13335 that initiated incentives for: the use of health information technology, the establishment of the position of the national health information technology coordinator, and the creation of the Office of the National Coordinator of Health Information Technology (ONC) [8]. (The ONC was renamed in 2024 to the Office of the Assistant Secretary for Technology Policy and Office of the National Coordinator for Health Information Technology (ASTP/ONC). All references in this chapter will remain as ONC). In 2009, the Affordable Care Act mandated that every health care institution migrate toward the use of a digital medical record system [8]. Also in 2009, the Health Information Technology for Economic and Clinical Health (HITECH) Act was passed by Congress that incentivized the rapid adoption of EHRs in health care and strengthened privacy standards for patient information privacy [8].

According to ONC, an *EHR* is a secure and historic as well as current real-time and patient-centered version of the patient's paper clinical and administrative record [9]. EHRs facilitate ready access to a patient's medical history, allergies, medications, treatment plans, immunizations, radiologic images, and laboratory test results and provide clinical decision support tools and analytics to support clinical decision-making [9]. Beyond the clinical environment at the point of care, EHR data can inform coalitions to mitigate population health disparities as well as to increase the quality and efficiency of health care [10]. Patient-reported outcomes stored in EHRs can prospectively inform research, quality health improvement initiatives, patient-centered care, and programs for improved population health [11]. Data reporting and information usage is becoming standard operating procedure such that the lines are blurring between traditionally reactive biosurveillance and emerging proactive public health prevention [12]. This is due, in part, to the rapid acceleration of EHR adoption described above. Methods to improve the timeliness, completeness, and accuracy of public health reporting could be exponentially streamlined with reporting straight from EHR data via regional and statewide health information exchanges. While this holds much promise to revolutionize the speed and quality of data received for public health reporting, interoperability must exist. That is to say that EHRs must be able to collect and send the correct data and the receiver (i.e., the public health department) of the data must be able to access and interpret the data as actionable information and knowledge such that every public health issue is not a battle [13].

Thus, in response to federal laws, the digitization of data collected across the health care ecosystem progressed to include some specialty areas. For example, laboratory technicians began to use laboratory information systems (LISs) and pharmacists began to use pharmacy information systems, primarily in terms of e-prescribing [14].

Table 16.1 Definitions

Term	Definition
Clinical informatics	The application of computer structures and algorithms and information technology to improve clinical communication and deliver health care services [17]
Data	Collected sequence(s) of facts, signs, and symbols [18, 19]
Data harmonization	The process of including data structures and modeling for recording semantics to facilitate data aggregation and reuse across disparate systems [20]
Electronic health record (EHR)	A historic, secure, and current real-time and patient-centered version of the patient's paper clinical and administrative record [9]
Health informatics	The science of information and an interprofessional field that studies and uses scientific inquiry, information, biomedical data, problem solving, and decision-making to improve human health and the delivery of health care services [8]
Information	Data with meaning [8]
Information system	A discrete set of information resources organized for the collection, processing, use, sharing, dissemination, maintenance, or disposition of information [21]
Interoperability	The ability of different information systems, applications (systems), and devices used to access, exchange, integrate, and cooperatively utilize data in a coordinated manner to optimize the health of individuals and populations globally [22]
Learning and knowledge health systems (LKHS)	When a health system with internal data and experience systematically integrates with external evidence and then that new knowledge is put into practice [23]
Protected health information (PHI)	Any type of health information that can identify an individual and is in the possession of or can be transmitted by a covered entity or its business associates [6]
Public health	Focuses on the population's health as a whole and is the science and art of preventing disease, prolonging life, and promoting health through organized efforts and informed choices of society, organizations, public and private communities, and individuals [1, 24]
Public health informatics	The application of health informatics to areas of prevention, preparedness, surveillance, health education, and health promotion [17]
Public health information system (PHIS)	Allows health departments to collect and maintain data to inform public health practice and they serve as foundational components for the infrastructure of public health [25]

The use of geographic information system (GIS) technologies in health care, and more specifically in public health, also increased. For example, GIS technologies are used by public health practitioners to model and map disease locations, surveillance, and movement including near real-time visualizations or hot spots of disease progression(s) [15, 16]. Other uses of GIS mapping include identification of access issues to essentials, such as food and health care, especially in zip codes that are known to have social determinant contributors to poor health outcomes [15, 16]. (See Chap. 15 on Population Health) (Table 16.1).

16.2 Definitions and Strategies

Public health focuses on the population's health as a whole and is the science and art of preventing disease, prolonging life, and promoting health through organized efforts and informed choices of society, organizations, public and private communities, and individuals [1, 24]. *Data* are collected sequence(s) of facts, signs, and symbols [18, 19]. *Information* is data with meaning [8]. An *information system* is a discrete set of information resources organized for the collection, processing, use, sharing, dissemination, maintenance, or disposition of information [21]. A *public health information system (PHIS)* facilitates the collation and maintenance of data contributing to the health of the public [25]. For example, emergency departments may have information systems that are specifically for disease surveillance detection (BioSense) by public health agencies [26, 27]. As of November 2022, there are seven main PHIS technologies with different capabilities that are available in the United States including Clinisys WorldCare, EpiTrax, Maven, NEDSS Base System (NBS), PRISM-

PHIS Technology Examples for Disease Surveillance					
Clinisys WorldCare	EpiTrax	Maven	National Electronic Disease Surveillance System (NEDSS) Systems	Prevention Impacts Simulation Model (PRISM) Systems	Sexually Transmitted Disease (STD*MIS) Management Information Systems

Fig. 16.1 Public Health Information Systems (PHIS) examples

Based, PRISM HDS, and the STD*MIS that can be adopted by states, territories, and project areas [26, 28, 29]. State health departments use the data from these systems to design health promotion programs to support the needs of the general public and oftentimes specific populations [25, 30]. The National Notifiable Diseases Surveillance System (NNDSS) is larger in scope and is used to store case surveillance data across the United States with approximately 3,000 health departments actively using its data to help keep populations in their local communities healthy [31] (Fig. 16.1).

The use of data from PHISs and the interoperability of these data with other disparate information systems requires the knowledge and skills of a health informaticist. The health informaticist assures data adequacy, accuracy, and relevancy for health decision-making, safety, and quality [32]. This decision-making is often augmented with data visualization efforts as an output of single or multiple data sources. Additionally, data and information stored in PHISs are useful to fields such as informatics. For context, *health informatics* is the science of information and an interprofessional field that studies and uses scientific inquiry, information, biomedical data, problem solving, and decision-making to improve human health [8]. *Clinical informatics* involves the application of computer structures and algorithms and information technology to improve clinical communication(s) and the delivery of health care services [17]. *Public health informatics* is the application of informatics to areas of public health including prevention, preparedness, surveillance, and health promotion [17].

16.3 Opportunities

16.3.1 Public Health Data Exchange

Data collection for public health purposes is not a new endeavor. Health care providers have been submitting patient data to public health agencies and the Centers for Disease Control and Prevention (CDC) for decades. However, these efforts, while mandated, were frequently misaligned, inconsistent, delayed, and lacked sustainability [33]. Such data collection efforts foster reactive rather than proactive visualization and decision-making. While some states are better than others at public health data exchange, at the convergence of deep-rooted practices and established technology is an opportunity for widespread data collection that holds the potential for public health analysts to "see" public health issues unfolding in near real-time, thereby enabling novel and strategic approaches to data analysis for disease prevention, detection, and management to advance public health practice and improvement outcomes [34]. While much of this was realized during the COVID-19 epidemic, the opportunity to broaden and deepen these efforts has yet to be realized [35].

16.3.2 Data Harmonization

Opportunities exist for better data harmonization across the field of public health. *Data harmonization* is the process of including data structures and modeling for recording semantics to facilitate data aggregation and reuse across disparate systems [20]. Doing so would broaden and deepen the primary or secondary use of health data that are collected at the point of care and then later used for public health purposes. The efficient use of such systems require shared, coordinated work among professionals from across the health care ecosystem. Public health practitioners must leverage data from disparate information systems to inform health promotion initiatives.

Interoperability is the ability of different information systems, applications (systems), and devices to: (a) access, (b) exchange, (c) integrate, and (d) cooperatively use data in a coordinated manner to optimize the health of individuals and populations globally [22]. More comprehensive interoperability among systems holds the opportunity to increase the ability for health information exchanges to disseminate aggregated information relative to disease prevention and surveillance efforts crucial to public health [10]. Interoperability advancements can propagate more efficient learning and knowledge health systems (LKHS) with shared goals among health care stakeholders for equitable health access, health practice changes, and continuous improvement [36, 37]. *Learning health systems (LHS)* exist when a health system with internal data and experience systematically integrates with external evidence and then the combined new knowledge is put into practice [23]. However, LHSs are not exclusive in the health system environment. While relatively new in the public health space, there is great opportunity for more widespread definitions of LHSs in public health. For example, quasi-LHSs were observed during the COVID-19 epidemic where data from multiple external sources from the field, rather than internal sources, were integrated internally and created new knowledge that changed practice [38].

Specific investigational needs drive data collection efforts such as for reporting, communications, or research purposes [13]. These needs influence the types of data that are collected and the methods through which data are obtained [13]. Public health analysts and epidemiological informaticists must do their due diligence to identify and follow up on the etiology of data that are missing or not accurate, adequate, of quality, or timely [39]. Some explanations may involve the lack of (a) data standards with shared specifications of meanings, (b) uniformity among how information is encoded in systems, as well as (c) semantic interoperability [13]. Semantic interoperability (SI) allows data to be interpretable by all parties involved during data sharing [40]. For example, SI is achieved when the meaning intended by the communicator is fully understood by the data receiver [13]. To glean meaning from the data stored in various systems, a scientific approach is needed during data collection, storage, management, and analysis. Such activities require the involvement of public health informaticist teams and data science subject matter experts as well as appropriate stakeholders, techniques, concepts, methods, and tools. The presence of accurate data is paramount in addition to the development, testing, and application of mental models of causality (i.e., theories) during contextual analyses [41]. Lastly, ethical data mining of public health data is a critical component to data use. Data mining is a process used to find features of interest, patterns, trends, anomalies, and correlations among data and it is increasingly being performed through artificial intelligence techniques [42–44].

16.3.3 Challenges

While it is the case that information systems can experience technical issues, have poor usage, or have data adequacy, accuracy, and currency lags, when those systems are used to retrieve health-related data for making health-related decisions, their monitoring must be more intense [13, 14, 45]. As providers across different specialties within the health care sector began using their own versions of health information systems (i.e., homegrown versions or condition specific), the heterogeneous nature and lack of interoperability among these systems needed to be addressed. The disparate nature of these systems require strong public health, population health, and clinical health care interprofessional collaborations and the interoperability of diverse health information systems to support the federal government's efforts toward streamlined health information technology per Executive Order 13335 [8]. These strong interprofessional collaborations can also lead to more cohesive actionable insights instead of stakeholders relying heavily on health informaticists as translators in the health care ecosystem [46]. Additionally, the act of storing and using large volumes of data (even if the data are accurate) does not guarantee meaningful answers to scientific or public health-related questions [41]. For example, the means through which the data are analyzed in conjunction with the accuracy of the underlying data determines whether data stored within information systems become meaningful [18]. Additional challenges exist in transporting public health data to the health information exchange. It is important to note that while health information exchanges bring value to public and population health efforts (e.g., improved and efficient aggregate data collection), accurate reporting by health care providers and their teams brings value to the health information exchange. Accurate reporting of interoperable data by interprofessional teams would contribute to health care providers and stakeholders accessing more expeditious information regarding public health testing and issues, more comprehensive public health reports, and improved quality data streams.

16.4 Case Study

Background*:

Bright Care is a health care facility in an urban area with a dense population. Within a week, five patients seeking care at the facility were diagnosed with pertussis (whooping cough) according to laboratory test results. As an infectious disease reportable to the Centers for Disease Control and Prevention (CDC), the staff at Bright Care have been treating the patients, actively reporting the pertussis cases to the CDC, and maintaining detailed patient records in the facility's electronic health record (EHR). Robert Smith is a lead health informaticist contracted by the CDC to review data from the testing institution's laboratory information system (LIS), Bright Care's EHR, and the BioSense platform to help monitor the incidence of emerging pertussis infections in the area alongside Barbara Campbell, an epidemiologist. To have more expeditious information, interprofessional stakeholders at bordering states' public health departments are collaborated with alongside nearby clinical health care institutions, data analysts, health journalists, population health professionals, contact tracing experts, as well as public health practitioners and public health communications specialists. The public health information systems (PHISs) that the bordering states' health departments utilize are not yet fully interoperable. Since the pertussis diagnoses at Bright Care are confirmed cases, the interprofessional stakeholders work together to stay informed with geographic information system (GIS) data and the latest data from the larger national notifiable diseases surveillance system (NNDSS) typically used for case surveillance. The public health practitioners on the team form a health coalition aimed to proactively prevent the spread of pertussis in nearby urban areas and other areas at risk for exposure. Press releases are issued to the public with health safety recommendations and guidelines. Overall, the stakeholders continue collaborating with each other and with health informatician subject matter experts to develop a robust learning and knowledge health system (LKHS) for data harmonization, interoperable information exchanges, enhanced disease surveillance, and risk evaluations for actionable insights against the spread of pertussis and other infectious agents. *This case study includes example scenarios for educational purposes and is not indicative of real-life occurrences.

Question:

Why are collaborations integral to the use of public health information systems?

16.5 Professional Organizations

16.5.1 American Medical Informatics Association® (AMIA®)

The mission of AMIA® is to lead the way in transforming health care through trusted science, education, and the practice of informatics. AMIA® connects a broad community of professionals and students interested in clinical and health informatics and is the bridge for knowledge and collaboration across a continuum, from basic and applied research to the consumer and public health arenas [47].

16.5.2 American Public Health Association (APHA)

The mission of APHA is to improve the health of the public and achieve equity in health status [48].

16.5.3 Healthcare Information and Management Systems Society (HIMSS)

The mission of HIMSS is to reform the global health ecosystem through the power of information and technology [49].

Knowledge Check Questions

1. What incentivized the widespread adoption of health information technology systems?
2. Name one example of a public health information system technology.
3. Name one opportunity for utilizing public health information systems.
4. Name one challenge to efficiently utilizing public health information systems.
5. Describe why interprofessional collaborations are needed to support the efficient use of public health information systems.

Answers

1. In 2004 Executive Order 13335 initiated incentives for the use of health information technology systems in healthcare.
2. BioSense is one example of a public health information system technology. BioSense is specifically used for disease surveillance detection.
3. Public health information systems allow public health analysts to surveil diseases that have the potential to become public health issues.
4. A lack of interoperability among public health information systems is a challenge against the streamlined use of these systems.
5. Interprofessional collaborations support the efficient use of public health information systems because these interactions can contribute to more cohesive actionable insights for health promotion.

References

1. Baba Z, Belinske S, Post D. Public health, population health, and planning:: ideas to improve communities. Dela J Public Health. 2018;4:14–8. https://doi.org/10.32481/djph.2018.03.004.
2. Johnson JA. Historical developments in public health and the 21st century. In: Novick & Morrow's Public Health Administration: Principles for Population-Based Management. Jones and Bartlett Learning; 2014. p. 11–31.
3. Tulchinsky TH. John snow, cholera, the broad street pump; waterborne diseases then and now. In: Case studies in public health. Elsevier; 2018. p. 77–99. https://doi.org/10.1016/B978-0-12-804571-8.00017-2.
4. Tulchinsky TH, Varavikova EA. A history of public health. In: The new public health. Elsevier; 2014. p. 1–42. https://doi.org/10.1016/B978-0-12-415766-8.00001-X.
5. Kruse CS, Smith B, Vanderlinden H, Nealand A. Security techniques for the electronic health records. J Med Syst. 2017;41:127. https://doi.org/10.1007/s10916-017-0778-4.
6. Isola S, Al Khalili Y. Protected health information. In: StatPearls. StatPearls Publishing; 2023.
7. Murphy SP. Healthcare information security and privacy. 1st ed. McGraw-Hill Education; 2015.
8. Jen MY, Mechanic OJ, Teoli D. Informatics. In: StatPearls. StatPearls Publishing; 2024.

9. HealthIT.gov. Frequently asked questions: what is an electronic health record (EHR)? 2019. https://www.healthit.gov/faq/what-electronic-health-record-ehr
10. Kruse CS, Stein A, Thomas H, Kaur H. The use of electronic health records to support population health: a systematic review of the literature. J Med Syst. 2018;42:214. https://doi.org/10.1007/s10916-018-1075-6.
11. Gensheimer SG, Wu AW, Snyder CF, PRO-EHR Users' Guide Steering Group, and PRO-EHR Users' Guide Working Group. Oh, the places we'll go: patient-reported outcomes and electronic health records. Patient. 2018;11:591–8. https://doi.org/10.1007/s40271-018-0321-9.
12. Wolicki SB, Nuzzo JB, Blazes DL, Pitts DL, Iskander JK, Tappero JW. Public health surveillance: at the core of the global health security agenda. Health Secur. 2016;14:185–8. https://doi.org/10.1089/hs.2016.0002.
13. Schulz S, Stegwee R, Chronaki C. Setandards in healthcare data. In: Kubben P, Dumontier M, Dekker A, editors. Fundamentals of clinical data science. Springer; 2019. https://doi.org/10.1007/978-3-319-99713-1_3.
14. Tummers J, Tekinerdogan B, Tobi H, Catal C, Schalk B. Obstacles and features of health information systems: a systematic literature review. Comput Biol Med. 2021;137:104785. https://doi.org/10.1016/j.compbiomed.2021.104785.
15. Tseng TS, Celestin MD, Yu Q, Li M, Luo T, Moody-Thomas S. Use of geographic information system technology to evaluate health disparities in smoking cessation class accessibility for patients in Louisiana Public Hospitals. Front Public Health. 2021;9:712635. https://doi.org/10.3389/fpubh.2021.712635.
16. Lyseen AK, Nøhr C, Sørensen EM, Gudes O, Geraghty EM, Shaw NT, Bivona-Tellez C, IMIA Health GIS Working Group. A review and framework for categorizing current research and development in health related geographical information systems (GIS) studies. Yearb Med Inform. 2014;9:110–24. https://doi.org/10.15265/IY-2014-0008.
17. American Medical Informatics Association ® (AMIA ®) Informatics: Research and Practice. https://amia.org/about-amia/why-informatics/informatics-research-and-practice
18. Van Meter HJ. Revising the DIKW pyramid and the real relationship between data, information, knowledge and wisdom. Law Tech Hum. 2020;2:69–80. https://doi.org/10.5204/lthj.1470.
19. Zins C. Conceptual approaches for defining data, information, and knowledge. J Am Soc Inf Sci. 2007;58:479–93. https://doi.org/10.1002/asi.20508.
20. Kush RD, Warzel D, Kush MA, Sherman A, Navarro EA, Fitzmartin R, Pétavy F, Galvez J, Becnel LB, Zhou FL, et al. FAIR data sharing: the roles of common data elements and harmonization. J Biomed Inform. 2020;107:103421. https://doi.org/10.1016/j.jbi.2020.103421.
21. National Institute of Standards and Technology (NIST) Information System. https://csrc.nist.gov/glossary/term/information_system
22. Healthcare Information and Management Systems Society (HIMSS) Interoperability in Healthcare. https://www.himss.org/resources/interoperability-healthcare
23. Agency for Healthcare Research and Quality (AHRQ). About Learning Health Systems. 2019. https://www.ahrq.gov/learning-health-systems/about.html
24. Winslow CE. The untilled fields of public health. Science. 1920;51:23–33. https://doi.org/10.1126/science.51.1306.23.
25. Roberts M. Successful public health information system database integration projects: a qualitative study. Online J Public Health Inform. 2018;10:e207. https://doi.org/10.5210/ojphi.v10i2.9221.
26. Centers for Disease Control and Prevention (CDC). Public Health Information Systems (PHIS). 2022. https://www.cdc.gov/std/informatics/public-health-information-systems.htm
27. Centers for Disease Control and Prevention (CDC) Biosense. https://www.cdc.gov/biosense/
28. Yarnoff B, Honeycutt A, Bradley C, Khavjou O, Bates L, Bass S, Kaufmann R, Barker L, Briss P. Validation of the prevention impacts simulation model (PRISM). Prev Chronic Dis. 2021;18:E09. https://doi.org/10.5888/pcd18.200225.
29. Shiver SA, Schmitt K, Cooksey A. Use of a business approach to improve disease surveillance data management systems and information technology process in Florida's Bureau of STD Prevention and Control. Public Health Rep. 2009;124(*Suppl 2*):98–102. https://doi.org/10.1177/00333549091240S214.
30. Yasnoff WA, O'Carroll PW, Koo D, Linkins RW, Kilbourne EM. Public health informatics: improving and transforming public health in the information age. J Public Health Manag Pract. 2000;6:67–75. https://doi.org/10.1097/00124784-200006060-00010.
31. Centers for Disease Control and Prevention (CDC) National Notifiable Diseases Surveillance System. https://www.cdc.gov/nndss/docs/NNDSS-Overview-Fact-Sheet-508.pdf
32. Veinot TC, Ancker JS, Bakken S. Health informatics and health equity: improving our reach and impact. J Am Med Inform Assoc. 2019;26:689–95. https://doi.org/10.1093/jamia/ocz132.
33. Doyle TJ, Glynn MK, Groseclose SL. Completeness of notifiable infectious disease reporting in the United States: an analytical literature review. Am J Epidemiol. 2002;155:866–74. https://doi.org/10.1093/aje/155.9.866.
34. Staes CJ, Xu W, LeFevre SD, Price RC, Narus SP, Gundlapalli A, Rolfs R, Nangle B, Samore M, Facelli JC. A case for using grid architecture for state public health informatics: the Utah perspective. BMC Med Inform Decis Mak. 2009;9:32. https://doi.org/10.1186/1472-6947-9-32.
35. Jiang JX, Cram P, Qi K, Bai G. Challenges and dynamics of public health reporting and data exchange dur-

ing COVID-19: insights from US hospitals. Health Aff Sch. 2024;2:qxad080. https://doi.org/10.1093/haschl/qxad080.
36. National Academy of Medicine. In: Whicher D, Ahmed M, Siddiqi S, Adams I, Zirkle M, Grossmann C, Carman KL, editors. Health data sharing to support better outcomes: building a foundation of stakeholder trust. National Academies Press; 2020. https://doi.org/10.17226/27110.
37. Platt JE, Raj M, Wienroth M. An analysis of the learning health system in its first decade in practice: scoping review. J Med Internet Res. 2020;22:e17026. https://doi.org/10.2196/17026.
38. Gustavson AM, Purnell A, Adly M, Awan O, Bräu N, Braus NA, Bryant MS, Chang L, Cyborski C, Darvish B, et al. A learning health system approach to long COVID care. Fed Pract. 2022;39:310–4. https://doi.org/10.12788/fp.0288.
39. Marino M, Lucas J, Latour E, Heintzman JD. Missing data in primary care research: importance, implications and approaches. Fam Pract. 2021;38:200–3. https://doi.org/10.1093/fampra/cmaa134.
40. de Mello BH, Rigo SJ, da Costa CA, da Rosa Righi R, Donida B, Bez MR, Schunke LC. Semantic interoperability in health records standards: a systematic literature review. Health Technol (Berl). 2022;12:255–72. https://doi.org/10.1007/s12553-022-00639-w.
41. Greenhalgh T. Miasmas, mental models and preventive public health: some philosophical reflections on science in the COVID-19 pandemic. Interface Focus. 2021;11:20210017. https://doi.org/10.1098/rsfs.2021.0017.
42. Benke K, Benke G. Artificial intelligence and big data in public health. Int J Environ Res Public Health. 2018;15 https://doi.org/10.3390/ijerph15122796.
43. Witten IH, Frank E, Hall MA, Pal CJ. Data mining: practical machine learning tools and techniques, Morgan Kaufmann series in data management systems. 4th ed. Morgan Kaufmann; 2016.
44. Han J, Kamber M, Pei J. Data mining: concepts and techniques. 3rd ed. Morgan Kaufmann; 2011.
45. Hersh WR, Weiner MG, Embi PJ, Logan JR, Payne PRO, Bernstam EV, Lehmann HP, Hripcsak G, Hartzog TH, Cimino JJ, et al. Caveats for the use of operational electronic health record data in comparative effectiveness research. Med Care. 2013;51:S30–7. https://doi.org/10.1097/MLR.0b013e31829b1dbd.
46. Meehan R. Health informatics workforce in the digital health ecosystem. Stud Health Technol Inform. 2024;310:1226–30. https://doi.org/10.3233/SHTI231160.
47. American Medical Informatics Association ® (AMIA ®) About AMIA. https://amia.org/about-amia
48. American Public Health Association (APHA) About APHA. https://apha.org/About-APHA
49. Healthcare Information and Management Systems Society (HIMSS) Who we are. https://www.himss.org/who-we-are

Genomics: Foundations, Applications, and Big Data in Health Informatics

17

Eugenia G. Giannopoulou, Chao Zhang, and Simon L. Lu

Foundational Domains

This chapter addresses the following AMIA Foundational Domains: F1—Health, F4—Health Information Science and Technology.

Learning Objectives

Upon completion of the chapter, students will be able to:

1. Explain basic concepts in genomics.
2. List some examples of widely used bioinformatics tools used in genomics.
3. Identify online genomics resources, such as databases and genomics browsers.
4. Summarize current challenges and opportunities in genomics.

E. G. Giannopoulou (✉)
Department of Biological Sciences, New York City College of Technology, City University of New York, New York, NY, USA
e-mail: Evgenia.Giannopoulou39@citytech.cuny.edu

C. Zhang · S. L. Lu
Department of Medicine, Boston University, Chobanian & Avedisian School of Medicine, Boston, MA, USA
e-mail: chz2009@bu.edu; slianglu@bu.edu

17.1 Introduction

Genomics, derived from "genome"—the complete genetic information in an organism's DNA—explores the structure, function, evolution, and interactions of genes and DNA elements. Beyond individual genes, it examines the holistic interplay of coding and non-coding regions and regulatory components. Its applications span medicine, healthcare, agriculture, and forensics.

The history of genomics spans decades, marked by key breakthroughs and technological advances (Fig. 17.1). The discovery of *DNA's double helix* in the 1950s was pivotal, laying the foundation for understanding genetic information. The *Human Genome Project* in the 1990s aimed to sequence the entire human genome, culminating in the early 2000s and providing a reference for future research. The emergence of *next-generation sequencing (NGS)* in 2005 revolutionized genomics by enabling faster, cheaper, and more efficient DNA sequencing. This led to large-scale high-throughput genomics projects, like the Encyclopedia of DNA Elements (ENCODE) [1, 2], the Cancer Genome Atlas (TCGA) [3], the 1000 Genomes project [4], genome-wide association studies (GWAS), and more, generating vast datasets to unravel biological complexities. The advances in DNA sequencing gave rise to the field of *personalized medicine*, an approach that provides tailored medical treatment according to the

C. Eldredge et al. (eds.), *Introductory Textbook in Health Informatics*, Health Informatics,
https://doi.org/10.1007/978-3-032-16657-9_17

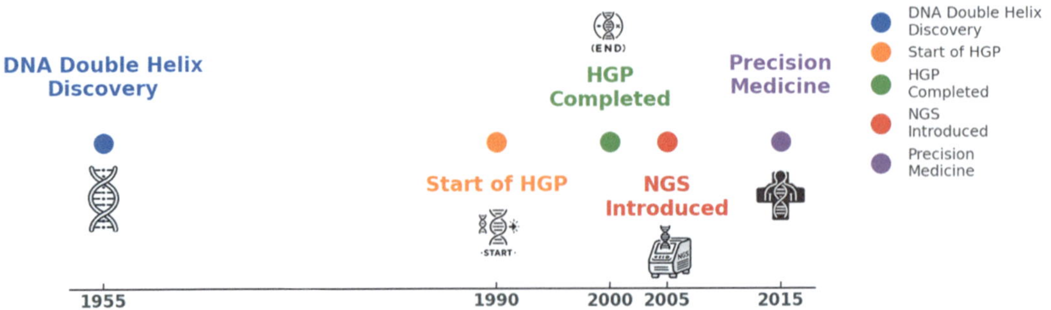

Fig. 17.1 Key milestones in genomics, including DNA double helix discovery, the Human Genome Project's start and completion, Next-Generation Sequencing, and Precision Medicine

genetic makeup of an individual. Personalized medicine (see Chap. 18), marked by the federally supported Precision Medicine Initiative in 2015, holds promise for improving patient outcomes, optimizing healthcare delivery, and advancing our understanding of diseases.

Advances in *genome editing technologies* have revolutionized genomics, enabling precise DNA modification across organisms and enhancing diagnostics, treatments, and patient outcomes. Genomics now plays a vital role in understanding genetic diversity, identifying disease-related genes, advancing personalized medicine, and improving healthcare. This chapter reviews genomics' history, technologies, applications, methods, and tools, while addressing future challenges and opportunities.

17.2 Basic Terminology in Genomics

DNA (deoxyribonucleic acid) consists of two intertwined strands forming the iconic double helix, with nucleotide bases (A, T, C, G) encoding an organism's genetic information. During *transcription*, DNA serves as a template to produce RNA (ribonucleic acid), which replaces thymine (T) with uracil (U). *RNA* then directs the assembly of amino acids into proteins during *translation*. This sequential pipeline of processes through which genetic information stored in DNA is converted into protein defines the *central dogma of molecular biology*, explaining how genetic instructions are stored, read, and utilized to build organisms. The unique sequence of nucleotides in DNA and RNA determines the diversity among organisms. *Genes* are DNA segments that contain the instructions for building specific proteins or functional RNA molecules. They are the basic units of heredity and play a fundamental role in determining the traits of an organism. *Transcripts* are RNA molecules that are synthesized from DNA during the process of transcription. There are several types of transcripts, including messenger RNA (mRNA), which carries the genetic information from DNA to the ribosome for protein synthesis, and non-coding RNAs (ncRNAs), which play regulatory roles in gene expression. *Proteins* are synthesized in the cytoplasm when the mRNA molecule is decoded to assemble a specific sequence of amino acids, forming a protein polypeptide chain. Proteins are large, complex molecules made up of amino acids that perform a wide variety of functions within cells, including catalyzing biochemical reactions, providing structural support, and serving as signaling molecules.

Single nucleotide polymorphisms, called *SNPs* (pronounced "snips"), are variations in a single nucleotide base at a specific position in the genome that occur within a population. They represent the most common type of genetic variation in humans and can influence traits, phenotypic characteristics, disease susceptibility, and drug response. Haplotypes are combinations of SNPs that are inherited together on the same chromosome. They are useful for studying the inheritance of genetic traits and understanding population genetics. Haplotypes can provide insights into genetic diversity, ancestry, and disease risk. The International HapMap Project [5] has investigated human haplotypes extensively.

These nucleotide sequences store biological information, regulate genes, and drive protein synthesis. In order to research the biological properties of life, these sequences needed to be measured and understood, leading to the research and development of sequencing technologies. *DNA sequencing* is the process of determining the precise order of nucleotide bases (A, T, C, G) in a DNA molecule. This technique allows scientists to read the genetic instructions encoded in an organism's genome. Sequencing provides insights into genetic variation, mutations, and the functional elements within DNA. By decoding these sequences, researchers can study genetic diversity, identify disease-causing mutations, and explore the molecular mechanisms that underpin life.

17.3 Evolution of Sequencing Technology

The evolution of sequencing technologies spans three generations, beginning with Fredrick Sanger's [6] breakthrough in 1977. *Sanger sequencing* involves dividing DNA into four reactions, incorporating radiolabeled ddNTPs that terminate synthesis, and analyzing DNA fragments via gel electrophoresis. While revolutionary, it was time-consuming and manual due to each sample needing to be processed individually. The introduction of automated sequencers in 1987 enabled simultaneous sequencing of hundreds of samples, paving the way for large-scale projects like the *Human Genome Project*, where the entire human genome was sequenced.

The next generation of sequencing emerged with *pyrosequencing* by Pål Nyrén in 1998, a method that detects light during DNA synthesis, allowing real-time monitoring. Unlike Sanger sequencing, it uses normal nucleotides and is faster and automated. Illumina sequencing, a key advancement, breaks DNA into fragments, amplifies them, and sequences by synthesis, generating millions of reads. Its automation by 454 Life Sciences facilitated large-scale DNA sequencing [7], heralding the advent of parallel sequencing techniques. This technology revolutionized genomics, making sequencing faster, cheaper, and widely accessible.

The third generation of sequencing focuses on *single-molecule sequencing (SMS)*, eliminating the need for DNA amplification. This was necessary because during DNA amplification, certain sequences are amplified over others, introducing potential mutations during the copying process. By removing the need for DNA amplification, these new techniques could better reduce bias and error, increase accuracy of capturing genetic information, and allow for a more streamlined and simplified workflow. Early SMS methods, like Stephen Quake's approach, attached DNA to a solid surface and used fluorescent nucleotides to capture sequences [8]. This first iteration of SMS techniques was considerably slow and costly but set the stage for the development of future SMS technologies. A breakthrough came with Pacific Biosciences' SMRT platform, where DNA polymerization occurs in tiny wells called zero-mode waveguides (ZMWs), allowing real-time, high-speed sequencing. Nanopore sequencing, led by Oxford Nanopore Technologies (ONT), represents another leap. DNA passes through nanopores [9], and changes in electrical conductivity reveal sequences. Devices like the portable MinION enable rapid, low-cost sequencing outside the lab. Despite some quality limitations, nanopore sequencing promises a faster, cheaper, and more accessible way to sequence DNA.

Sequencing technology has advanced dramatically, transforming biological research. Early methods took years to sequence a few hundred nucleotides, but today millions can be sequenced quickly. These innovations have accelerated discoveries and enabled breakthroughs across fields, with even greater potential as sequencing continues to evolve.

17.3.1 The Human Genome Project

The idea of the Human Genome Project (HGP) [10–12] started to attract attention in the mid-1980s when scientists realized the vast possibilities of human genome sequencing in deciphering the secrets of human biology and disease. The HGP launched in 1990 as a collaborative international [13] effort aimed at determining the complete sequence of the approximately three billion DNA base pairs in the human genome, discovering the entire set of human genes and making them accessible for further research studies. Sanger sequencing was the sequencing method of choice for the HGP. The first draft, completed in June 2000, was a preliminary version of the complete sequence and covered approximately 90% of the human genome with high accuracy. Although not complete or fully accurate, the draft sequence was a significant milestone providing researchers with a valuable resource to begin exploring the human DNA. Importantly, the sequence of the human genome generated by HGP was not from a single person, but from multiple volunteers recruited by the project researchers. The HGP was completed in 2003, reporting several findings that transformed our understanding of genetics and its implications in biology and medicine. Two of these findings are (1) the fact that humans are 99.9% genetically identical, and (2) that there are only 20,000–25,000 human genes (while less complex organisms have a higher number of genes, and popular earlier predictions stated that humans had up to 100,000 genes). Concurrently with the HGP [14], a private company called Celera Genomics [15] also pursued sequencing of the human genome. HGP and Celera followed different strategies both in how they sequenced the DNA, but also in data sharing. HGP's openness in making their results publicly accessible has facilitated numerous discoveries in genetics and medicine, while also having raised awareness of the ethical, legal, and social implications of genomic research and use of genetic information. Overall, the HGP has had a profound impact on medicine, science, and our society, shaping the way we interact with our genetic blueprint [11, 16].

17.3.2 Other Genomes Sequenced

The success of the Human Genome Project (HGP) spurred interest in sequencing other organisms. The mouse genome, sequenced in 2002 [17] by the Mouse Genome Sequencing Consortium, was pivotal due to its genetic similarity to humans, advancing human biology research. Another genome that was sequenced in 2009 [18] is the giant panda, an iconic and endangered species native to China. While not as important to the research and understanding of humans, the sequencing of the giant panda has allowed for insights to panda evolution, adaptation, and conservation. Sequencing of plants (e.g., maize, tomato, coffee sequenced in 2009, 2012, 2014, respectively) has also provided valuable insights into their genetic makeup and evolutionary history, as well as opportunities for agricultural research, and crop improvement through breeding and genetic engineering. From humans to plants, the sequencing of other genomes has provided significant insights to our understanding of the genetic code within each and every organism.

17.4 Sequence Alignment

Bioinformatics, a subfield of health informatics, combines biology, computer science, and statistics to analyze and interpret biological data. Sequence alignment, a key step in bioinformatics, arranges DNA, RNA, or protein sequences to identify regions of similarity, helping infer functional, structural, or evolutionary relationships. Over the past three decades, numerous sequence alignment methods have been developed to address various challenges. Here, we briefly introduce three major methods widely used today, showcasing the evolution of sequence alignment algorithms.

17.4.1 BLAST

In 1990, before the *Human Genome Project (HGP)* launched, scientists recognized the need for efficient tools to compare genomic sequences. This led to the development of the Basic Local Alignment Search Tool (BLAST) at the *National Center for Biotechnology Information (NCBI)*. BLAST [19] enables rapid comparison of biological sequences against databases, identifying sequences with significant similarity to a query. Prior to BLAST, the Smith–Waterman [20] algorithm was the primary method for local sequence alignment. While highly accurate, it was computationally intensive and slow, as it exhaustively searched all possible alignments. In contrast, BLAST uses a heuristic approach to quickly identify local alignments. It begins by generating short "k-letter" words (e.g., for "GTREF," the words are "GTR," "TRE," and "REF") called seeds, identifying common words between the query and database sequences. BLAST then extends these alignments bidirectionally, adjusting scores based on alignment quality. Extensions stop when scores fall below a threshold, retaining only high-scoring alignments. Results are ranked using an Expect value (E-value), which measures the significance of the High-Scoring Segment Pair (HSP) score, factoring in query length and database size. BLAST is faster than Smith–Waterman, though with approximated accuracy, and offers specialized versions tailored for DNA or protein database searches.

17.4.2 STAR: RNA-seq Aligner

In the new millennium, *RNA sequencing (RNA-seq)* advanced significantly, replacing microarrays for studying the transcriptome. This advancement required the development of RNA-seq aligners. This was because during transcription, RNA splicing occurs, removing non-coding sequences (introns) and leaving only the coding sequences (exons) that ultimately join together, forming exon-exon junctions that will encode for a specific protein. Traditional aligners like BLAST struggled with aligning RNA-seq reads that connect the different parts of a gene (exon-exon junctions) making them less effective for analyzing RNA data. *STAR* [21] *(Spliced Transcripts Alignment to a Reference)* was developed to address this, providing fast and accurate mapping of RNA-seq reads to a reference genome. STAR works in two steps: first, it indexes the reference genome for rapid mapping, and then it aligns reads while accounting for splice junctions and gene structures. Its efficiency comes from parallelization and multi-threading, allowing it to process large datasets quickly. STAR also generates outputs like read counts per gene, enabling downstream analyses such as gene expression studies, differential expression, and the discovery of novel transcripts or fusion genes.

17.4.3 Kraken

In the 2010s, the advent of advanced sequencing technologies heralded a new era in microbiome research, providing researchers with unprecedented insights into the complex microbial communities inhabiting various environments. Large-scale initiatives such as the *Human Microbiome Project* [22] generated massive datasets, requiring tools to identify sequences and assign them to different taxonomic levels, often amidst a backdrop of taxonomic uncertainty inherent in microbiome studies. While the BLAST has been adapted to address this challenge, its efficiency may wane when confronted with the sheer magnitude of modern metagenomic datasets. Kraken [23] is a specialized tool designed for metagenomic analysis, offering fast and accurate taxonomic classification of DNA sequences. Using a curated database of k-mers from diverse genomes, it achieves sensitivity and specificity comparable to BLAST but with much greater speed and scalability. Kraken processes millions of sequences per minute, making it efficient for both desktop and high-performance computing, even with limited resources. Thus, in the era of big data microbiology, Kraken emerges as an indispensable tool, offering unparalleled efficiency, accuracy, and scalability for metagenomic analysis and microbiome studies.

17.5 Repositories and Data Visualization Tools

17.5.1 Data Repositories

Genomics databases are repositories of genomic data, including DNA sequences, gene annotations, genetic variations, and other related information. Representative examples of well-known genomics databases include NCBI's GenBank [24], Ensembl [25], Protein Data Bank (PDB) [26], HapMap project [5], 1000 genomes project [27–29], ENCODE [1, 2], dbSNP [30], and TCGA [3]. These databases are valuable resources for researchers studying various aspects of genomics, including gene expression, protein function, and disease genetics. A reference genome is a complete representation of a species' genetic material, and serves as a standard against which other individual genomes can be compared and analyzed. Reference genomes exist for various species, including viruses, bacteria, fungi, plants, and animals. They are essential for various genomic studies, such as identifying genetic variants, annotating genes, understanding evolutionary relationships, and more. The majority of reference genomes are available online through browsers such as the UCSC Genome Browser [31].

Understanding these terms provides a foundation for comprehending genomics processes, including how genetic information is stored, expressed, and translated into functional proteins, and how genomics data are stored, analyzed, and visualized.

Repositories for genomic data play critical roles in biomedical research by providing access to high-quality genomic, transcriptomic, and structural data for various organisms and biological processes. NCBI hosts several databases, such as GenBank for DNA sequences, PubMed for biomedical literature, dbSNP for genetic variations, the Sequence Read Archive (SRA) [32] for raw sequencing data, and ClinVar [33, 34] for clinical interpretations of genetic variants. The Gene Expression Omnibus (GEO) [35], also hosted by NCBI, is a public repository for gene expression data, including microarray and RNA sequencing data. It enables researchers to freely access and analyze gene expression profiles from various organisms and experimental conditions. The European Bioinformatics Institute (EBI) also offers a wide range of databases and tools for biological data storage and analysis, such as Ensembl [25] for genome annotations and variation data, ArrayExpress for functional genomics data, and European Nucleotide Archive (ENA) [36] for nucleotide sequences.

17.5.2 Genome Browsers

Annotated genomes are genomes where specific regions, such as genes, regulatory elements, or other functional sequences, have been identified and labeled. These annotations offer detailed insights into the functions of different genomic regions, including protein-coding sequences and gene regulatory elements. They have enhanced our understanding of an organism's genetic blueprint and facilitated comparisons of potential genetic changes influenced by various factors. *Genome browsers* use these annotations to help researchers visualize the genome, making it easier to explore and understand the function and organization of DNA in a user-friendly, interactive way.

The UCSC Genome Browser [31] provides access to a great collection of genome assemblies and annotations for various organisms. Users can visualize genomic data, such as DNA sequences, gene annotations, genetic variations, conservation tracks, and epigenomic marks, in customizable tracks, as well as to upload their own experimental genomic data for further analysis and comparison. The Ensembl [25] Genome Browser is another browser that offers access to annotated genomes, gene predictions, genetic variations, and comparative genomics data for a wide range of species. It provides interactive tools for visualizing and analyzing genomic data, including gene expression, regulatory elements, and evolutionary conservation. The Integrative Genomics Viewer (IGV) [37] is a high-performance genomics viewer developed by the Broad Institute, that allows users to visualize and analyze genomic data, including aligned sequencing reads, gene annotations, copy number variations, and structural variants. IGV supports a wide range of data formats and provides tools for data exploration. Other browsers available for genomics visualization are JBrowse [38], WashU Epigenome Browser [39], and the NCBI Genome Data Viewer [40].

17.6 Applications of Genomics

17.6.1 Big Data Analytics, Machine Learning, and Genomics in Healthcare

Advances in sequencing technologies have made it feasible to generate vast amounts of genomic data quickly and cost-effectively, while computer science and big data analytics, such as machine learning, data mining, natural language processing, and statistical analysis, assist in processing, analyzing, and deriving insights from large and complex datasets. Integration of genomics with clinical data from electronic health records (EHRs) and other diverse data sources allows for a more comprehensive understanding of disease mechanisms, treatment responses, and patient outcomes. Along the same lines, predictive modeling can be used to identify individuals at risk for certain diseases based on their genomic profiles, and to inform personalized treatment strategies. Big data analytics can also accelerate the drug discovery process by analyzing large datasets to identify potential drug candidates and predict their efficacy and safety profiles. In the area of population/public health, analyzing large-scale genomic and clinical datasets can identify patterns and trends in disease prevalence, risk factors, and treatment responses, thus informing public health interventions and policies aimed at preventing and managing diseases more effectively. In summary, combining machine learning and big data analytics with genomics in healthcare holds immense potential for advancing medicine and healthcare. However, addressing technical, ethical, and regulatory challenges is essential to realizing the full benefits of this integration.

17.6.2 Genomic Medicine

Genomic medicine is the integration of an individual's genetic information into clinical practice for the purpose of predicting, diagnosing, treating, and preventing disease. The field has evolved rapidly with advances in genomics and has the potential to revolutionize healthcare by enabling more personalized and effective treatments tailored to each individual's genetic makeup. Precision or personalized medicine [41, 42] allows healthcare providers to customize treatment plans based on specific genetic characteristics of patients revealed by genetic testing: analyzing an individual's DNA to identify variations or mutations that may be associated with certain diseases or conditions. This can further help in diagnosing genetic disorders, predicting the risk of developing certain diseases, and guiding treatment decisions. Genomic medicine also encompasses gene therapy, which involves modifying a person's genes to treat or prevent disease. This approach is powerful for treating genetic disorders and certain types of cancer by correcting or replacing faulty genes. Pharmacogenomics is another vital component in genomic medicine that studies how an individual's genetic makeup influences their response to drugs. By understanding genetic variations that affect drug metabolism, efficacy, and toxicity, healthcare providers can prescribe medications that are most likely to be safe and effective for each patient. As genomic technologies continue to advance and become more accessible, their integration with medicine is expected to improve patient care and outcomes across a wide range of medical conditions. However, the widespread use of genomic information in medicine raises various ethical, legal, and social issues, including privacy concerns, informed consent, equitable access to genomic technologies, and the potential for genetic discrimination.

17.6.3 Transcriptomics, Epigenomics, and Metagenomics

Transcriptomics studies the transcriptome, which includes all RNA molecules like mRNA, tRNA, and rRNA. While only a small part of the genome codes for proteins, most research focuses on mRNA due to its link with diseases. Early methods like microarrays (introduced in 1995 [43]) quantified known mRNA levels using fluorescent probes but were limited to detecting predefined genes. RNA sequencing (RNA-seq) [44], introduced later, replaced microarrays by providing a more comprehensive view of the transcriptome, including novel transcripts and different gene isoforms. More recently, single-cell RNA sequencing has allowed researchers to measure gene expression in individual cells, revealing cell-specific changes during aging, disease progression, or treatment.

Epigenomics [45] is the study of the heritable post-translational modifications and regulatory mechanisms that control gene expression. Importantly, the prefix "epi" refers to changes that occur "on" or "above" the genome, meaning without altering the DNA sequence. These chemical modifications occur on a cell's DNA or histones (proteins associated with DNA packaging necessary for fitting the genetic material within the cell nucleus) and include DNA methylation, histone modifications, chromatin remodeling, and non-coding RNA-mediated regulation. Studying epigenomics helps uncover mechanisms of gene regulation, cellular differentiation, and disease, with potential for developing epigenetic therapies and diagnostic tools for various diseases [14, 46].

Metagenomics [47], also known as microbiomics, is another genomics subfield and studies the microbial communities associated with a particular host organism or environment. In metagenomics, researchers study and analyze the genetic material recovered directly from environmental samples (e.g., soil, water, air) or the human microbiome extracted from specific organs. It characterizes the genetic composition and functional potential of these communities, with applications ranging from basic to environmental monitoring [48] and biotechnology [49].

17.6.4 Structural and Comparative Genomics

Structural genomics focuses on understanding the 3D structures of proteins encoded by mRNA. Traditional methods like X-ray crystallography, NMR, and cryo-EM provide accurate measurements of protein structures [50] but are costly, time-consuming, and limited to partial proteins. Over the past three decades, scientists have employed various computational methods, including physical, statistical, and machine learning-based approaches, to model 3D protein structures [51]. In 2020, Google's AlphaFold2 revolutionized the field with highly accurate predictions [52], enabling the study of proteins unattainable by experiments and the design of novel proteins [53]. Structural genomics also studies RNA structure [54] and uses high-throughput genomic and epigenomic techniques to capture chromatin conformation or genomic structural variants [55].

Comparative genomics studies genomic similarities and differences across species, conditions, or diseases, often used in evolutionary research. A phylogenetic tree is a graphical representation of the evolutionary history of species, which has been employed since Charles Darwin's "On the Origin of Species." After 1990, scientists redefined the phylogenetic tree using molecular criteria to replace classic phenotypic criteria [56]. Computational tools, especially multiple sequence alignment, have been used to determine the evolutionary relationships between species. In microbiology or virology, comparative genomics has been used to understand microbial variants under different conditions or diseases. For example, comparing the COVID-19 virus genome with other coronaviruses helped identify its highly pathogenic regions and facilitate vaccine development by targeting specific regions of the virus [57, 58].

17.6.5 Genomic Variation Projects

Genomic variations are differences in DNA sequences among populations that influence genome function, evolution, and disease. Studying these variations often requires substantial resources, which are scarcely affordable by one or two labs. Therefore, many large-scale consortium studies have been conducted to address various important biomedical problems. *ENCODE* [1, 2] is a public research project that has systematically mapped transcription, chromatin structure, and histone modifications, assigning biochemical functions to 80% of the human genome. Later, ENCODE was extended to other model organisms. The *HapMap* Project [5] is an international effort that collected DNA samples from global populations to link genotypes with over a million variants, particularly SNPs. The project developed a freely available resource for exploring SNPs, facilitated the development of diagnostic tools, and enhanced our understanding of the relationship between SNPs and diseases. Although SNPs are associated with phenotypes and diseases, they only contribute to a small proportion of the human genome. To comprehensively understand common human genetic variation, the *1000 Genomes* Project [27–29] set out to reconstruct the genomes of 2504 individuals from 26 populations by applying whole-genome sequencing. This project established the most detailed catalogue of human genetic variation at the time. The *All of Us Research Program* is a large-scale, US-based initiative aimed at advancing precision medicine by collecting genetic, but also environmental, and health data from one million diverse participants. Its goal is to understand how differences in lifestyle, biology, and environment influence health and disease, enabling personalized approaches to prevention, treatment, and care.

17.7 Case Study

In this section, we will walk through a case study analyzing public databases using GEO2R [59], an interactive web tool from NCBI that performs sample comparison and differential expression analysis. The RNA-seq dataset we will use is human dermal fibroblasts derived from 133 healthy individuals ranging from 1 to 94 years old, and 10 patients with Hutchinson-Gilford Progeria Syndrome (HGPS), a premature aging disease [60]. The dataset's accession number is GSE113957 [61].

In the GEO2R website, we first enter the GSE113957 accession number into the GEO accession box and click "Set." After entering the accession number, all samples belonging to this dataset will be loaded. We then define the two groups to analyze, healthy and HGPS, since we want to compare gene expression between the control and diseased patients. We click "Define groups" and enter "healthy" and "HGPS." Next, we assign specific samples to each of the groups. For this case study, we perform a 4 versus 4 sample comparison; for each group, we select the samples and then click on the group that the samples belong to (e.g., samples GSM3124631, GSM3124632, GSM3124633, GSM3124634 belong to the healthy group, and samples GSM3124693, GSM3124694, GSM3124698, GSM3124701 to the HGPS group). The samples are then group color-coded (Fig. 17.2), and ready to be analyzed. We click "Analyze" to run the analysis.

The results of the GEO2R analysis are shown as visualizations and as a table, which displays the most significant and differentially expressed genes between the healthy and HGPS groups. The table is sorted by the highest significance (lowest p-value) of the genes. Clicking on each entry of the table displays a graph of the gene expression profile across all analyzed samples (Fig. 17.3).

Healthy	GSM3124633	87_8yr_Male_Caucasian	Skin; Unspecified	GM00499	Normal	Male	8	Caucasian
Healthy	GSM3124634	88_8yr_Male_Caucasian	Skin; Inguinal area	GM08398	Normal	Male	8	Caucasian
HPGS	GSM3124693	139_8_Female-HGPS_Caucasian	Skin; Leg	AG11513	HGPS	Female	8yr	Caucasian
HPGS	GSM3124694	141_8_Male-HGPS_Unknown	Unknown	PRF167	HGPS	Male	8yr	Unknown
HPGS	GSM3124698	200_8yr6mos_M_Unknown	Unknown	HGADFN169	HGPS	Male	8yr6mos	Unknown
HPGS	GSM3124701	203_8yr10mos_M_Unknown	Unknown	HGADFN143	HGPS	Male	8yr10mos	Unknown
Healthy	GSM3124631	85_7yr_Male_Black	Skin; inguinal area	GM05757	Normal	Male	7	Black
Healthy	GSM3124632	86_7yr_Male_Caucasian	Skin; Unspecified	GM00409	Normal	Male	7	Caucasian

Fig. 17.2 Sample selection in GEO2R using the GSE113957 dataset. Four samples were selected for each group

a Top differentially expressed genes

Download full table Select columns

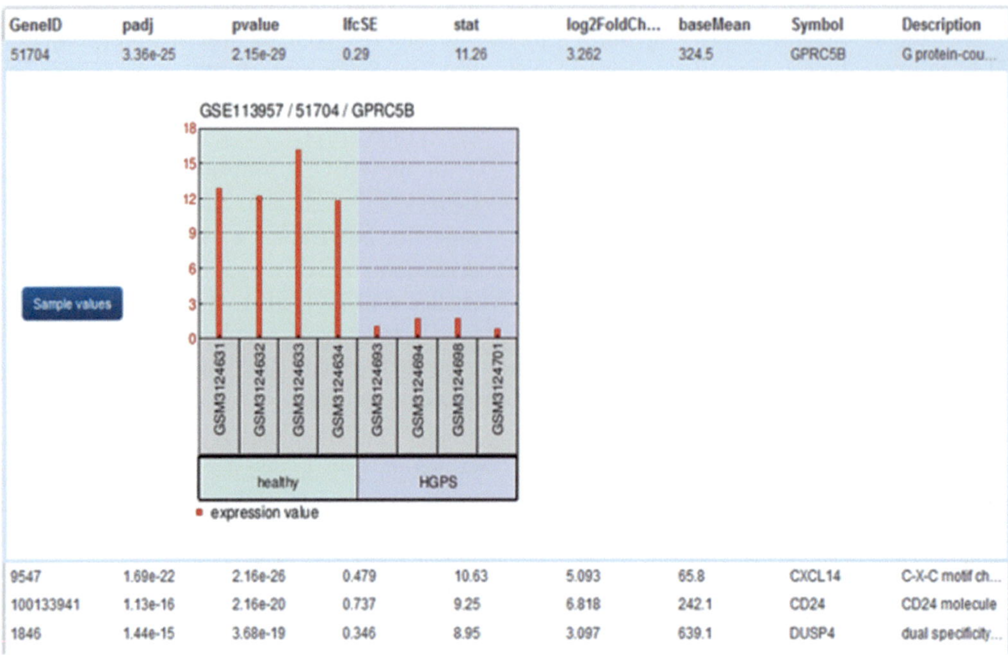

GeneID	padj	pvalue	lfcSE	stat	log2FoldCh...	baseMean	Symbol	Description
51704	3.36e-25	2.15e-29	0.29	11.26	3.262	324.5	GPRC5B	G protein-cou...
9547	1.69e-22	2.16e-26	0.479	10.63	5.093	65.8	CXCL14	C-X-C motif ch...
100133941	1.13e-16	2.16e-20	0.737	9.25	6.818	242.1	CD24	CD24 molecule
1846	1.44e-15	3.68e-19	0.346	8.95	3.097	639.1	DUSP4	dual specificity...

b

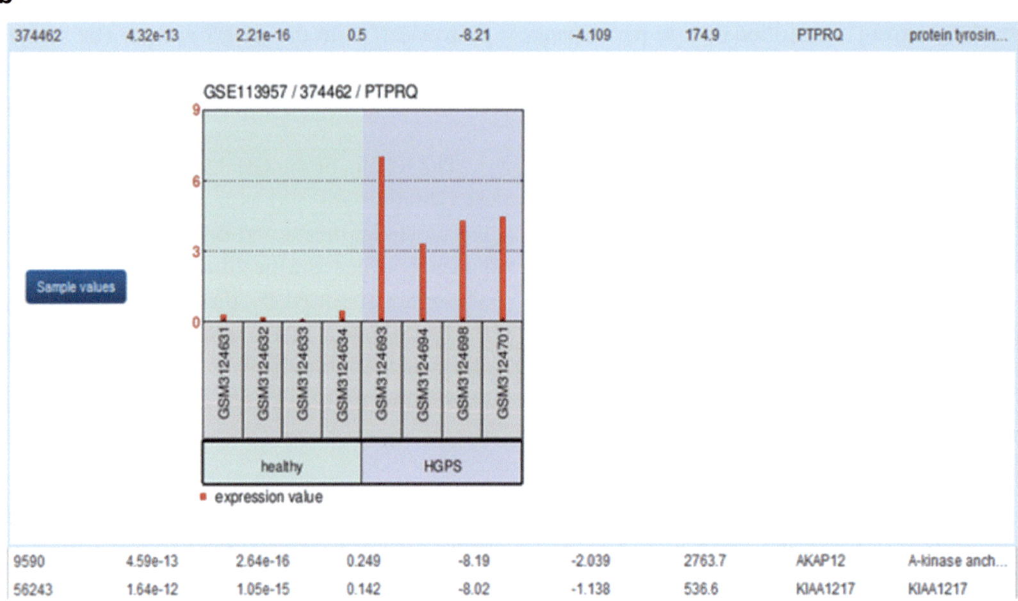

GeneID	padj	pvalue	lfcSE	stat	log2FoldCh...	baseMean	Symbol	Description
374462	4.32e-13	2.21e-16	0.5	-8.21	-4.109	174.9	PTPRQ	protein tyrosin...
9590	4.59e-13	2.64e-16	0.249	-8.19	-2.039	2763.7	AKAP12	A-kinase anch...
56243	1.64e-12	1.05e-15	0.142	-8.02	-1.138	536.6	KIAA1217	KIAA1217

Fig. 17.3 Table of top differentially expressed genes from GEO2R analysis with gene expression profile graph for (**a**) GPRC5B and (**b**) PTPRQ genes

In our example, the GPRC5B gene is expressed significantly higher in healthy patients when compared to HGPS patients, while the PTPRQ gene is expressed significantly higher in HGPS. The differential expression level for each gene is found in the log2FoldChange column, which represents the magnitude of change of a gene's expression between the compared groups. A positive log2FoldChange indicates higher expression in the first group (healthy) and a negative log2FoldChange indicates higher expression in the second group (HGPS). Of the numerous visualizations that GEO2R generates during analysis, the volcano plot is one of the most used visualizations for differential expression analysis (Fig. 17.4). It displays statistical significance (-log10 p-value) versus magnitude of change (log2 fold change) between the compared groups. Clicking on a gene on the volcano plot creates a pop-up of the graph showing details for that gene. Click on "Explore and download" to further interact with the volcano plot. In this interactive plot, you can mouse over data points to see the exact gene annotation and data. The highlighted data points are significantly differentially expressed based on an adjusted *p*-value cutoff of 0.05. Red highlighted points belong to the healthy group and blue to the HGPS group. As seen in the example, the most significantly differentially expressed (lowest p-value) gene, GPRC5B, is the highest point in the plot and highlighted in red, corresponding to the healthy group. GEO2R is a useful tool for the preliminary exploration of differentially expressed genes between different experimental conditions. Downstream analysis can follow to extract meaningful biological information from the genomics dataset.

17.7.1 Downstream Analysis

RNA-seq data can be further explored by looking for underlying biological processes and molecular functions, associated with the observed gene expression changes. This process is called functional enrichment analysis and will be performed

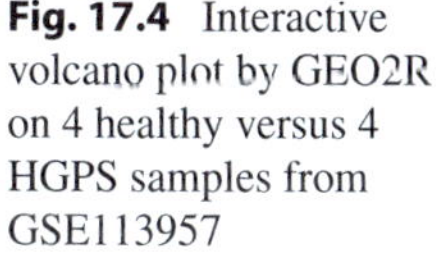

Fig. 17.4 Interactive volcano plot by GEO2R on 4 healthy versus 4 HGPS samples from GSE113957

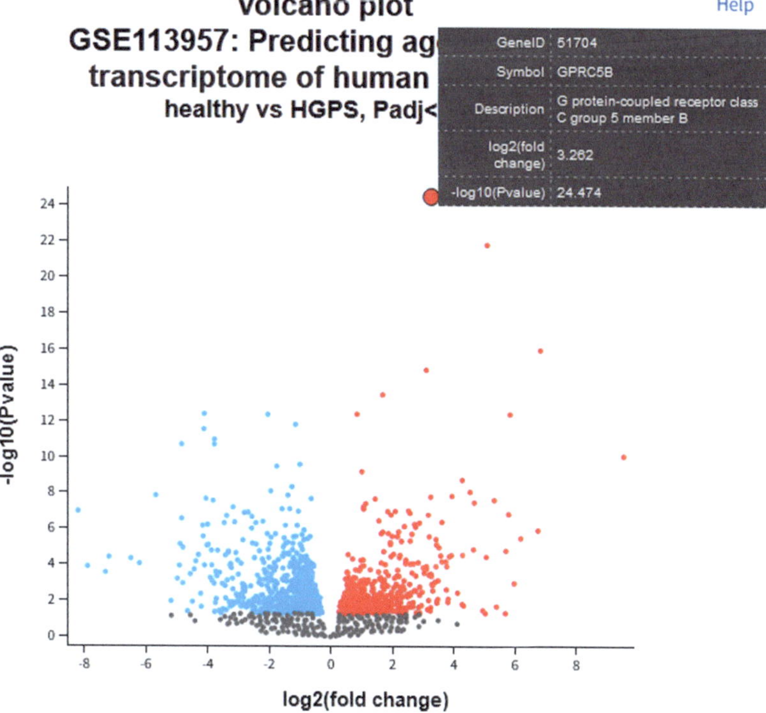

using DAVID [62] (Database for Annotation, Visualization, and Integrated Discovery), a web service for functional annotation and enrichment analysis of gene lists, and R programming language and software environment. First, we download the table of the top differentially expressed genes by clicking "Download full table." This will download the table shown in GEO2R as a TSV file, which can be opened and viewed in a spreadsheet software. Before moving to R, we need to register via email address for an account on the DAVID website (https://david.ncifcrf.gov/webservice/register.htm), in order to be able to use this web service later through R, and map the differentially expressed genes to significantly enriched functions and pathways for each of our groups. The following part requires familiarity in R programming. In a new R script in RStudio, we load the packages needed and define a few parameters as shown in the figure below. We then load the differentially expressed gene list downloaded previously from GEO2R.

```
# Load packages
library("RDAVIDWebService")
library('AnnotationDbi')
library("org.Hs.eg.db")
```

```
name <- "healthy_vs_HGSP"
file <- "GSE113957.top.table.tsv"
num_genes <- 3500

DEG.list <- read.table(file, header = TRUE, stringsAsFactors = FALSE, check.names = FALSE, sep = "\t")
```

The next step is to filter the genes by setting a cutoff where the expression of genes (log two fold change) is greater than or equal to the absolute value of 1.

```
# UPREGULATED: Filtered by diff >= 1
DEG.list.UP <- DEG.list[DEG.list$log2FoldChange>=1,]

# DOWNREGULATED: Filtered by diff <= -1
DEG.list.DOWN <- DEG.list[DEG.list$log2FoldChange<=-1,]
DEG.list.DOWN$log2FoldChange <- DEG.list.DOWN$log2FoldChange*-1
```

For each group, we assign the filtered gene lists and use the AnnotationDbi package to map the EntrezIDs for each respective gene. An EntrezID is a gene identifier according to the NCBI Entrez database.

```
group_1_marker <- DEG.list.UP
group_1_marker <- group_1_marker[order(group_1_marker$pvalue),]
keys_1=group_1_marker$Symbol[1:num_genes]
keys_1_upper <- tools::toTitleCase(toupper(keys_1))
egids_1 <- AnnotationDbi::select(org.Hs.eg.db, keys=keys_1_upper, columns=c("SYMBOL", "ENTREZID"), keytype="SYMBOL")

group_2_marker <- DEG.list.DOWN
group_2_marker <- group_2_marker[order(group_2_marker$pvalue),]
keys_2=group_2_marker$Symbol[1:num_genes]
keys_2_upper <- tools::toTitleCase(toupper(keys_2))
egids_2 <- AnnotationDbi::select(org.Hs.eg.db, keys=keys_2_upper, columns=c("SYMBOL", "ENTREZID"), keytype="SYMBOL")
```

We then use the DAVIDWebService to connect to DAVID. We enter the email used for registration at the location of the black box (Fig. 17.5). The EntrezIDs generated previously are now used to map functions and pathways from DAVID. The results can be saved as csv files, which can then be used to plot the top ten enriched functions in each of the groups.

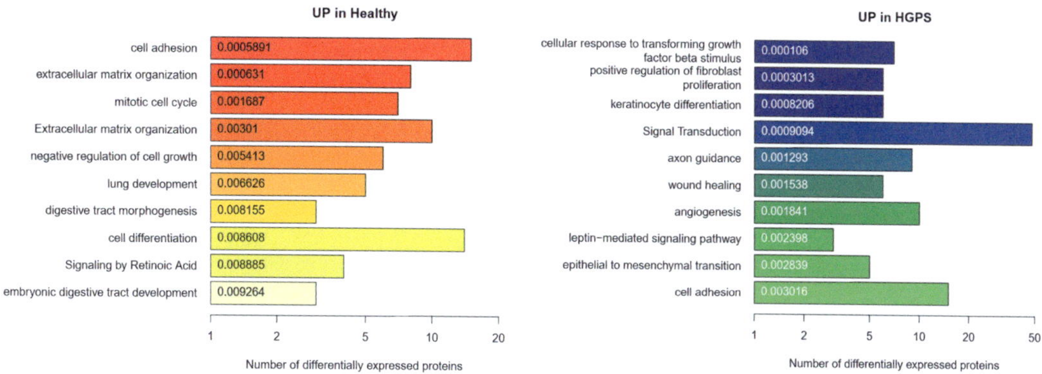

Fig. 17.5 Barplots of the top ten enriched pathways and functions for healthy (left) and HGPS (right) patients

```
replacENTREZID <- function(functionMatrix, mapping) {
  for(i in 1:nrow(functionMatrix)) {
    genelist <- trimws(strsplit(functionMatrix[i,]$Genes, ",")[[1]])
    geneName <- mapping[match(genelist, mapping$ENTREZID), 1]
    functionMatrix[i,]$Genes <- paste(geneName, collapse = ",")
  }
  return(functionMatrix)
}

enrichment_fn <- function(gene_names) {
  david <- DAVIDWebService$new(email=██████████, url="https://david.ncifcrf.gov/webservice/services/DAVIDWebService.DAVIDWebServiceHttpSoap12Endpoint/")
  result <- addList(david, gene_names[,2], idType = "ENTREZ_GENE_ID", listName = "L1.UP", listType = "Gene")
  setAnnotationCategories(david, c("GOTERM_BP_DIRECT", "KEGG_PATHWAY", "REACTOME_PATHWAY"))
  gene_functions_df <- getFunctionalAnnotationChart(david)
  gene_functions_df <- replacENTREZID(gene_functions_df, gene_names)

  return(gene_functions_df)
}

group_1_functions = enrichment_fn(egids_1)
write.csv(group_1_functions, file=paste(name,'_data_gene_enrichment_UP.csv', sep = ""))

group_2_functions = enrichment_fn(egids_2)
write.csv(group_2_functions, file=paste(name, '_data_gene_enrichment_DOWN.csv', sep = ""))
```

```
library(dplyr)
library(colorRamps)

wrap.it <- function(x, len)
{
  sapply(x, function(y) paste(strwrap(y, len),
                              collapse = "\n"),
         USE.NAMES = FALSE)
}

# Call this function with a list or vector
wrap.labels <- function(x, len)
{
  if (is.list(x))
  {
    lapply(x, wrap.it, len)
  } else {
    wrap.it(x, len)
  }
}

pdf("healthy_vs_HGPS.pdf", width=8,height=11)

n=45
par(mar=c(5,17,2,2))
layout(matrix(c(1:2), 2, 1, byrow = TRUE),
       widths=c(1,1), heights=c(1,1))

UP <- read.csv("healthy_vs_HGSP_data_gene_enrichment_UP.csv", stringsAsFactors=FALSE)
DOWN <- read.csv("healthy_vs_HGSP_data_gene_enrichment_DOWN.csv", stringsAsFactors=FALSE)

top10UP <- UP[1:10, c("Term", "Count","PValue")]
top10UP["Group"] = c(rep("Healthy",10))
top10UP <- top10UP %>% mutate(Term = sub(".*[:~]", "", Term))
top10UP <- top10UP[order(-top10UP$PValue),]
top10UP <- top10UP %>% mutate(PValue = signif(PValue, digits=4))
par(las=2)

xx <- barplot(height=top10UP$Count, names.arg=wrap.labels(top10UP$Term, n), horiz=TRUE, main="UP in Healthy", xlab = "Number of
differentially expressed proteins", col= rev(heat.colors(10)), log="x", xlim = c(1, 20), xaxt="n")
axis(1, las=1)
text(x = 1, y = xx, label = top10UP$PValue, col = "black", cex=1, pos=4)

top10DOWN <- DOWN[1:10, c("Term", "Count","PValue")]
top10DOWN["Group"] = c(rep("HGPS",10))
top10DOWN <- top10DOWN %>% mutate(Term = sub(".*[:~]", "", Term))
top10DOWN <- top10DOWN[order(-top10DOWN$PValue),]
top10DOWN <- top10DOWN %>% mutate(PValue = signif(PValue, digits=4))
par(las=2)

xx <- barplot(height=top10DOWN$Count, names.arg=wrap.labels(top10DOWN$Term, n), horiz=TRUE, main="UP in HGPS", xlab = "Number o
f differentially expressed proteins", col= rev(blue2green(10)), log="x", xlim = c(1, 50), xaxt="n")
axis(1, las=1)
text(x = 1, y = xx, label = top10DOWN$PValue, col = "white", cex=1, pos=4)

dev.off()
```

17.8 Challenges in Genomics Research

Although genomics research presents a wealth of opportunities for advancing our understanding of genetics, human health, and disease, it also comes with several challenges. The multi-dimensional nature of genomic data requires sophisticated computational tools for storage, analysis, and interpretation. Managing and analyzing big genomic datasets is challenging in terms of scalability, computational resources, and bioinformatics expertise. Interpreting genetic variants and their clinical significance, as well as differentiating between benign and pathogenic variants are complex tasks, requiring integration of diverse data sources and knowledge from a diverse group of professionals. Translating genomic discoveries into clinical practice also faces challenges related to validation, standardization, and integration into healthcare systems, as well as to training clinicians to effectively incorporate genomics into patient care decisions. Ethical concerns are also raised in genomic research, regarding privacy, informed consent, data sharing, potential misuse of genetic information, and protection of participant confidentiality. These issues need careful consideration to ensure responsible conduct of research. Finally, lack of diversity in genomics research nowadays is addressed more systematically [63–65], since in the past it has led to underrepresentation of diverse populations. Taking into consideration health disparities and diversity in genomic studies is crucial for developing generalizable findings.

Knowledge Check Questions

1. Describe the difference between a DNA fragment and a sequenced read.
2. What are the advantages of pyrosequencing over Sanger sequencing?
3. What is the reason that BLAST was not suitable for alignment of RNA-seq reads?
4. What is the purpose of a genome browser?
5. Explain the difference between a gene, a transcript, and a protein.
6. Describe in which ways genomics has been integrated in the healthcare system.
7. Does the study of the organismal population of a lake belong to epi- or meta-genomics?

References

1. A user's guide to the encyclopedia of DNA elements (ENCODE). PubMed. https://pubmed.ncbi.nlm.nih.gov/21526222/.
2. Qu H, Fang X. A brief review on the human encyclopedia of DNA elements (ENCODE) project. Genomics Proteomics Bioinformatics. 2013;11:135–41.
3. The Cancer Genome Atlas Pan-Cancer analysis project. Nat Genet. https://www.nature.com/articles/ng.2764.
4. Durbin RM, et al. A map of human genome variation from population-scale sequencing. Nature. 2010;467:1061–73.
5. International HapMap Consortium. The International HapMap Project. Nature. 2003;426:789–96.
6. Sanger F, Nicklen S, Coulson AR. DNA sequencing with chain-terminating inhibitors. Proc Natl Acad Sci USA. 1977;74:5463–7.
7. A sequencing method based on real-time pyrophosphate. Science. https://www.science.org/doi/10.1126/science.281.5375.363.
8. Sequence information can be obtained from single DNA molecules. Proc Natl Acad Sci U S A. https://www.pnas.org/doi/abs/10.1073/pnas.0230489100.
9. Continuous base identification for single-molecule nanopore DNA sequencing. Nat Nanotechnol. https://www.nature.com/articles/nnano.2009.12.
10. Collins FS, Fink L. The human genome project. Alcohol Health Res World. 1995;19:190–5.
11. Hood L, Rowen L. The Human Genome Project: big science transforms biology and medicine. Genome Med. 2013;5:79.
12. Waterston RH, Lander ES, Sulston JE. On the sequencing of the human genome. Proc Natl Acad Sci. 2002;99:3712–6.
13. Birney E. The International Human Genome Project. Hum Mol Genet. 2021;30:R161–3.
14. Lander ES, et al. Initial sequencing and analysis of the human genome. Nature. 2001;409:860–921.
15. Venter JC, et al. The sequence of the human genome. Science. 2001;291:1304–51.
16. Gibbs RA. The Human Genome Project changed everything. Nat Rev Genet. 2020;21:575–6.
17. Mouse Genome Sequencing Consortium, et al. Initial sequencing and comparative analysis of the mouse genome. Nature. 2002;420:520–62.

18. The sequence and de novo assembly of the giant panda genome. Nature. https://www.nature.com/articles/nature08696.
19. BLAST programs — BLASTHelp documentation. https://blast.ncbi.nlm.nih.gov/doc/blast-help/references.html#references.
20. Smith TF, Waterman MS. Identification of common molecular subsequences. J Mol Biol. 1981;147:195–7.
21. Dobin A, et al. STAR: ultrafast universal RNA-seq aligner. Bioinformatics. 2013;29:15–21.
22. Peterson J, et al. The NIH Human Microbiome Project. Genome Res. 2009;19:2317–23.
23. Wood DE, Lu J, Langmead B. Improved metagenomic analysis with Kraken 2. Genome Biol. 2019;20:257.
24. Clark K, Karsch-Mizrachi I, Lipman DJ, Ostell J, Sayers EW. GenBank. Nucleic Acids Res. 2016;44:D67–72.
25. The Ensembl genome database project. PubMed. https://pubmed.ncbi.nlm.nih.gov/11752248/.
26. Berman HM, et al. The protein data bank. Nucleic Acids Res. 2000;28:235–42.
27. 1000 Genomes Project Consortium, et al. A map of human genome variation from population-scale sequencing. Nature. 2010;467:1061–73.
28. 1000 Genomes Project Consortium, et al. A global reference for human genetic variation. Nature. 2015;526:68–74.
29. Devuyst O. The 1000 Genomes Project: welcome to a new world. Perit Dial Int. 2015;35:676–7.
30. Smigielski EM, Sirotkin K, Ward M, Sherry ST. dbSNP: a database of single nucleotide polymorphisms. Nucleic Acids Res. 2000;28:352–5.
31. Kent WJ, et al. The human genome browser at UCSC. Genome Res. 2002;12:996–1006.
32. Leinonen R, Sugawara H, Shumway M, International Nucleotide Sequence Database Collaboration. The sequence read archive. Nucleic Acids Res. 2011;39:D19–21.
33. Landrum MJ, et al. ClinVar: public archive of relationships among sequence variation and human phenotype. Nucleic Acids Res. 2014;42:D980–5.
34. Landrum MJ, et al. ClinVar: improvements to accessing data. Nucleic Acids Res. 2020;48:D835–44.
35. Clough E, Barrett T. The Gene Expression Omnibus database. Methods Mol Biol. 2016;1418:93–110.
36. Leinonen R, et al. The European Nucleotide Archive. Nucleic Acids Res. 2011;39:D28–31.
37. Integrative genomics viewer. Nat Biotechnol. https://www.nature.com/articles/nbt.1754.
38. JBrowse 2: a modular genome browser with views of synteny and structural variation. Genome Biol | Full Text. https://genomebiology.biomedcentral.com/articles/10.1186/s13059-023-02914-z.
39. The Human Epigenome Browser at Washington University. Nat Methods. https://www.nature.com/articles/nmeth.1772.
40. Rangwala SH, et al. Accessing NCBI data using the NCBI Sequence Viewer and Genome Data Viewer (GDV). Genome Res. 2021;31:159–69.
41. Collins FS, Varmus H. A new initiative on precision medicine. N Engl J Med. 2015;372:793–5.
42. Yang J, Nittala MR, Velazquez AE, Buddala V, Vijayakumar S. An overview of the use of precision population medicine in cancer care: first of a series. Cureus. 2023;15:e37889.
43. Petersen DW, Kawasaki ES. Manufacturing of microarrays. Adv Exp Med Biol. 2007;593:1–11.
44. Wang Z, Gerstein M, Snyder M. RNA-Seq: a revolutionary tool for transcriptomics. Nat Rev Genet. 2009;10:57–63.
45. Romanoski CE, Glass CK, Stunnenberg HG, Wilson L, Almouzni G. Roadmap for regulation. Nature. 2015;518:314–6.
46. López-Camarillo C, Gallardo-Rincón D, Álvarez-Sánchez ME, Marchat LA. Pharmaco-epigenomics: on the road of translation medicine. Adv Exp Med Biol. 2019;1168:31–42.
47. Riesenfeld CS, Schloss PD, Handelsman J. Metagenomics: genomic analysis of microbial communities. Annu Rev Genet. 2004;38:525–52.
48. Taş N, et al. Metagenomic tools in microbial ecology research. Curr Opin Biotechnol. 2021;67:184–91.
49. Chistoserdova L. Recent progress and new challenges in metagenomics for biotechnology. Biotechnol Lett. 2010;32:1351–9.
50. Structural genomics and the Protein Data Bank. PubMed. https://pubmed.ncbi.nlm.nih.gov/33957120/.
51. Kuhlman B, Bradley P. Advances in protein structure prediction and design. Nat Rev Mol Cell Biol. 2019;20:681–97.
52. Jumper J, et al. Highly accurate protein structure prediction with AlphaFold. Nature. 2021;596:583–9.
53. Watson JL, et al. De novo design of protein structure and function with RFdiffusion. Nature. 2023;620:1089–100.
54. Zhang J, Fei Y, Sun L, Zhang QC. Advances and opportunities in RNA structure experimental determination and computational modeling. Nat Methods. 2022;19:1193–207.
55. Bienko M. How Hi-C ignited the era of 3D genome biology. Nat Rev Genet. 2023;24:418.
56. Kapli P, Yang Z, Telford MJ. Phylogenetic tree building in the genomic age. Nat Rev Genet. 2020;21:428–44.
57. Suardana IBK, et al. Whole-genome comparison of representatives of all variants of SARS-CoV-2, including subvariant BA.2 and the GKA clade. Adv Virol. 2023;2023:6476626.
58. Hu B, Guo H, Zhou P, Shi Z-L. Characteristics of SARS-CoV-2 and COVID-19. Nat Rev Microbiol. 2021;19:141–54.
59. GEO2R – GEO. NCBI. https://www.ncbi.nlm.nih.gov/geo/geo2r/.
60. Fleischer JG, et al. Predicting age from the transcriptome of human dermal fibroblasts. Genome Biol. 2018;19:221.
61. GEO Accession viewer. https://www.ncbi.nlm.nih.gov/geo/query/acc.cgi?acc=GSE113957.

62. Dennis G, et al. DAVID: database for annotation, visualization, and integrated discovery. Genome Biol. 2003;4:R60.
63. Chong HY, Allotey PA, Chaiyakunapruk N. Current landscape of personalized medicine adoption and implementation in Southeast Asia. BMC Med Genet. 2018;11:94.
64. Peprah E, Wiley K, Sampson U, Narula J. A new age for African-driven genomics research: human heredity and health in Africa (H3Africa). Glob Heart. 2017;12:67–8.
65. Genotyping and population characteristics of the China Kadoorie Biobank. PubMed. https://pubmed.ncbi.nlm.nih.gov/37601966/.

Precision Medicine

18

Eugenia G. Giannopoulou and Andrea Sboner

Foundational Domains

This chapter addresses the following AMIA Foundational Domains: F1—Health, F4—Health Information Science and Technology.

Learning Objectives

Upon completion of the chapter, the students will be able to:

1. Summarize the history of precision medicine and its healthcare applications.
2. Explain the theory of next-generation sequencing and its role in precision medicine.
3. Describe specific methodologies used in the analysis of precision medicine datasets.
4. Identify online resources used in precision medicine.
5. Summarize current challenges in precision medicine and identify potential solutions.

E. G. Giannopoulou
Department of Biological Sciences, New York City College of Technology, City University of New York, New York, NY, USA
e-mail: Evgenia.Giannopoulou39@citytech.cuny.edu

A. Sboner (✉)
Department of Pathology and Laboratory Medicine, Englander Institute for Precision Medicine, Institute for Computational Biology, Meyer Cancer Center, Weill Cornell Medicine, New York, NY, USA
e-mail: ans2077@med.cornell.edu

18.1 History of Genomics and Its Relation to Precision Medicine

The completion of the human genome reference in 2001 marked a turning point in genetics and medicine. Advances like next-generation sequencing (NGS) dramatically reduced sequencing costs and time, enabling large-scale studies to uncover the genetic basis of diseases. Projects such as the 1000 Genomes Project, ENCODE, UK Biobank, TCGA, and HapMap significantly advanced understanding of the human genome's functional aspects. The insights gained from these projects have enabled the establishment of *precision medicine* as alterations of the genome can now "precisely" explain the biology of a disease. Precision medicine aims to tailor medical treatments and interventions to individual patients, taking into account their gene variability, the environment, and lifestyle of each person [1]. By elucidating the genetic basis of diseases, including both rare and common disorders, precision medicine holds promise for more accurate diagnosis, targeted therapies, and improved patient outcomes.

The time is right for precision medicine due to several converging factors. The breakthroughs in genomic technologies have made it faster, more affordable, and more accurate to sequence entire genome or specific regions of interest. Additionally, the aforementioned initiatives have

C. Eldredge et al. (eds.), *Introductory Textbook in Health Informatics*, Health Informatics,
https://doi.org/10.1007/978-3-032-16657-9_18

generated vast amounts of data from diverse populations and diseases. These big datasets provide valuable resources for identifying genetic variants associated with specific diseases and disorders. As a consequence, sophisticated algorithms and computational tools have been developed to assist in the analysis and interpretation of these complex genomic data at scale. The era of big data and artificial intelligence (AI) is now characterized by applications that integrate electronic health records, genomic data, and real-time patient monitoring data, identify complex patterns, and use predictive modeling techniques to help guide clinical decision-making. At the same time, the identification of genetic mutations and disease biomarkers has led to the development of targeted therapies. Precision medicine stands at the crossroads of all these critical factors, forcing a shift from the traditional "one-size-fits-all" approach in healthcare to an individualized treatment and intervention according to a patient's unique genetic makeup. In this chapter, we describe the field of precision medicine and its healthcare applications, present specific methodologies used in the analysis of precision medicine datasets, and discuss current challenges.

18.2 Genetic Variations and Their Role on Diseases

Every human cell contains about 3.1 billion nucleotides—adenine (A), cytosine (C), thymine (T), and guanine (G)—that encode life's instructions. While 99% of the genome is shared among humans [2] and ~98% with chimpanzees [3], small genetic differences drive individual traits (e.g., height, eye color, facial features), disease susceptibility, behavioral traits, response to drugs and therapies, immune response, and more. These variations range from single nucleotide changes to large structural alterations in the genome.

Single nucleotide polymorphisms, frequently called *SNPs* (pronounced "snips"), are DNA sequence variations occurring when a single nucleotide in the genome differs between individuals of a species or between paired chromosomes in an individual. For example, the DNA sequence AAGC*C*TA has a SNP where cytosine (C) is replaced by thymine (T), resulting in AAGC*T*TA. SNPs can occur naturally within populations through mechanisms like mutations, inheritance, and genetic drift. *Genetic drift* refers to random changes in the frequency of genetic variants, including SNPs, within a population. Unlike mutations, which introduce new changes, genetic drift happens by chance, especially in small populations. For instance, if a small group of individuals with a specific SNP becomes isolated or produces more offspring than others, that SNP may become more common over generations, not because it provides any advantage, but due to random chance. For a variant to be classified as SNP, it must be found in at least 1% of the population; otherwise it is considered a rare mutation. The average frequency of SNPs in the human genome is one SNP for every 1000 nucleotides, which means there are approximately five million different SNPs in a person's genome [4], while more than 600 million SNPs have been found in populations around the world [5]. *Single nucleotide variants* (SNVs) refer to any single nucleotide difference in the DNA sequence, regardless of its frequency in the population. SNVs include SNPs, but also other types of single-nucleotide changes, such as de novo mutations or somatic mutations that occur during an individual's lifetime in specific cells. Insertions and deletions, frequently called *indels*, are genetic variations involving the addition or removal of nucleotides in the DNA sequence. They range from a single base pair to several nucleotides and can disrupt protein-coding sequences or regulatory elements. *Copy Number Variations* (CNVs) are structural changes involving the duplication or deletion of large segments of DNA, ranging in size from kilobases to megabases. CNVs can affect gene dosage, leading to changes in gene expression levels, and may contribute to phenotypic diversity and disease susceptibility. Structural Variations are large-scale alterations in the genome, including inversions, translocations, and chromosomal rearrangements and can have significant consequences for gene function and genome stability. Finally, *repetitive*

DNA sequences occur when short DNA sequences, known as tandem repeats, are abnormally expanded in the genome. These expansions can lead to various genetic disorders. For example, Huntington's disease and fragile X syndrome are associated with instability in repetitive DNA regions (Table 18.1).

There have been numerous studies and projects aimed at cataloging human genetic variations, such as the *1000 Genomes Project* [4] and the *Genome Aggregation Database* (gnomAD) [6]. The 1000 Genomes Project was an international collaboration that aimed to create a comprehensive catalog of human genetic variation, including SNPs, insertions, deletions, and structural variants, by sequencing the genomes of thousands of individuals from diverse populations worldwide. The project started in 2007 and sequenced the genomes of approximately 2500 individuals [7] from 26 populations across the globe. NGS technologies were used in combination with computational methods to identify genetic variants by comparing the sequenced genomes to the reference human genome sequence. The data, including variant calls and genotype data, were made freely available to the scientific community to facilitate further research in genetics and genomics. The 1000 Genomes Project has had a significant impact on understanding of human genetic diversity, evolution, and disease. The gnomAD aggregates and harmonizes whole exome (WES) (i.e., sequencing of the protein-coding regions of the genome) and whole genome sequencing (WGS) (i.e., sequencing of the entire genome) data from diverse human populations to create a reference dataset of genetic variation. It supports human genomics research, such as the identification of rare and common genetic variants associated with human diseases and traits, the estimation of allele frequencies and population-specific patterns of genetic variation, and the assessment of the functional impact of genetic variants on protein structure and function.

Table 18.1 Key genetic variation types and their characteristics

Genomic variation	Definition	Key features
SNP (Single Nucleotide Polymorphism)	DNA variation where a single nucleotide differs between individuals or paired chromosomes.	Occurs in at least 1% of the population; average frequency: 1 SNP per 1000 nucleotides (~5 million per person).
Indels (Insertions and Deletions)	Genetic variations involving the addition or removal of small numbers of nucleotides in the DNA sequence.	Range in size from 1 base pair to several nucleotides; can disrupt coding or regulatory regions.
CNVs (Copy Number Variations)	Structural variations involving duplication or deletion of large DNA segments.	Can affect gene dosage, gene expression, and contribute to phenotypic diversity or disease susceptibility.
Repetitive DNA	DNA sequences that are repeated multiple times (tandem repeats), often abnormally expanded.	Associated with genetic disorders like Huntington's disease and fragile X syndrome; impacts genome stability.

While most genetic variants are "harmless", some can cause diseases or disorders. The genome contains regions that organize and encode the biological information essential for life. The ENCODE [8, 9] project aimed to identify all the elements present in the genomes of humans and model species. The most important of these are *protein coding genes*, which contain the information to produce proteins—the functional elements of cells, responsible for all of its activities. Humans have approximately 20,000 protein-coding genes, covering about 1–2% of the entire genome. However, other non-coding regions play crucial roles in regulation and control, such as promoters, enhancers [10], insulators, and regions encoding long-non-coding RNAs, small RNAs, and more. These regions are known as regulatory elements [9] and are the vast majority of the human genome.

Given the important role of protein-coding genes, variations in their nucleotide sequence may disrupt their function, hence natural selection helps keep the functional sequence, by either removing potential deleterious variations (*purifying* or *negative selection*) or favoring advantageous variations (*positive selection*). However, deleterious variations can still occur and lead to diseases or disorders. Each cell contains two copies (alleles) of DNA. In many cases, a defective allele is compensated by the healthy one. However, in some cases, a single defective allele is sufficient to confer a specific trait (dominant), whereas sometimes both alleles need to carry the specific variation to cause a particular phenotype (recessive). Sickle cell anemia, for example, is a condition that affects red blood cells, responsible for carrying oxygen throughout the body (i.e., red blood cells have a sickle shape and are less efficient in moving around blood vessels). People with a homozygous (in both alleles) variation in the gene encoding for hemoglobin suffer from this condition (recessive). However, people with only one allele affected (heterozygous) are healthy, and more resistant to malaria. Not surprisingly, people living in areas where malaria is endemic tend to have a heterozygous allele. Notably, sickle cell disease incidence in the United States affects predominantly people of West African ancestry [11], where malaria is more common than in East Africa. Sickle cell disease is one of the Mendelian (or monogenic) diseases, characterized by a mutation in a single gene. Other examples of Mendelian diseases [12] are: cystic fibrosis, Huntington's disease, Duchenne muscular dystrophy, and hemophilia. In addition to SNPs, other small insertions and deletions [13, 14] can occur and disrupt the function of a gene. One example is cystic fibrosis, where a 3 nucleotide deletion in the CFTR gene causes the disease. Fragile-X syndrome is caused by repeated duplication of 3 nucleotides in the promoter region of FMR1. Several of the more common diseases are not caused by a single gene mutation. For example, diabetes, cardiovascular, and neurological diseases are not defined by alterations of single genes or regulatory regions, but likely, by the combined effect of multi-gene mutations, as well as environmental factors affecting their regulation.

Cancer is primarily a polygenic disease, which means that it is triggered by alteration in multiple genetic loci. Since the completion of the human genome, projects like TCGA [15] and the International Cancer Genome Consortium (ICGC) [16] and others have sought to identify the key driver alterations that occur in normal cells and drive them to transform into cancer cells. These types of alterations are called *somatic* because they are limited to the tumor cells only. Several SNVs, indels, and *somatic copy number alterations* (SCNAs, extra copies of areas in the genome or losses of genetic material) have been identified as drivers of cancer or as mechanisms of therapeutic resistance. In many cases, these variations affect genes that are involved in specific biological pathways, indicating their important role for cancer cell survival, such as PIK3CA, BRAF, KRAS, and more. For example, the gene ERBB2 (and its protein Her2) is commonly amplified in a subset of breast, gastric, bladder, endometrial, and other cancers; the gene EGFR shows both SNVs and SCNAs in lung cancers, and some mutations occur as a result of the initial targeted therapy.

Gene fusions are also common in cancer. They typically occur when two regions of the genome are rearranged such that are in proximity and may give rise to a new protein, such in the case of BCR-ABL1 in certain cases of blood cancer (where parts of chromosome 2 are "swapped" with chromosome 9) [17, 18], or over-express a gene that normally is not active in that cell, such as TMPRSS2-ERG in prostate cancer (where ERG is a transcription factor that is normally not expressed in prostate cell, and TMPRSS2 is highly androgen regulated) [19, 20].

Regardless of the nature of the alterations, whether germline (occurring in the parent's reproductive cells and getting incorporated into the DNA of every cell in the body of the offspring) or somatic (occurring in tumor cells only), modern DNA sequencing technologies can help identify them. In fact, testing for mutations is nowadays recommended for many types of cancer as molecular profiling provides indications to the clinicians on how to best treat patients, fulfilling the precision medicine mantra of administering the right drug to the right patient at the right time. Similarly, molecular profiling of germline can help geneticists to better diagnose and treat patients with rare conditions.

18.3 From Bench to Bedside

Precision medicine is a multidisciplinary effort that involves various professionals collaborating across different domains, such as physicians, laboratory technicians, pathologists, bioinformatics analysts, software engineers, genetic counselors, clinical researchers, and more. Here, we discuss a typical clinical workflow in a precision medicine institute that begins when a physician requests a sequencing test for a patient. The laboratory then acquires the patient's samples and sequences the DNA or RNA, followed by bioinformatics pipelines that perform computational analysis on the sequenced data and provide results to the molecular pathologists, who then reviews the results and issue a report to the clinicians.

18.3.1 Cancer Treatments

Nowadays, when a patient is diagnosed with cancer, several treatment options may be available, in addition to the traditional ones (e.g., surgery, radiation, chemotherapy). One of the most promising treatments in the context of our increased knowledge of tumor development and progression is *targeted therapy*, where a specific drug is "designed" to affect only the cells that harbor a specific molecular alteration. The first of this type was imatinib, a kinase inhibitor targeting BCR-ABL1 fusions in chronic myeloid leukemia (CML) in the early 2000s. Imatinib increased survival rate at 5 years in patients with CML of about 40% and is now around 80–90% [21, 22]. Since then, many drugs have been developed to target the specific alterations discovered. More recently, a new paradigm shift happened in the context of targeted therapies. Cancer drugs were typically tested in the context of the specific organ (e.g., breast cancer). At the end of 2018, the US Food and Drug Administration (FDA) approved a cancer drug, larotrectinib, targeting NTRK1 gene fusion [23, 24], regardless of the site of the tumor. Since then, other drugs have been approved by the FDA only based on the molecular alterations and not the site of origin, such as trastuzumab [25] in both breast and bladder cancer. However, in some cases, the tumor site does make a difference, as is the case of BRAF mutations, common in melanoma and colorectal cancer: targeted treatments successful in melanoma do not affect colorectal cancer cells, suggesting that the tumor microenvironment plays a role indeed.

Another type of renewed optimism for cancer treatment is the advent of *immunotherapy*. This approach, instead of targeting cancer cells, focuses on harnessing each patient's immune system to attack and kill tumor cells. This therapeutic option has been successful in some cancer types and less so in others. One of the issues is to ensure that the immune system recognizes tumor cells as invaders. In order to do so, tumor cells need to present on their surface a sufficient number of neoantigens, structures different from the adjacent normal cells. Thus, one way to identify patients who may respond to immunotherapy is to find tumors with several mutations that, statistically, increase the likelihood of generating more antigens.

18.3.2 Clinical Genomics Workflow

Either in targeted therapies or immunotherapy, it is important to molecularly characterize each patient's tumor. Hence, in the precision medicine context, once a cancer diagnosis is rendered, clinicians request molecular testing. This process is outlined in Fig. 18.1, which illustrates the typical workflow followed by clinical genomics laboratories for molecular testing. After the specimen (surgical specimen or biopsy) is collected and transferred to the clinical genomic laboratory. Depending on the type of test, a normal control can also be acquired by the laboratory for processing. Clinical laboratories may offer different types of assays, from targeted ones, where only a

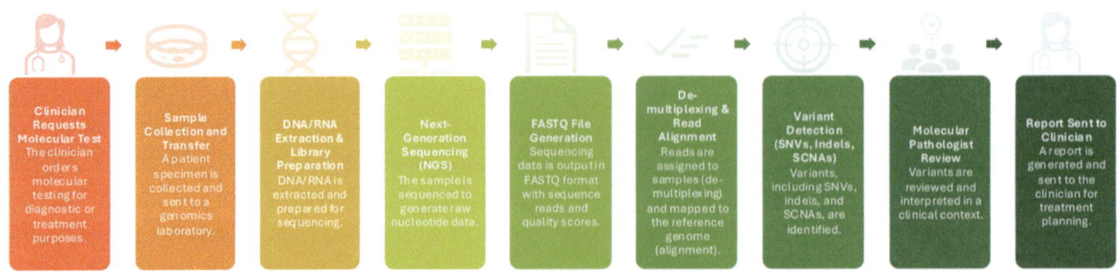

Fig. 18.1 Workflow for molecular testing in clinical genomics laboratories within the context of precision medicine

limited set of genes and genomic areas are evaluated, to WES or WGS sequencing tests, where all protein-coding genes, or the entire genome are evaluated, respectively. With broader assays (e.g., WES/WGS), a normal sample from the same individual is usually sequenced at the same time to remove all mutations that are not tumor-specific. With smaller assays, sequencing the tumor may be sufficient, but there is always a higher risk of reporting rare non-pathogenic SNPs instead of SNVs.

The laboratory then extracts the DNA and/or RNA samples and prepares them for sequencing following the specific protocols of the assay (i.e., library preparation). Once the library of DNA/RNA molecules is ready, NGS occurs, which "translates" the biological material into a digital sequence of A, C, T, and Gs. The output of a sequencer is typically recorded in FASTQ files, a specific format that encodes a header, the sequence, an optional line, and the quality of the identified nucleotides. A FASTQ file may contain millions of DNA sequences, called reads. Bioinformatics tools are then used to perform a series of computational tasks that identify the genetic variations in the sequenced reads of the original samples. The first computational step is *de-multiplexing* and it is required because during library preparation, samples from multiple individuals are pooled together to decrease the cost of sequencing. With de-multiplexing we recognize which molecule belongs to which individual, by leveraging an artificial short tag (typically a combination of 6 nucleotides) that is added to each molecule during library preparation. Once the sequencing is completed, the reads are grouped together by reading the patient-specific tags and FASTQ files are generated to contain reads of only one patient.

The next step is to identify the genomic location of those reads (i.e., chromosome number and base pairs position), in a process called *alignment*. Alignment has been simplified by the availability of the human genome reference sequence. Several computational tools have been developed over the years to address the task of read alignment [26] (e.g., BWA, Bowtie2, STAR). To simplify the goal of the alignment process, one can consider it as a sophisticated search of a text string or a group of characters in a book. The text string is the sequenced read and the book is the human reference genome sequence, which is indexed [27] a priori to make the search more efficient. Alignment methods have been optimized for speed, as millions of reads need to be searched (aligned) as fast as possible. Additionally, the alignment methods need to be aware of the presence of "typos" in the text searching, which means the presence of genomic variations in the reads, such as SNVs or indels. The alignment step results in a file formatted as Sequence Alignment Map (SAM) [27] or its binary version (BAM). *Variant detection* follows, identifying differences between the reference genome and the patient sample. Each nucleotide that is different from the reference genome is a putative single nucleotide variant or, if more than one nucleotide, an indel. For matched normal controls, the same analysis is performed, but a comparison between the tumor results and the matched normal results takes place, thus excluding events that are not tumor-specific. SCNAs are detected by comparing read counts between tumor and normal samples, identifying amplifications or deletions in specific regions. Several tools are available and could be used for detecting, manipulating, and annotating SNVs, indels, and SCNAs (e.g., GATK, Vardict, CNVkit, VCFTools, SnpEff) [28–31]. However, the ultimate evaluation in a clinical laboratory comes from the molecular pathologist who is trained to evaluate and interpret the raw results of the *bioinformatics pipelines* in the context of the questions raised by the clinician: Which subtype of tumor is this? What is the first choice of treatment? Is there evidence of a resistance mutation? Can the patient be treated with immunotherapy? To aid the molecular pathologist in evaluating the results of the bioinformatic pipeline in the precision medicine context, several knowledge bases have been developed that classify cancer variants in severity (e.g., ClinVar [32], COSMIC [33], ClinGen [34]). However, continuously maintaining and updating a knowledge base for precision medicine and cancer variants presents several challenges, primarily due to the rapidly evolving nature of genomic research and the continuous influx of new data. Once the molecular pathologist has reviewed the data, a report is sent back to the clinician, who now has more information on how to treat the patient.

18.3.3 Challenges of Molecular Testing in Cancer Treatment

While molecular testing is becoming a necessity for cancer treatment, it is worth mentioning that the accessibility of molecular testing for cancer diagnosis and treatment is a critical issue that can significantly impact patient care and outcomes. The cost of sequencing technology is decreasing, but the cost of interpreting the results in the context of the most current medical knowledge remains high, as the constant influx of new discoveries requires molecular pathologists and oncologists to continually maintain up-to-date knowledge. Thus, the high cost of testing may present a barrier, especially for patients without adequate insurance coverage or financial resources. Additionally, some tests may not be covered by insurance, further limiting access for certain patient populations. Access to molecular testing may also be limited in regions with inadequate healthcare infrastructure, limited availability of specialized laboratories, trained personnel, and equipment necessary for conducting molecular testing. Finally, lack of awareness among healthcare providers and patients about the importance and utility of molecular testing for cancer diagnosis and treatment can lead to underutilization of these services. Although educational initiatives can assist to increase awareness regarding molecular testing, a multifaceted approach involving collaboration among healthcare providers, policymakers and all professionals involved in the precision medicine industry is needed to address those challenges and ultimately improve patient care and outcomes. While cancer molecular testing is quite common and sometimes required nowadays, germline testing is also being utilized for precision medicine for diagnostic or prognostic purposes. The process in the lab is similar, however the interpretation of the results requires genetic counselors to properly determine the relationships between genotype (an individual's genetic makeup) and phenotype [35] (the observable traits).

18.4 Technologies for Precision Medicine

Precision medicine relies on various technologies that allow for the customization of healthcare, treatment, and prevention strategies. Here we discuss sequencing technologies enabling precision medicine, tools that simplify the execution of bioinformatics pipelines, and the recent advances on AI that will have an impact in the near future. We also discuss the integration of smart devices for patient monitoring, and the development of virtual/mixed reality applications as emerging fields in healthcare.

18.4.1 Sequencing Technologies

The advent of massively parallel sequencing has revolutionized the way we investigate the changes that happen at the molecular level, shedding a deeper light into the mechanisms of disease formation and progression. Much like the historic introduction of microscopy in the late 1500s, which revealed the hidden world of microbes and bacteria, sequencing technologies have allowed us to peer into the intricate molecular landscape of patient samples, leading into the precision medicine era.

The past two decades have witnessed remarkable advancements in NGS technology, unraveling the intricate tapestry of our genetic information. Bulk RNA sequencing (RNA-seq) and DNA sequencing (e.g., WES, WGS, targeted sequencing) have been foundational in uncovering common mutations and functional alterations in various diseases. However, NGS has also been applied to more complex applications, such as Hi-C to understand the 3D structure of the genome, or the emerging field of spatial biology, where sequencing is associated with a physical location on a glass slide. Illumina NGS, also known as sequencing by synthesis (SBS), has been widely adopted and has played a pivotal role in advancing genomics research and personalized medicine. Beyond Illumina NGS, other sequencing platforms have emerged, each with unique features and applications [36] (e.g., IonTorrent, PacBio, Nanopore).

Regardless of the specific sequencing platform used, the essence of sequencing lies in translating biological specimens, whether DNA or RNA, into a common language based on a four-letter alphabet (A, T, G, C for DNA; A, U, G, C for RNA). This universality of the nucleotide alphabet enables the development of diverse experimental protocols to address a wide range of biological questions. Importantly, bioinformatics pipelines and tools, mostly available in the public domain, allow for standardizing sample processing and analysis, thereby further facilitating researchers in their quest to understand biomedical processes.

From bulk sequencing, where a collection of cells in a tissue are evaluated, experimental protocols have evolved to single-cell sequencing, where each cell is evaluated for mutations, gene expression, or chromatin accessibility. This improvement enabled the precise interrogation of how cells evolve and communicate. In hematological malignancies (e.g., leukemia, lymphoma, multiple myeloma), single-cell sequencing has emerged as a powerful tool to monitor how sub-clones (i.e., subset of cells) evolve in the context of drug treatment. In solid tumors, the spatial location of cells also carries important information. For example, if T-cells are "infiltrated" within tumor cells, it is more likely that the patient would respond to immunotherapy, which is in contrast to cases where T-cells are only present "around" the tumor. The more recent evolution of the technology now allows to interrogate spatial localization, thus providing new precise insights into basic biology, disease development, and progression.

Sequencing has brought a revolution in our interrogation of basic molecular mechanisms and will likely continue to do so. While this technology has mostly been used as a "molecular microscope" by providing unprecedented views into molecular mechanisms, it is worth noting that its use in combination with CRISPR (clustered regularly interspaced short palindromic repeats), another revolutionary technology that allows to "manipulate" the genome, will further our understanding of biology and improve our amelioration of diseases and disorders [37].

18.4.2 Big Genomic Data and AI

Sequencing technologies are at the backbone of precision medicine and produce a vast amount of data that is processed, summarized, and analyzed [38]. Bioinformatics pipelines typically perform a "deterministic" analysis of the genome in order to identify important patterns of disease, such as cancer-specific mutations, pharmacogenomics variants, or variations that confer a risk to develop a disorder. In the context of cancer, TCGA [15] and ICGC [39] in the past couple of decades sought out to catalog all alterations that drive the disease. The hypothesis is that recurrent alterations (i.e., those occurring in several patients) likely play a key role. Indeed, many of them have now been identified and well-characterized and, as a result, targeted treatments are now available. However, a somber picture has emerged: only a few genes have mutations conferring a growth advantage, i.e., cancer drivers, common to many tumors. There is a long tail of alterations specific to an ever smaller subpopulation of patients [40, 41]. Understanding which of these rarer alterations are causal for the development of the disease is becoming critical for precision oncology. One way to address this is to accumulate as much information on these not-so-common mutations and to develop methods to predict their severity, either in silico or via functional studies. While large consortia focused on sequencing many patients, others started interrogating the functional aspects of those mutations. Efforts such as DepMap try to evaluate them via probing cancer models with a plethora of functional studies [42, 43].

Whether sequencing patients or cancer models, it has been clear that the vast amount of data generated needs to be made available to the larger scientific community. Tools for the secure and ethical sharing of data have been developed (e.g., cBioPortal, Cosmic, UK Biobank, All of Us) leading to an acceleration of the discoveries in the field [44–46]. Many datasets are available in centralized repositories such as dbGaP in the US, EGA in Europe, DDBJ in Japan and the Genome Sequence Archive in China which now contain exabytes of data [47–51]. Clearly, novel technologies for processing and analyzing these huge datasets are needed. The recent advances in the field of AI coupled with enhanced computational power and data availability have dramatically increased the interest of applying AI tools to biomedical questions. Machine learning (ML), a branch of AI which learns from data, has been very successfully applied in the medical field, especially when processing and analyzing digital images in radiology and pathology [52–56]. One of the most common ML applications is classification, where the model predicts a specific class based on input features (e.g., predicting a breast cancer lesion from a mammography [57]). For such an analysis, ML methods require a set of labeled data to train from (i.e., data where the answer is known). The current era of big data provides the amount of information that is needed, and increasingly more algorithms and methods are applied in the fields of biomedicine and healthcare.

AI has also been successful in advancing the field of protein folding, where a structure of a protein can be predicted in silico [58], as well as drug discovery, with ML models used to predict the binding of small-molecule ligands to protein targets of biological and pharmaceutical interest (e.g., DNA encoded libraries) [59]. Very recently, improvements in generative AI (such as GPT-4o, Claude, Gemini, BERT, LLaMA, Stable Diffusion) have reached the public. Models that can generate new text, images, or videos based on a request of the user (i.e., the prompt) are currently being evaluated on their ability to answer complex medical questions [60]. They can be used to search and summarize the overwhelming corpus of medical knowledge that is generated nowadays, or even to explain complex medical knowledge to patients themselves. Those generative models can also create new synthetic data in order to augment the training sets for ML learning models, although careful considerations for ethical use, biases are required. We are still at the infancy of the AI revolution, and thorough evaluations of AI tools are absolutely necessary, especially when applied to the biomedical field [61].

18.4.3 mHealth and VR

When considering big data in precision medicine, one typically thinks of the massive data generated by sequencing machines that profile patients' genomes. Several other technologies, however, also contribute to the generation of health data, even outside traditional care facilities. Many of us use monitoring devices, such as a smartwatch, which records lots of health and wellness information. Others also wear devices that constantly monitor vitals, such as heart rate or blood oxygen, and provide information about stress or sleep. The constant monitoring during day and night can provide rich information on the health status of the individual. The location of a smartphone for example can indicate whether someone stayed at home all day or went out for a walk; this can help determine the effect of chemotherapy for a cancer patient. Mobile applications allow tracking an individual's fitness or health status, and provide valuable information to researchers, clinicians, and healthcare providers, in order to, in turn, optimize care. Moreover, personalized interventions can be delivered via mobile apps, such as dietary reminders, scheduling tools, and more [62–64]. Wearable devices can also offer some type of intervention, in addition to providing monitoring capabilities, such as smartwatches that calm people before public speaking by vibrating at a certain time [65].

Spatial computing is another application made possible by advances in computing powers. With this term, we consider the entire spectrum that goes from virtual reality (VR), that is a full-immersion digital world, to extended or mixed reality, where digital objects are overlaid on top of the real world. Although VR applications have been mainly developed for the gaming industry, spatial computing has also been used in medical applications to treat mental health issues, such as addiction, fear, and to provide medical education to patients and training to medical students [66, 67]. Mixed reality applications can make healthcare delivery more efficient by providing information to clinicians in a novel way, especially in situations where a traditional keyboard and monitor cannot be used (e.g., in an operating room), thus fulfilling the "at the right time" component in the precision medicine mantra. In a laboratory, mixed reality can help process samples by facilitating training of new lab technologists and provide remote assistance by being hands-free. The combination of generative AI and VR/XR application can further expand on these applications by providing solutions tailored to the specific patient, such as an avatar explaining medical concepts to the patient in a culturally sensitive way.

18.5 Integration with Clinical Informatics

The integration of sequencing technology, AI, and wearable/smart devices into clinical practice holds immense promise for advancing precision medicine. However, thorough evaluation is crucial to ensure their effectiveness, reliability, safety, and ethical implications. The scientific process requires testing a hypothesis by conducting controlled experiments and repeated measurements. Typically, there is a comparison of two (or more) groups, each one as homogenous as possible to avoid any confounding factors. The more data available, the better the statistical power to detect the effect under study. In a clinical setting, this may not be possible as a decision needs to be taken for one patient. This is known as the N-of-1 problem of precision medicine [68].

One way to address this issue is to make sure that the models developed in research are robust enough to be applied to clinical care. In the case of sequencing technology, rigorous evaluation of the entire process, from the lab protocols to the bioinformatics pipelines, is requested before a sequencing assay can be used in the clinic. Moreover, the assays need to be continuously monitored and evaluated to guarantee that they maintain the original standards [69].

Furthermore, provenance of samples and data (i.e., the documentation of the origin, collection process, and handling of biological samples and associated data) is crucial for clinical operations. It is the role of clinical informatics to make sure that at every step of the entire process, there is clear identification of the origin of all samples and data. Typically, in a laboratory, this is ensured by a Laboratory Information Management System (LIMS) that records every information at every step. Laboratory personnel are trained to use LIMS to trace the steps performed. Clinical informatics is crucial to identify not only which LIMS to use, but also how different systems may interact with LIMS (e.g., the test ordering system, a sequencing machine, the electronic health record system). An efficient precision medicine clinical system is one that ensures the optimal delivery of care to the patients by ensuring that all components are well tested and integrated. The more digital integration, the faster the delivery of the information to clinicians.

18.6 Future of Precision Medicine

We are now at the cusp of another revolution in precision medicine. The combination of advances in sequencing technologies, the collection of massive amounts of data, and the enhanced computational power that enables both AI and spatial computing are poised to drastically change the practice of medicine. AI applied to imaging data can now perform at the same level of a trained physician in many fields [55, 70, 71]. In fact, the optimal use of AI could support a physician's efforts in treating patients, facilitate the discovery of new drugs and treatments, and improve teaching of the new generation of physicians and researchers. Along the same lines, spatial biology can help better understand the basic biological mechanisms of a disease. The field is still in its infancy, but has already provided insights into the evolution of diseases, the susceptibility of cancer cells to treatments, and the interplay between cancer cells and their microenvironment. These advances have already shifted the paradigm of homogeneous cancer cells, highlighting instead their diversity and time dependency.

One aspect that needs to be addressed in the near future is the role of different genetic ancestries in the development and progression of diseases. In fact, most of our knowledge is based on studies that included mainly people of European descent. The vast majority of the human population, however, is of a different ancestry. To fill this gap, recent initiatives such as Human Heredity and Health in Africa (H3Africa) [72], China Kadoorie Biobank [73, 74], Southeast Asia Genomic Research Partnership (SEAP) [75], and All of Us [46], have been established. The new discoveries that the initial results provided are outstanding [76, 77]. Increasing the diversity of our genomic databases is critical to truly provide precision medicine to all patients. Indeed, the future of precision medicine is in our ability to include as many diverse people as possible, a challenge that would require engaging the different communities that make up our human family [78].

Knowledge Check Questions

1. Describe the difference between SNPs and SNVs.
2. In which cases WES can be used instead of WGS in the context of precision medicine?
3. How many protein-coding genes are there in the human genome? How many nucleotides does the human DNA consist of?
4. Is cancer a monogenic or polygenic disease? Why?
5. What is the difference between somatic and germline mutations?
6. What has been the shift in cancer drugs after 2018?
7. What process is performed with the computational step of sequence alignment?
8. What are the challenges regarding the accessibility of molecular testing?
9. In which cases single-cell sequencing is preferred over bulk RNA-sequencing?

References

1. Garrido P, et al. Proposal for the creation of a national strategy for precision medicine in cancer: a position statement of SEOM, SEAP, and SEFH. Clin Transl Oncol. 2018;20:443–7.
2. Lander ES, et al. Initial sequencing and analysis of the human genome. Nature. 2001;409:860–921.
3. Waterson RH, Lander ES, Wilson RK, The Chimpanzee Sequencing and Analysis Consortium. Initial sequence of the chimpanzee genome and comparison with the human genome. Nature. 2005;437:69–87.
4. 1000 Genomes Project Consortium, et al. A map of human genome variation from population-scale sequencing. Nature. 2010;467:1061–73.
5. Home – SNP – NCBI. https://www.ncbi.nlm.nih.gov/snp/.
6. Chen S, et al. A genomic mutational constraint map using variation in 76,156 human genomes. Nature. 2024;625:92–100.
7. 1000 Genomes Project Consortium, et al. A global reference for human genetic variation. Nature. 2015;526:68–74.
8. An integrated encyclopedia of DNA elements in the human genome. Nature. https://www.nature.com/articles/nature11247.

9. A user's guide to the encyclopedia of DNA elements (ENCODE). PubMed. https://pubmed.ncbi.nlm.nih.gov/21526222/.
10. Ernst J, Kellis M. Discovery and characterization of chromatin states for systematic annotation of the human genome. Nat Biotechnol. 2010;28:817–25.
11. CDC. Data & statistics on sickle cell disease | CDC. Centers for Disease Control and Prevention. 2022. https://www.cdc.gov/ncbddd/sicklecell/data.html.
12. Chong JX, et al. The genetic basis of Mendelian phenotypes: discoveries, challenges, and opportunities. Am J Hum Genet. 2015;97:199–215.
13. Chen W, Zhang L. The pattern of DNA cleavage intensity around indels. Sci Rep. 2015;5:8333.
14. Lin M, et al. Effects of short indels on protein structure and function in human genomes. Sci Rep. 2017;7:9313.
15. The Cancer Genome Atlas Pan-Cancer analysis project. Nat Genet. https://www.nature.com/articles/ng.2764.
16. International Cancer Genome Consortium, et al. International network of cancer genome projects. Nature. 2010;464:993–8.
17. Quintás-Cardama A, Cortes JE. Chronic myeloid leukemia: diagnosis and treatment. Mayo Clin Proc. 2006;81:973–88.
18. Quintás-Cardama A, Cortes J. Molecular biology of bcr-abl1–positive chronic myeloid leukemia. Blood. 2009;113:1619–30.
19. Tomlins SA, et al. Recurrent fusion of TMPRSS2 and ETS transcription factor genes in prostate cancer. Science. 2005;310:644–8.
20. Fang L, et al. TMPRSS2-ERG promotes the initiation of prostate cancer by suppressing oncogene-induced senescence. Cancer Gene Ther. 2022;29:1463–76.
21. Hochhaus A, et al. Long-term outcomes of imatinib treatment for chronic myeloid leukemia. N Engl J Med. 2017;376:917.
22. Di Felice E, et al. The impact of introducing tyrosine kinase inhibitors on chronic myeloid leukemia survival: a population-based study. BMC Cancer. 2018;18:1069.
23. Manea CA, et al. A review of NTRK fusions in cancer. Ann Med Surg (Lond). 2022;79:103893.
24. Drilon A, et al. Efficacy of larotrectinib in TRK fusion–positive cancers in adults and children. N Engl J Med. 2018;378:731–9.
25. Maximiano S, Magalhães P, Guerreiro MP, Morgado M. Trastuzumab in the treatment of breast cancer. BioDrugs. 2016;30:75–86.
26. Zanti M, et al. Performance evaluation of pipelines for mapping, variant calling and interval padding, for the analysis of NGS germline panels. BMC Bioinformatics. 2021;22:218.
27. Li H, et al. The sequence alignment/map format and SAMtools. Bioinformatics. 2009;25:2078–9.
28. Liu F, et al. Systematic comparative analysis of single-nucleotide variant detection methods from single-cell RNA sequencing data. Genome Biol. 2019;20:242.
29. Quinn EM, et al. Development of strategies for SNP detection in RNA-seq data: application to lymphoblastoid cell lines and evaluation using 1000 Genomes data. PLoS One. 2013;8:e58815.
30. Lai Z, et al. VarDict: a novel and versatile variant caller for next-generation sequencing in cancer research. Nucleic Acids Res. 2016;44:e108.
31. Talevich E, Shain AH, Botton T, Bastian BC. CNVkit: genome-wide copy number detection and visualization from targeted DNA sequencing. PLoS Comput Biol. 2016;12:e1004873.
32. Landrum MJ, et al. ClinVar: public archive of relationships among sequence variation and human phenotype. Nucleic Acids Res. 2014;42:D980–5.
33. COSMIC: the Catalogue Of Somatic Mutations In Cancer. PubMed. https://pubmed.ncbi.nlm.nih.gov/30371878/.
34. Welcome to ClinGen. https://clinicalgenome.org/.
35. Richards S, et al. Standards and guidelines for the interpretation of sequence variants: a joint consensus recommendation of the American College of Medical Genetics and Genomics and the Association for Molecular Pathology. Genet Med. 2015;17:405–23.
36. Next-generation sequencing technologies: an overview. ScienceDirect. https://www.sciencedirect.com/science/article/pii/S0198885921000628?via%3Dihub.
37. Frangoul H, et al. CRISPR-Cas9 gene editing for sickle cell disease and β-thalassemia. N Engl J Med. 2021;384:252–60.
38. Stephens ZD, et al. Big data: astronomical or genomical? PLoS Biol. 2015;13:e1002195.
39. Zhang J, et al. The international cancer genome consortium data portal. Nat Biotechnol. 2019;37:367–9.
40. Armenia J, et al. The long tail of oncogenic drivers in prostate cancer. Nat Genet. 2018;50:645–51.
41. Scholl C, Fröhling S. Exploiting rare driver mutations for precision cancer medicine. Curr Opin Genet Dev. 2019;54:1–6.
42. Ghandi M, et al. Next-generation characterization of the cancer cell line encyclopedia. Nature. 2019;569:503–8.
43. Tsherniak A, et al. Defining a cancer dependency map. Cell. 2017;170:564–576.e16.
44. Gao J, et al. Integrative analysis of complex cancer genomics and clinical profiles using the cBioPortal. Sci Signal. 2013;6:pl1.
45. Sudlow C, et al. UK biobank: an open access resource for identifying the causes of a wide range of complex diseases of middle and old age. PLoS Med. 2015;12:e1001779.
46. Ramirez AH, et al. The All of Us Research Program: data quality, utility, and diversity. Patterns (NY). 2022;3:100570.
47. Mailman MD, et al. The NCBI dbGaP database of genotypes and phenotypes. Nat Genet. 2007;39:1181–6.
48. Tryka KA, et al. NCBI's database of genotypes and phenotypes: dbGaP. Nucleic Acids Res. 2014;42:D975–9.

49. DDBJ update: streamlining submission and access of human data. Nucleic Acids Res | Oxford Academic. https://academic.oup.com/nar/article/49/D1/D71/5958489.
50. Lappalainen I, et al. The European Genome-phenome Archive of human data consented for biomedical research. Nat Genet. 2015;47:692–5.
51. Zhang S-S, et al. GSA-human: genome sequence archive for human. Yi Chuan. 2021;43:988–93.
52. Bahadir CD, et al. Artificial intelligence applications in histopathology. Nat Rev Electr Eng. 2024;1:93–108.
53. Ahmad R. Reviewing the relationship between machines and radiology: the application of artificial intelligence. Acta Radiol Open. 2021;10:2058460121990296.
54. Challen R, et al. Artificial intelligence, bias and clinical safety. BMJ Qual Saf. 2019;28:231–7.
55. Khosravi P, et al. Deep learning enables robust assessment and selection of human blastocysts after in vitro fertilization. NPJ Digit Med. 2019;2:21.
56. Najjar R. Redefining radiology: a review of artificial intelligence integration in medical imaging. Diagnostics (Basel). 2023;13:2760.
57. McKinney SM, et al. International evaluation of an AI system for breast cancer screening. Nature. 2020;577:89–94.
58. Jumper J, et al. Highly accurate protein structure prediction with AlphaFold. Nature. 2021;596:583–9.
59. McCloskey K, et al. Machine learning on DNA-encoded libraries: a new paradigm for hit finding. J Med Chem. 2020;63:8857–66.
60. Stenzl A, et al. Application of artificial intelligence to overcome clinical information overload in urological cancer. BJU Int. 2022;130:291–300.
61. Dr. Eric Topol on How AI is transforming health and medicine. Clinical Center. https://www.cc.nih.gov/news/2024/nov-dec/eric-topol-ai.
62. Free C, et al. The effectiveness of mobile-health technology-based health behaviour change or disease management interventions for health care consumers: a systematic review. PLoS Med. 2013;10:e1001362.
63. Aung MH, Matthews M, Choudhury T. Sensing behavioral symptoms of mental health and delivering personalized interventions using mobile technologies. Depress Anxiety. 2017;34:603–9.
64. Aung MSH, et al. Leveraging multi-modal sensing for mobile health: a case review in chronic pain. IEEE J Sel Top Signal Process. 2016;10:962–74.
65. Azevedo RT, et al. The calming effect of a new wearable device during the anticipation of public speech. Sci Rep. 2017;7:2285.
66. Hu H-Z, et al. Application and prospect of mixed reality technology in medical field. Curr Med Sci. 2019;39:1–6.
67. Lungu AJ, et al. A review on the applications of virtual reality, augmented reality and mixed reality in surgical simulation: an extension to different kinds of surgery. Expert Rev Med Devices. 2021;18:47–62.
68. Samuel JP, Wootton SH, Tyson JE. N-of-1 trials: the epitome of personalized medicine? J Clin Transl Sci. 2023;7:e161.
69. Roy S, et al. Standards and guidelines for validating next-generation sequencing bioinformatics pipelines: a joint recommendation of the Association for Molecular Pathology and the College of American Pathologists. J Mol Diagn. 2018;20:4–27.
70. Ardila D, et al. End-to-end lung cancer screening with three-dimensional deep learning on low-dose chest computed tomography. Nat Med. 2019;25:954–61.
71. Gulshan V, et al. Development and validation of a deep learning algorithm for detection of diabetic retinopathy in retinal fundus photographs. JAMA. 2016;316:2402–10.
72. Peprah E, Wiley K, Sampson U, Narula J. A new age for African-driven genomics research: human heredity and health in Africa (H3Africa). Glob Heart. 2017;12:67–8.
73. China Kadoorie Biobank of 0.5 million people: survey methods, baseline characteristics and long-term follow-up. PubMed. https://pubmed.ncbi.nlm.nih.gov/22158673/.
74. Genotyping and population characteristics of the China Kadoorie Biobank. PubMed. https://pubmed.ncbi.nlm.nih.gov/37601966/.
75. Chong HY, Allotey PA, Chaiyakunapruk N. Current landscape of personalized medicine adoption and implementation in Southeast Asia. BMC Med Genet. 2018;11:94.
76. Bergström A, et al. Insights into human genetic variation and population history from 929 diverse genomes. Science. 2020;367:eaay5012.
77. Bick AG, et al. Genomic data in the All of Us Research Program. Nature. 2024;627:340–6.
78. Fatumo S, et al. A roadmap to increase diversity in genomic studies. Nat Med. 2022;28:243–50.

Translational Informatics

19

Philip Barrison and Rachel Richesson

Foundational Domains

This chapter addresses the following AMIA Foundational Domains: F1—Health, F3—Social and Behavioral Science, F7—Social, Behavioral, and Information Science Applied to Health.

Learning Objectives

After reading this chapter, you should be able to

1. Describe the knowledge-to-practice gap and identify barriers to reducing it.
2. Define the fields of translational science and informatics and explain their relationship with other fields or disciplines of health informatics.
3. Explain the translational research spectrum and its application to health informatics.
4. Understand the relationship between translational informatics and implementation science and identify relevant implementation frameworks.
5. Explain the relationship between translational informatics and learning health systems.

P. Barrison (✉)
Department of Learning Health Sciences, The University of Michigan Medical School, Ann Arbor, MI, USA

Medical Scientist Training Program, The University of Michigan Medical School, Ann Arbor, MI, USA
e-mail: phbarris@med.umich.edu

R. Richesson
Department of Learning Health Sciences, The University of Michigan Medical School, Ann Arbor, MI, USA
e-mail: richessr@med.umich.edu

19.1 Introduction

Over the past 50 years, research and innovation in health care have continued to accelerate at unprecedented rates. The doubling rate of medical knowledge (the amount of time it takes for the total amount of biomedical knowledge to double in size) has exponentially increased. It is estimated that in 1950 the doubling rate was 50 years, 7 years in 1980, 3.5 years in 2010, and just 73 days in 2020 [17]. Despite the rapid growth in new medical knowledge, it takes far longer for new scientific discoveries to make it to the patient's bedside. It has been estimated that, on average, it takes 17 years for scientific discoveries to be implemented into clinical practice [6, 28]. This delay is often referred to as the *knowledge-to-practice gap* or the *gap from bench-to-bedside* [36, 60]. While the rate of discovery in health care is moving at a record-breaking pace, this 17-year knowledge-to-practice gap remains stubbornly fixed. Healthcare systems, providers, and patients have been stuck in a growing ocean of biomedical knowledge, fighting to keep their heads above water and ensure that the care delivered is based on the best available evidence.

C. Eldredge et al. (eds.), *Introductory Textbook in Health Informatics*, Health Informatics,
https://doi.org/10.1007/978-3-032-16657-9_19

Translational science and its associated field in biomedical informatics, translational informatics, have emerged in response to the continued knowledge-to-practice gap. While the practice of translational informatics is complex and broad, its focus adheres to foundational principles related to data-driven evidence generation and practice change—more specifically, on using information technology to access data quickly and effectively from the clinical environment, facilitate new knowledge generation, and implement new knowledge into clinical practice. Translational informatics offers a diverse set of theories and methods that allow experts in health informatics to collaborate in multidisciplinary teams and work to reduce the knowledge-to-practice gap. In this chapter, we will explore how translational informatics emerged in the complex health informatics ecosystem, introduce some key frameworks and theories that guide translational informatics, and discuss future opportunities and challenges for experts looking to facilitate translational informatics research.

19.2 History: How Did We End Up Where We Are?

In the following section, we review why the knowledge-to-practice gap has become a significant obstacle, explore the origins of translational science, and discuss the motivating factors that have led to the development of translational informatics.

19.2.1 The Knowledge-to-Practice Gap

As we introduced at the outset of this chapter, the biomedical community is increasingly glutted by an influx of new knowledge that is often impossible for humans to keep pace with without the use of information technology and tools. Despite this massive influx of new knowledge, it still takes long periods for that knowledge to broadly influence how clinical medicine is practiced. This discrepancy between an increasing base of biomedical knowledge and the length of time it takes for that knowledge to make it into clinical practice means that healthcare systems and providers must struggle more than ever to assess the strength and integrity of evidence, determine its relevance, and make decisions on how it will change the way that they practice. The time from bench to bedside can be conceptualized as a pipeline with successive leakage points [29]. In the knowledge-to-practice pipeline, there are numerous steps along the way that slow down the ability for new knowledge to reach clinical practice. This process can be thought of as a series of leakage points in the flow of original research into practice. Leakage points can occur at multiple points across the knowledge-to-practice pipeline, as enumerated below:

- *From original research to journal submission.* Before research is published, various factors impact what research ideas are pursued and deemed worthy of publication. Funding mechanisms and funders' priorities, alongside the pressure of academic appointments, promotions, and tenure criteria on researchers, can influence what research is prioritized, what data is collected, and what knowledge is generated. Negative research results are often not prioritized and reported by investigators, and this "publication bias" can lead to duplication of work by new investigators unaware of previous efforts [19].
- *From submission to publication.* The peer-review process for academic journals provides a form of rigor that protects the internal validity of what gets published. However, decisions made by peer reviewers and journal editors may influence how results are reported and prioritized, along with decisions to deemphasize negative results, qualitative results, and results that do not conform to the gold standard of randomized controlled trials. This results in publication biases that do not accurately represent the extent of biomedical research being performed [10, 41].
- *From publication to implementation.* The longest part of the knowledge-to-practice pipeline. If newly discovered knowledge makes its way into a publication, many years may pass

before it is taken up for wide-scale use. This is influenced by the decision for that knowledge to be incorporated into reviews, guidelines, textbooks, and novel technologies, as well as the decision of knowledge users to adopt the new knowledge into clinical practice.

In the final stage of the knowledge-to-practice pipeline described above, many factors influence whether new knowledge, while valid, is considered and applied by its intended audience. It is incorrect to assume that just because knowledge is put out into the publishing landscape, end users, such as physicians, nurse practitioners, and other advanced practice and allied health professionals, will readily uptake that knowledge. This assumption is sometimes referred to as the *empty vessel fallacy*—the expectation that the end user is an empty vessel into which information and knowledge can be added and, once full, will spill over into action [29, 47]. The recipient of new knowledge approaches that knowledge with their preexisting experiences, value systems, attitudes, beliefs, and contextual constraints. Additional barriers to implementing knowledge include information limitations, clinical workload/workflows, underdeveloped implementation plans, inadequate training, organizational hurdles, and a lack of supporting infrastructure [44]. [Note that the complexities and challenges of moving knowledge into practice stimulated the development of a new research discipline, *Implementation Science*, which is the scientific study of methods and strategies to promote the systematic uptake of research findings and evidence-based practice by practitioners into routine practice [7].]

19.2.2 Translational Science

In recent decades, translational science has emerged and adapted to meet the growing demands of the knowledge-to-practice gap. Translational science is the process and rigorous study of bridging the gap between scientific studies and their practical applications in real-world healthcare settings [4, 15, 59]. Translational science includes work investigating scientific, operational, financial, and administrative innovations that transform research, altering its implementation and dissemination and improving its uptake rate into practice. In other words, translation science aims to investigate methods to minimize the time it takes for research discoveries to be used at the patient's bedside and for public health more broadly.

In 2012, the U.S. National Institutes of Health (NIH) established the *National Center for Advancing Translational Sciences* (NCATS) in an effort to address the cultural and infrastructural bottlenecks preventing the movement of biomedical knowledge into practice. The mission of NCATS was to act as a catalytic hub for generating innovative methods and technologies to enhance the development, evaluation, and implementation of diagnostics and therapeutics across health conditions [13]. Under NCATS, the Clinical and Translational Science Awards (CTSA) Program now supports more than 60 medical institutions attempting to advance clinical and translational science [37, 62].

The former director of NCATS, Christopher P. Austin, broadly defined biomedical translation as "the process of turning observation in the laboratory, clinic, and community into interventions that improve the health of individuals and the public" [4]. In summary, we can broadly define translational science as the field of investigation that seeks to understand the scientific and operational principles underlying each step of the translational process.

19.2.3 Translational Informatics

Translational science is inherently broad but can be further divided to better address the various types of work it encompasses. Translational informatics has arisen as one such subdivision of translational science. It is an interdisciplinary field at the intersection of health care, information technology, and biomedical research [45]. It focuses on harnessing the power of data, information systems, computational methods, and biomedical knowledge to facilitate the translation of scientific discoveries and findings into practical applications and solutions that can enhance healthcare delivery and improve patient outcomes. It is the practice of translational science through the lens of information science. In other words, translational informatics is the practice of using information technology to facilitate the work of translational science.

As a result, translational informatics focuses on effectively using data, information systems, computational methods, and computable biomedical knowledge to facilitate the translation of scientific discoveries and research findings into practical applications and solutions that improve healthcare delivery and patient outcomes. Translation informatics, hence, leverages tools and techniques from a variety of disciplines in health informatics to accomplish tasks across the research lifecycle, such as

- *Data querying, aggregation, and quality assessment.* Methods for accessing, retrieving, and verifying data quality from sources such as biorepositories, electronic health records, and patient registries.
- *Data integration and harmonization.* Tools and methods for combining data from multiple sources and unifying disparate data fields to ensure complete, accurate, and up-to-date data sets.
- *Hypothesis discovery and testing.* Working alongside experts in other health informatics and biomedical research domains to use health data to generate new knowledge from experimentation, modeling, and system development.
- *Knowledge management.* Tools and methods for stewarding computable biomedical knowledge generated as research products. Knowledge management methods account for the long-term findability, accessibility, interoperability, reusability, and trustworthiness of computable biomedical knowledge.
- *Knowledge implementation.* Using tools and theories from across the spectrum of implementation science, user-centered design, and human–computer interactions to facilitate the movement of computable biomedical knowledge into practice.

19.3 How Does Translational Informatics Relate to Other Disciplines of Health Informatics?

Translational informatics cannot stand alone. It is an inherently interdisciplinary field of health informatics that relies on theories and methods from across health informatics. There is a strong overlap between translational informatics and clinical informatics, clinical research informatics, and public health informatics. In each of these disciplines, translational informatics can play a role in integrating information technologies and novel computable biomedical knowledge generated by them into broader practice.

During its early inception, the field of translational informatics focused specifically on *translational bioinformatics*, which, in turn, focused specifically on the advancement of computable knowledge generated from biological and genomic data for diagnosis and drug discovery [57]. The field of translational informatics has since moved past this limited scope to cover the application and discovery of all kinds of evidence, resulting in applications ranging from guideline development, behavior interventions, technical platforms, and policy change.

As the premier professional society for informatics professionals, the American Medical Informatics Association (AMIA) should be a first stop for definitions of the subdomains of informatics and research and training around evolving methods and emerging topics (amia.org).

19.4 Theories and Frameworks to Support Translational Informatics

With a focus on developing evidence-based principles for ensuring appropriate clinical data acquisition, knowledge generation, and deployment of knowledge into wide-scale, context-sensitive use, theoretical frameworks are helpful for experts working in translational informatics to identify barriers and facilitators to their work, track their work overtime, and communicate the interests of their work across organizational stakeholders. In the following section, we describe some high-level theories and frameworks that can guide research teams and organizations as they approach novel questions that may require informatics solutions.

19.4.1 From Data to Information to Knowledge

The broad goal of all health and biomedical informatics is to transform raw data into information by providing relevant context, followed by the subsequent generation of actionable new knowledge [45]. All work in information science begins with *data*, which can be thought of as recorded words, numbers, diagrams, and images. On its own, data is meaningless. For example, if a group of information scientists is building a clinical decision support system, providing them with a list of numbers on their own has no value. In this case, they have raw data but no information to act on. With appropriate context, data becomes *information*. Suppose the same information scientists are now provided with additional context to the list of numbers they received, such as patient identifiers, units of measurement, and dates of data collection. In that case, they are now being provided with information. Meanwhile, *knowledge* results from deliberate and/or analytic processes in which individuals use information to draw new conclusions and insights into their world. With the available information in the data set, the information scientists may develop a new clinical decision support system for alerting doctors in the intensive care unit that a patient is at a higher risk of developing an acute kidney injury. The development of this new model is the development of new knowledge, and the clinical decision support system persists as an informatics tool to deliver that knowledge to a clinical user who can act upon it [63].

No matter the topic—genomics, clinical decision support, machine learning, natural language processing, or population health informatics—experts in information science must address and overcome the challenges inherent in moving across the data to information to knowledge spectrum. When experts agree on a task, questions must be resolved to understand how data will be acquired from a particular source, how enough context will be provided to yield sufficient information, and how the information will be used to make new and actionable knowledge.

New knowledge is often presented and disseminated in several different ways. Traditionally, knowledge would be spread through academic research papers and books. However, the outputs of informatics work frequently yield computable artifacts that may contain newly developed knowledge embedded in machine-readable (and often executable) formats that can be readily shared. This is referred to as *computable biomedical knowledge* (CBK). CBK is "the result of analytic and/or deliberative process about human health or affecting human health, that is explicit and, therefore, can be represented and reasoned upon using logic, formal standards, and mathematical approaches" [42]. Some examples of CBK include algorithms, clinical calculators, practice guidelines, message tailoring models, order sets, and predictive models [21].

Developing CBK is not the end of the story in informatics. After information technology experts develop CBK, many questions remain regarding the appropriate methods of validating, disseminating, implementing, and stewarding CBK. Ensuring that CBK is findable, accessible, interoperable, reusable, and trusted (FAIR-T) is a challenge that requires knowledge engineers to determine appropriate standards of knowledge representation and packaging, define adequate metadata, and ensure that there is sufficient infrastructure to support the management and dissemination of the CBK [1, 20, 35, 61].

19.4.2 The Translational Research Spectrum

As expressed up to this point, moving research into practice is a socio-technical problem within a complex health and IT ecosystem. Frameworks can help researchers, organizations, and policymakers disambiguate the different processes for developing new insights, generating evidence from research, and moving from data to knowledge to practice. One way of doing this is by using the five-category *translational research spectrum* outlined by the National Institute of Health (T0-T4) [22, 37]. This spectrum outlines the complexity of translation research, ranging from lab bench research to large-scale clinical implementation and public health outcomes. While there is some disagreement on the margins of each of the phases of the translational research spectrum, research under this spectrum can generally be categorized into one of five domains based on the overall goal and data sources (Table 19.1, column A). We use a similar framework of discovery to application to implementation at scale to describe the phases (activities and methods) of translational informatics (Table 19.1, column B).

Table 19.1 The translational research spectrum: a comparison of goals and data sources between translational science and translational informatics

Translational phase	Translational science	Translational informatics
T0—*Basic science discovery*	*Goal:* To uncover the "how" and "why" of biomedical discovery by investigating the foundational basic science of health and human disease. This may include investigating biochemical mechanisms and protein structures *Data source:* Data from wet lab, nonanimal research	*Goal:* In informatics, T0 research focuses on developing new computational health and human disease models. This includes developing computational models of physiology and pathology outside of a direct clinical use case *Data source:* Genomics, proteomics, metabolomics, EHR data, and patient registry data
T1—*Basic science to initial human testing*	*Goal:* Focuses on the early effectiveness of basic science models in humans to understand possible applications and implications of T0 research *Data source:* Data from animal model research	*Goal:* In informatics, T1 research explores the early application of computational knowledge to complete a certain task in patient care effectively. This is done in a low-stakes environment that will not directly impact clinical workflows or decision-making and focuses primarily on the targeted populations and use cases of a given intervention *Data source:* Retrospective collections of patient data and other relevant model inputs
T2—*Translation to patients*	*Goal:* Performance of early clinical trials to assess the efficacy of new biomedical interventions. During T2 research, investigators are interested in how interventions perform in the "ideal patient" and the general patient population they are targeting *Data source:* Data from clinical trials	*Goal:* In informatics, T2 research is focused on the early, prospective application of computable knowledge and technologies in the clinical care environment. It is concerned with seeing the direct primary outcome of the intended tool or intervention when provided to the intended end users *Data source:* Data from prospective tool, technology, or intervention effectiveness trials

(continued)

Table 19.1 (continued)

Translational phase	Translational science	Translational informatics
T3—*Translation to practice*	*Goal:* To understand the implementation and dissemination outcomes related to scientific discovery. While T0-T2 research heavily focuses on assessing the mechanisms, efficacy, and effectiveness of scientific findings, T3 research focuses more on understanding the context and mechanisms for best implementing and disseminating research outcomes *Data source:* Implementation data, often for large, multicenter hybrid design clinical trials	*Goal:* To understand the implementation and dissemination outcomes of informatics interventions and computable biomedical knowledge. Rather than focusing on the effectiveness of a tool, such as a model, researchers are interested in learning more about the socio-technical factors that impact its use, uptake, and efficacy *Data source:* Data from studies of implementation science, user experience, and human–computer interactions
T4—*Translation to communities*	*Goal:* T4 research focuses on large-scale outcomes and the effectiveness of interventions at the population level. It requires scientific interventions to be disseminated and implemented across a large population. This allows researchers to better understand the long-term impacts of interventions across diverse groups of people and inform guidelines and policies based on these outcomes *Data source:* Population health data, including data from electronic health records, patient registries, and insurance companies	*Goal:* In informatics, T4 research focuses on the large-scale outcomes and effectiveness of informatics interventions and technologies at the population level. The technology or computable knowledge has to be widely adopted and implemented into more extensive socio-technical infrastructures to be able to adequate assess for the long-term impacts of informatics interventions *Data source:* Population health data, including data from electronic health records, patient registries, and insurance companies

Although the translational research spectrum presented in Table 19.1 is often represented with discrete and linear phases, in reality, these practices intersect without clearly defined margins. Additionally, the goals and data sources for translational science are not mutually exclusive to the goals and data sources of translational informatics. Translational informatics may also aid researchers in completing tasks across the translational science spectrum, as was traditionally the case in its original inception as translational bioinformatics. Researchers may frequently move iteratively back and forth between stages of the translational research spectrum. In many cases, researchers may work in one or two of these phases of the research spectrum. Siloed from the larger context in which their work evolves over time. Breaking down these silos and ensuring that organizations and research communities can map their efforts to this pipeline is an essential aspect of translation science [39].

19.4.3 Data Quality for Translational Informatics

Whether biological or clinical researchers are working on early foundational research (T0/1/2) or exploring implementation and public health outcomes (T3/4), the data's relevance, quality, and integrity are essential. The first step any investigator needs to take is to access the appropriate data and assess its fitness. Researchers need to determine not only what data is necessary to approach the problem they seek to solve but also what additional context is necessary to yield sufficient information. Whether that data is coming from pathology records of biopsy specimens, live data from the electronic health record, or large population registries, researchers must wrestle with not only ensuring that the data they desire is available but that the data quality is sufficient to ensure highly reliable, replicable, and trustworthy results. This is where informatics professionals can contribute to supporting the science of translation, new discoveries, and knowledge/evidence generation in informatics itself.

Data quality is broadly defined as fitness for use [46]. The National Academy of Medicine defines data quality as "data strong enough to support conclusions and interpretations equivalent to those derived from error-free data" [33]. Data quality may be impacted by data accuracy, consistency, completeness, contextual validity, accessibility, and currency [56]. Electronic health record data is notorious for lacking accuracy, consistency, and completeness. This is due to multiple challenges, including constraints placed on end users by data entry processes, the predominance of natural language text fields across the EHR, inconsistent and variable workflows among healthcare providers, variable expectations regarding best practices for data entry, and human error [31]. Other forms of patient-related health data, such as patient-reported outcomes and patient registries, may present unique data quality issues that information scientists must grapple with when determining the best approaches to ensuring accurate and usable data [2, 12, 27].

Methods for ensuring data quality are discussed in this book's separate chapter. To learn more about methods for ensuring data quality, consult Chap. 30 on Data Management.

19.4.4 Implementation Science

Translational science, and hence translational informatics, overlaps with another emerging and rapidly evolving field, implementation science. *Implementation science* is the systematic study of best practices for implementing and disseminating scientific discoveries into practice [7]. Regarding translational informatics, implementation science concerns how CBK can best be moved from online repositories and publications to clinical acceptance and use. Implementation science divides the work of implementation into various areas of study, each with its own frameworks, theories, and models [43]. While the exact details of these theories and methods are beyond the scope of this chapter, we would like to briefly introduce three of the foundational theoretical approaches of implementation science.

Process models are used to describe or guide the process of translation. They often specify the steps that need to be taken to implement knowledge into practice and can be helpful when looking for ways to structure implementation projects. One of the most widely used process frameworks is the Implementation Research Logic Model (IRLM), which breaks down the implementation processes into the assessment of determinants, selection of implementation strategies, description of implementation strategy mechanisms, and selection of implementation outcomes [55]. While models like the IRLM are broadly applicable to any topic in health care, other process models are more specific. For example, the SALIENT framework is explicitly for outlining the process of implementing clinical artificial intelligence into practice [58].

Determinant frameworks explore the barriers and facilitators that may influence stakeholders' decisions regarding intervention uptake and implementation outcomes. Classic determinant frameworks include the Consolidated Framework for Implementation Research (CFIR) [16] and the Theoretical Domains Framework (TDF) [3]. Similar to process models, informatics-specific determinant frameworks have been created, such as the Behavior and Acceptance Framework (BEAR), which is designed to help investigators assess barriers and facilitators to implementing clinical decision support systems [11].

Evaluation frameworks specify aspects of implementation that should be evaluated to determine the "success" of implementation. Evaluation frameworks often differentiate implementation outcomes from effectiveness outcomes. *Effectiveness outcomes* can be thought of as outcomes that focus on outcomes directly related to the intervention, answering questions such as, Did the intervention work? What are the possible side effects of the intervention? Who did the intervention perform best for?

Effectiveness outcomes are often associated with the T0–T2 phases of the translational research spectrum. *Implementation outcomes* concern the reach, adoption, implementation, and sustainability of interventions. Commonly used frameworks for outlining implementation outcomes include the RE-AIM framework [26] and the Proctor framework [49].

19.4.5 Learning Health Systems

The interdisciplinary breadth of translational science and informatics raises the question, "How can health systems best incorporate translational informatics in a way that utilizes the interdisciplinary nature of the field to best improve the health system's ability to provide up-to-date, high-quality evidence in their clinical practice?" While translational informatics can be embedded across various research teams, information technology teams, and research teams in a health system, to reach its true potential, it must be organized in a way that reaches across stakeholders in an organization to help facilitate improvements in health care. One proposed way to do this that has garnered attention in recent years is the learning health system (LHS).

An LHS is an organization that is committed to continuous learning that improves its ability to provide evidence-based health care [23]. The Institute of Medicine and its successor, the National Academy of Medicine, have promoted the following broad definition of learning health systems:

> In a learning health care system, science, informatics, incentives, and culture are aligned for continuous improvement and innovation, with best practices seamlessly embedded in the delivery process; patients and family are active participants in all elements; and new knowledge is captured as an integral by-product of the delivery experience. [14]

An LHS is committed to performing continuous *learning cycles* in which the organization identifies a problem of interest, collects data, generates knowledge from that data, moves that knowledge into practice, and continues to collect data about that intervention after it has been implemented to inform continued improvement. In other words, LHSs are built on continuous cycles of practice-to-data (P → D), data-to-knowledge (D → K), knowledge-to-practice (K → P), and practice-back-to-data (P → D) (Fig. 19.1).

To carry out successful learning cycles, robust social and technical infrastructure services need to be interconnected to support the continuous actions of data acquisition, knowledge generation, and knowledge implementation [25]. This infrastructure includes the people, policies, technologies, and processes that support the goals of the LHS. Importantly, this infrastructure should be multiuse and support multiple successive learning cycles around different problems/interventions that occur at the same time. The sociotechnical infrastructural services aligning with and supporting each stage of the improvement cycle include: [24]

1. Services supporting the development and function of learning communities (communities of practice dedicated to improving health care quality around a central topic(s))
2. Services to develop and apply tools that measure performance and performance outcomes
3. Services to provide health information as analyzable data
4. Services to enable and govern access to and use of data
5. Services to share and analyze data
6. Services to access and evaluate external knowledge
7. Services to merge and interpret internal and external knowledge
8. Services to codify and persist new knowledge in human and computer-readable forms
9. Services to enable the delivery of knowledge-directed interventions
10. Services to promote and support performance changes

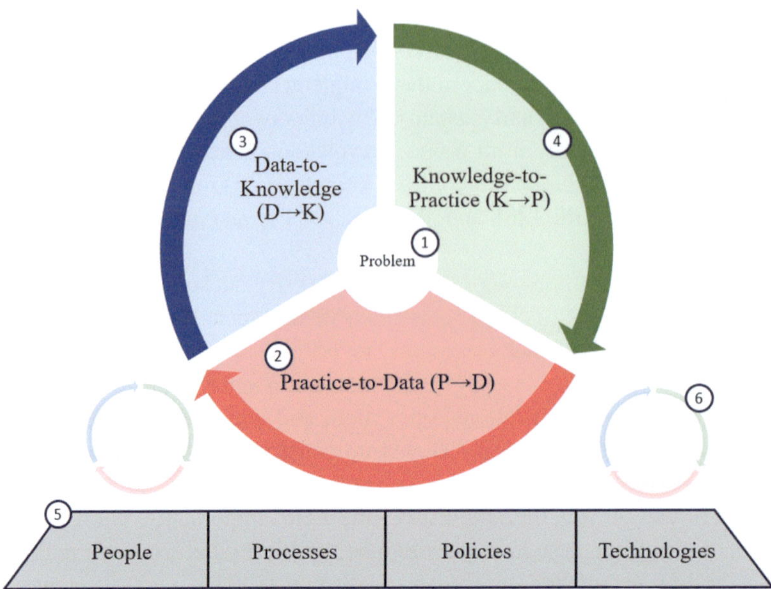

Fig. 19.1 Learning Health Systems [LHSs] can be conceptualized as continuous cycles. In an LHS, a community of practice comes together around a common problem in healthcare (1). This community of practice seeks to continuously generate knew knowledge (3), move that knowledge into practice (4), and evaluate and derive knew data from practice (2). By combining various infrastructural services, including combinations of people, processes, policies, and technologies (5), an LHS can work to facilitate continuous learning and improvement. These infrastructural services may be organized in such a way to allow for them to support multiple learning cycles performed around different healthcare problems (6)

The technologies, people, processes, and policies supporting each of these services may vary between LHSs. Experts in translational informatics can contribute to developing these services by bringing expertise in data quality, data integration, model development, knowledge management, knowledge stewardship, and implementation science.

19.5 Example: Preventing Pediatric Falls; A Learning Health System

Pediatric falls and fall-related injuries in healthcare facilities have been identified as a significant sentinel event responsible for pediatric morbidity and mortality [48]. More than half of the reported falls in the hospital result in injuries [38, 50, 53].

A group of doctors, nurses, patient advocates, and quality improvement experts at a major Midwestern Health Center are interested in developing an LHS dedicated to reducing pediatric fall rates. One intervention of interest among this emergent LHS is developing and implementing a fall risk prediction model. Many existing pediatric fall risk prediction models have been developed independently by different health systems, with minimal external validation [34]. Additionally, many of these models are based on metrics for adult fall risk assessment tools, which raises concerns because many of the risk factors for pediatric patients are unique [18]. Due to these concerns, the emergent LHS is interested in developing its own risk prediction model. The newly minted LHS decides to partner with a team of information scientists to explore how to create the necessary technical infrastructure to support improvement cycles related to this goal.

Some of the technical hurdles the LHS will have to work with the information technology to overcome include

- *P → D:* The team will have to identify the necessary data to collect to understand the current fall rates in their health system, assess trends over time, and develop a helpful fall prediction model. This data may include data from the EHR such as patient fall rates, fall rate stratified by unit, date of falls, patient identifiers for each fall, carefully selected patient characteristics that may influence fall rate, and any other data the LHS finds important. Information technologists will have to work to understand the appropriate pipelines and governance processes for reliably and consistently accessing this data, assessing data quality, and providing it to the necessary parties.
- *D → K*: The team will have to develop a new model for fall prediction. This may include interdisciplinary collaboration between information scientists, data analysts, and domain experts (such as pediatricians and nurses) to guide the development and in vivo development of models.
- *K → P:* Once the team has developed a fall prediction model, they will have to work together to create an implementation plan for integrating the model into the existing IT stack running at their children's hospital, outline effectiveness and implementation outcomes, and develop the necessary procedures for implementing and using the new fall prediction model.

By the time the LHS has completed an initial learning cycle from data to knowledge to practice, its work has only just begun. It is now imperative for the LHS to continue evaluating how their computable knowledge is performing in practice and continuing through successive learning cycles to ensure the sustainability and improvement of their intervention. The infrastructure that information technologists have networked to support these tasks should be robust enough to be reused under various circumstances so that the LHS can more effectively complete future learning cycles.

19.6 Opportunities and Challenges for the Future of Translational Informatics

Despite the potential for translational informatics to improve the rate of integrating scientific knowledge into practice, an ever-stubborn, multi-year knowledge-to-practice gap persists. As discussed in this chapter, various barriers exist in the knowledge-to-practice pipeline that result in the leakage of scientific evidence and delay the translation of new knowledge into practice. These barriers are deeply entrenched in existing practices around the publication, stewardship, and adoption of new biomedical knowledge and will require interdisciplinary collaboration and system-level thinking to overcome.

Despite the large-scale adoption of electronic health records and other health information technology into the healthcare ecosystem since the turn of the twenty-first century, the healthcare ecosystem remains plagued by disparate information technology ecosystems [32]. The limited interoperability between information technology systems has been a persistent problem facing healthcare systems and can severely limit the ability of experts in translational informatics to access high-quality data successfully; integrate and harmonize data sets across IT stacks; perform timely hypothesis testing; implement computable biomedical knowledge back into the local IT environment; and ensure their computable biomedical knowledge is findable, accessible, interoperable, and reusable [9].

Developing and adopting standards are important areas of work that will be critical to enabling translational informatics. Data standards cover a wide variety of applications and uses. Whether it be common data models, such as OMOP [51], exchange standards, such as HL7 FHIR [5], or more domain-specific standards, such as LOINC for lab data [40] or ICD-10 for diagnostic codes [30], standards can play a valuable role in ensuring data and computable knowledge are interoperable and easily accessible [See Chap. 23-Introduction to standards and interoperability for more information on data standards]. Despite the increased adoption of such standards, such as HL7 FHIR in the wake of the twenty-first Century Cures Act [52], we are still far from true interoperability among IT systems in the healthcare setting. Many IT professionals and researchers have commented on the persistent challenges of assigning labels associated with implementing HL7 FHIR [54]. These challenges are not specific to HL7 FHIR but instead reflect more considerable challenges in the development and implementation of standards [8].

The vision of LHSs offers a potential route for integrating translational informatics as an operationalized part of healthcare organizations. However, the disparate nature of health information technologies presents an infrastructural challenge to developing LHSs. Before the reality of LHSs can be realized, work needs to be done to identify the socio-technical services (people, processes, technologies, and workflows) that can facilitate learning health activities. Currently, many of these services exist in isolation, with early work being done to provide standard methods for linking services. Translational informatics can play a crucial role in building out these services to better facilitate translating knowledge into practice.

19.7 Future Directions

The need for high-quality evidence to answer pressing clinical questions is growing. Consequently, the need for informatics professionals throughout knowledge generation and implementation, from T0 to T4 research, is immense. Translational informatics can play important roles in the emergence of pragmatic clinical trials, precision medicine, and learning health systems. Many future career opportunities will present themselves for experts in translational informatics looking to make an impact in these fields, among many others in health care. While the challenges facing the reduction of the knowledge-to-practice gap are immense, these challenges also provide bountiful areas for future investigation for informaticians interested in translational informatics.

References

1. Alper BS, Flynn A, Bray BE, Conte ML, Eldredge C, Gold S, Greenes RA, Haug P, Jacoby K, Koru G, McClay J, Sainvil ML, Sottara D, Tuttle M, Visweswaran S, Yurk RA. Categorizing metadata to help mobilize computable biomedical knowledge. Learn Health Syst. 2021;6:e10271. https://doi.org/10.1002/lrh2.10271.
2. Arts DGT, de Keizer NF, Scheffer G-J. Defining and improving data quality in medical registries: a literature review, case study, and generic framework. J Am Med Inform Assoc. 2002;9:600–11. https://doi.org/10.1197/jamia.M1087.
3. Atkins L, Francis J, Islam R, O'Connor D, Patey A, Ivers N, Foy R, Duncan EM, Colquhoun H, Grimshaw JM, Lawton R, Michie S. A guide to using the theoretical domains framework of behaviour change to investigate implementation problems. Implement Sci. 2017;12:77. https://doi.org/10.1186/s13012-017-0605-9.
4. Austin CP. Translating translation. Nat Rev Drug Discov. 2018;17:455–6. https://doi.org/10.1038/nrd.2018.27.
5. Ayaz M, Pasha MF, Alzahrani MY, Budiarto R, Stiawan D. The fast health interoperability resources (FHIR) standard: systematic literature review of implementations, applications, challenges and opportunities. JMIR Med Inform. 2021;9:e21929. https://doi.org/10.2196/21929.
6. Balas EA, Weingarten S, Garb CT, Blumenthal D, Boren SA, Brown GD. Improving preventive care by prompting physicians. Arch Intern Med. 2000;160:301–8. https://doi.org/10.1001/archinte.160.3.301.
7. Bauer MS, Kirchner J. Implementation science: what is it and why should I care? Psychiatry Res. 2020;283:112376. https://doi.org/10.1016/j.psychres.2019.04.025.
8. Bowker G, Star SL. Sorting things out: classification and its consequences. The MIT Press; 2000.
9. Braunstein ML. Health Care in the age of interoperability: the potential and challenges. IEEE Pulse. 2018;9:34–6. https://doi.org/10.1109/MPUL.2018.2856941.
10. Callaham M, Wears RL, Weber E. Journal prestige, publication bias, and other characteristics associated with citation of published studies in peer-reviewed journals. JAMA. 2002;287:2847–50. https://doi.org/10.1001/jama.287.21.2847.
11. Camacho J, Zanoletti-Mannello M, Landis-Lewis Z, Kane-Gill SL, Boyce RD. A conceptual framework to study the implementation of clinical decision support systems (BEAR): literature review and concept mapping. J Med Internet Res. 2020;22:e18388. https://doi.org/10.2196/18388.
12. Chang EM, Gillespie EF, Shaverdian N. Truthfulness in patient-reported outcomes: factors affecting patients' responses and impact on data quality. Patient

Relat Outcome Meas. 2019;10:171–86. https://doi.org/10.2147/PROM.S178344.

13. Collins FS. Reengineering translational science: the time is right. Sci Transl Med. 2011;3:90cm17-90cm17. https://doi.org/10.1126/scitranslmed.3002747.
14. Committee on the Learning Health Care System in America, Institute of Medicine. Best care at lower cost: the path to continuously learning health care in America. Washington (DC): National Academies Press (US); 2013.
15. Curry SH. Translational science: past, present, and future. BioTechniques. 2008;44:ii–viii. https://doi.org/10.2144/000112749.
16. Damschroder LJ, Reardon CM, Widerquist MAO, Lowery J. The updated consolidated framework for implementation research based on user feedback. Implement Sci. 2022;17:75. https://doi.org/10.1186/s13012-022-01245-0.
17. Densen P. Challenges and opportunities facing medical education. Trans Am Clin Climatol Assoc. 2011;122:48–58.
18. DiGerolamo K, Davis KF. An integrative review of pediatric fall risk assessment tools. J Pediatr Nurs. 2017;34:23–8. https://doi.org/10.1016/j.pedn.2017.02.036.
19. Fanelli D. Negative results are disappearing from most disciplines and countries. Scientometrics. 2011;90(2012):891–904. https://doi.org/10.1007/s11192-011-0494-7.
20. Flynn A, Conte M, Boisvert P, Richesson R, Landis-Lewis Z, Friedman C. Linked metadata for FAIR digital objects carrying computable Knowledge. RIO. 2022;8:e94438. https://doi.org/10.3897/rio.8.e94438.
21. Flynn A, Shi W, Fischer R, Friedman C. Digital knowledge objects and digital knowledge object clusters: unit holdings in a learning health system knowledge repository, In: Annual Hawaii international conference on system sciences (HICSS). Presented at the 2016 49th annual Hawaii international conference on system sciences (HICSS). 2016.
22. Fort DG, Herr TM, Shaw PL, Gutzman KE, Starren JB. Mapping the evolving definitions of translational research. J Clin Transl Sci. 2017;1:60–6. https://doi.org/10.1017/cts.2016.10.
23. Friedman C, Rubin J, Brown J, Buntin M, Corn M, Etheredge L, Gunter C, Musen M, Platt R, Stead W, Sullivan K, Van Houweling D. Toward a science of learning systems: a research agenda for the high-functioning learning health system. J Am Med Inform Assoc. 2015;22:43–50. https://doi.org/10.1136/amiajnl-2014-002977.
24. Friedman CP, Lomotan EA, Richardson JE, Ridgeway JL. Socio-technical infrastructure for a learning health system. Learn Health Syst. 2024;8:e10405. https://doi.org/10.1002/lrh2.10405.
25. Friedman CP, Macy J. Infrastructure and the learning health system. Learn Health Syst. 2022;8(1):e10405.
26. Glasgow RE, Vogt TM, Boles SM. Evaluating the public health impact of health promotion interventions: the RE-AIM framework. Am J Public Health. 1999;89:1322–7. https://doi.org/10.2105/ajph.89.9.1322.
27. Gliklich RE, Leavy MB, Dreyer NA. Obtaining data and quality assurance, in: registries for evaluating patient outcomes: a user's guide [Internet]. 4th ed. Agency for Healthcare Research and Quality (US); 2020.
28. Green LW. Closing the chasm between research and practice: evidence of and for change. Health Promot J Austr. 2014;25:25–9. https://doi.org/10.1071/HE13101.
29. Green LW. Making research relevant: if it is an evidence-based practice, where's the practice-based evidence? Fam Pract. 2008;25:i20–4. https://doi.org/10.1093/fampra/cmn055.
30. Hirsch JA, Nicola G, McGinty G, Liu RW, Barr RM, Chittle MD, Manchikanti L. ICD-10: history and context. Am J Neuroradiol. 2016;37:596–9. https://doi.org/10.3174/ajnr.A4696.
31. Honeyford K, Expert P, Mendelsohn EE, Post B, Faisal AA, Glampson B, Mayer EK, Costelloe CE. Challenges and recommendations for high quality research using electronic health records. Front Digit Health. 2022;4:940330. https://doi.org/10.3389/fdgth.2022.940330.
32. Information Technology and the U.S. Workforce: Where Are We and Where Do We Go from Here?. National Academies Press, Washington, DC.. 2017. https://doi.org/10.17226/24649.
33. Institute of Medicine (US) Roundtable on Research and Development of Drugs, Biologics, and Medical Devices, 1999. Assuring data quality and validity in clinical trials for regulatory decision making: workshop report. National Academies Press (US), Washington (DC).
34. Kim E-J, Kim G-M, Lim J-Y. A systematic review and meta-analysis of fall prevention programs for pediatric inpatients. Int J Environ Res Public Health. 2021;18:5853. https://doi.org/10.3390/ijerph18115853.
35. Lamprecht A-L, Garcia L, Kuzak M, Martinez C, Arcila R, Martin Del Pico E, Dominguez Del Angel V, van de Sandt S, Ison J, Martinez PA, McQuilton P, Valencia A, Harrow J, Psomopoulos F, Gelpi JL, Chue Hong N, Goble C, Capella-Gutierrez S. Towards FAIR principles for research software. DS. 2020;3:37–59. https://doi.org/10.3233/DS-190026.
36. Lang ES, Wyer PC, Haynes RB. Knowledge translation: closing the evidence-to-practice gap. Ann Emerg Med. 2007;49:355–63. https://doi.org/10.1016/j.annemergmed.2006.08.022.
37. Leshner AI, Terry SF, Shultz AM, Liverman CT. The CTSA program at NIH: opportunities for advancing clinical and translational research. National Academies Press; 2013.
38. Levene S, Bonfield G. Accidents on hospital wards. Arch Dis Child. 1991;66:1047–9. https://doi.org/10.1136/adc.66.9.1047.
39. Luke DA, Carothers BJ, Dhand A, Bell RA, Moreland-Russell S, Sarli CC, Evanoff BA. Breaking down silos: mapping growth of cross-disciplinary collaboration in a translational science initiative. Clin Transl Sci. 2015;8:143–9. https://doi.org/10.1111/cts.12248.

40. McDonald CJ, Huff SM, Suico JG, Hill G, Leavelle D, Aller R, Forrey A, Mercer K, DeMoor G, Hook J, Williams W, Case J, Maloney P, for the Laboratory LOINC Developers. LOINC, a universal standard for identifying laboratory observations: a 5-year update. Clin Chem. 2003;49:624–33. https://doi.org/10.1373/49.4.624.
41. Mlinarić A, Horvat M, Šupak Smolčić V. Dealing with the positive publication bias: why you should really publish your negative results. Biochem Med. 2017;27:447–52. https://doi.org/10.11613/BM.2017.030201.
42. Mobilizing Computable Biomedical Knowledge (MCBK) [WWW Document], 2023. MCBK. https://mobilizecbk.med.umich.edu/home. Accessed 21 Jan 23.
43. Nilsen P. Making sense of implementation theories, models and frameworks. Implement Sci. 2015;10:53. https://doi.org/10.1186/s13012-015-0242-0.
44. Parmar J, Sacrey LA, Anderson S, Charles L, Dobbs B, McGhan G, Shapkin K, Tian P, Triscott J. Facilitators, barriers and considerations for the implementation of healthcare innovation: a qualitative rapid systematic review. Health Soc Care Community. 2022;30:856–68. https://doi.org/10.1111/hsc.13578.
45. Payne P, Embi P. An introduction to translational informatics and the future of knowledge-driven healthcare. In: Translational informatics. London: Springer-Verlag; 2015. p. 3–19.
46. Pipino LL, Wang RY, Funk JD, Lee YW. Journey to data quality. The MIT Press; 2006.
47. Polgar S, Freeman H, Levine S, Reader L. Health actions in cross-cultural perspectives. In: Handbook of medical sociology. Englewood Cliffs: Prentice Hall; 1963.
48. Preventing falls and fall-related injuries in healthcare facilities (No. 55), 2015. Sentinal event alert. The Joint Commission.
49. Proctor E, Silmere H, Raghavan R, Hovmand P, Aarons G, Bunger A, Griffey R, Hensley M. Outcomes for implementation research: conceptual distinctions, measurement challenges, and research agenda. Admin Pol Ment Health. 2011;38:65–76. https://doi.org/10.1007/s10488-010-0319-7.
50. Razmus I, Davis D. The epidemiology of falls in hospitalized children. Pediatr Nurs. 2012;38:31–5.
51. Reinecke I, Zoch M, le, Reich C, Sedlmayr M, Bathelt F. The usage of OHDSI OMOP—a scoping review. In: German medical data sciences 2021: digital medicine: recognize—understand—heal. IOS Press; 2021. p. 95–103. https://doi.org/10.3233/SHTI210546.
52. Rep. Bonamici, S. [D-O.-1, 2016. H.R.34 - 114th Congress (2015–2016): 21st century cures act [WWW Document]. http://www.congress.gov/. Accessed 24 Feb 23.
53. Schaffer PL, Daraiseh NM, Daum L, Mendez E, Lin L, Huth MM. Pediatric inpatient falls and injuries: a descriptive analysis of risk factors. J Spec Pediatr Nurs. 2012;17:10–8. https://doi.org/10.1111/j.1744-6155.2011.00315.x.
54. Setyawan R, Hidayanto AN, Sensuse DI, Kautsarina, Suryono RR, Abilowo K. Data integration and interoperability problems of HL7 FHIR implementation and potential solutions: a systematic literature review. In: 2021 5th international conference on informatics and computational sciences (ICICoS). Presented at the 2021 5th International Conference on Informatics and Computational Sciences (ICICoS); 2021. p. 293–8. https://doi.org/10.1109/ICICoS53627.2021.9651762.
55. Smith JD, Li DH, Rafferty MR. The implementation research logic model: a method for planning, executing, reporting, and synthesizing implementation projects. Implement Sci. 2020;15:84. https://doi.org/10.1186/s13012-020-01041-8.
56. Syed R, Eden R, Makasi T, Chukwudi I, Mamudu A, Kamalpour M, Kapugama Geeganage D, Sadeghianasl S, Leemans SJJ, Goel K, Andrews R, Wynn MT, ter Hofstede A, Myers T. Digital health data quality issues: systematic review. J Med Internet Res. 2023;25:e42615. https://doi.org/10.2196/42615.
57. Tenenbaum JD. Translational bioinformatics: past, present, and future. Genomics Proteomics Bioinformatics. 2016;14:31–41. https://doi.org/10.1016/j.gpb.2016.01.003.
58. van der Vegt AH, Scott IA, Dermawan K, Schnetler RJ, Kalke VR, Lane PJ. Implementation frameworks for end-to-end clinical AI: derivation of the SALIENT framework. J Am Med Inform Assoc. 2023;30:1503–15. https://doi.org/10.1093/jamia/ocad088.
59. Waldman SA, Terzic A. Clinical and translational science: from bench-bedside to Global Village. Clin Transl Sci. 2010;3:254–7. https://doi.org/10.1111/j.1752-8062.2010.00227.x.
60. Westerlund A, Nilsen P, Sundberg L. Implementation of implementation science Knowledge: the research-practice gap paradox. Worldviews Evid-Based Nurs. 2019;16:332–4. https://doi.org/10.1111/wvn.12403.
61. Wilkinson MD, Dumontier M, Aalbersberg IJ, Appleton G, Axton M, Baak A, Blomberg N, Boiten J-W, da Silva Santos LB, Bourne PE, Bouwman J, Brookes AJ, Clark T, Crosas M, Dillo I, Dumon O, Edmunds S, Evelo CT, Finkers R, Gonzalez-Beltran A, Gray AJG, Groth P, Goble C, Grethe JS, Heringa J, 't Hoen PAC, Hooft R, Kuhn T, Kok R, Kok J, Lusher SJ, Martone ME, Mons A, Packer AL, Persson B, Rocca-Serra P, Roos M, van Schaik R, Sansone S-A, Schultes E, Sengstag T, Slater T, Strawn G, Swertz MA, Thompson M, van der Lei J, van Mulligen E, Velterop J, Waagmeester A, Wittenburg P, Wolstencroft K, Zhao J, Mons B. The FAIR guiding principles for scientific data management and stewardship. Sci Data. 2016;3:160018. https://doi.org/10.1038/sdata.2016.18.
62. Zerhouni EA. Translational and clinical science — time for a new vision. N Engl J Med. 2005;353:1621–3. https://doi.org/10.1056/NEJMsb053723.
63. Zins C. Conceptual approaches for defining data, information, and knowledge. J Am Soc Inf Sci Technol. 2007;58:479–93. https://doi.org/10.1002/asi.20508.

Patient Safety

20

Harrison Mohr, Julie K. Johnson, and Paul Barach

Foundational Domains

This chapter addresses the following AMIA Foundational Domains: F1—Health, F5—Human Factors and Sociotechnical Systems.

Learning Objectives

After reading this chapter, you should be able to.

1. Define patient safety and become aware of its impact on global health.
2. Understand key tools and frameworks for assessing and improving patient safety.
3. Identify illustrative examples of how patient harm may occur in the context of health informatics technologies.
4. Describe the relationship of patient safety to other areas of healthcare and health informatics.
5. Consider how the changing technological landscape will create new opportunities and challenges for the future of patient safety.

H. Mohr
Illinois Institute of Technology, Chicago, IL, USA

J. K. Johnson
Northwestern University Feinberg School of Medicine, Chicago, IL, USA

P. Barach (✉)
Thomas Jefferson University, Philadelphia, PA, USA

Imperial College, London, UK

University of North Carolina, Chapel Hill, USA

The medical profession has become a major threat to health.
—Ivan Illich, 1977, *Limits of Medicine*

20.1 Introduction

Imagine it is your first day on the job as a health informatics consultant for a regional healthcare system. You just completed a coveted degree in clinical informatics and you walk into the office excited to tackle your employer's most pressing data science problems. You feel confident, armed with your polished toolkit of regression models, neural networks, and data visualization proficiencies. Your new boss greets you warmly and then details your first project. The healthcare system has had a series of adverse patient events that led to significant patient harm and the clinicians blame the electronic medical record. Your boss asks you to uncover the root causes of the problem and use a data-driven approach to implement a systemic change in the use of medical records to help stop further patient harm. Your boss asks you to assess your solution for the potential risks of causing future patient harm and wants you to outline recommendations related to common frameworks for medical harm reduction. You are taken off guard and are at a loss for how to connect your newly honed data analysis skills to this real world problem.

Your boss looks at you for a few moments of awkward silence and then says, "So what do you know about patient safety?" It is at this moment

C. Eldredge et al. (eds.), *Introductory Textbook in Health Informatics*, Health Informatics,
https://doi.org/10.1007/978-3-032-16657-9_20

that you realize that without a thorough understanding of the systemic factors leading to patient harm and listening to the lived experience of patients and hospital staff, and even with your data analytic skills there are still glaring gaps in your understanding of how to improve outcomes for patients. You walk to your cubicle and download a textbook chapter on patient safety for health informatics.

The Agency for Healthcare Research and Quality (AHRQ) defines patient safety as the "freedom from accidental or preventable injuries produced by medical care" (Table 20.1) [36]. Thus, practices or interventions that improve patient safety are those that reduce the occurrence of preventable adverse events. Adverse events and medical errors are healthcare's most pervasive violation of the Hippocratic Oath, medicine's foundational tenet of "first do no harm." Such events cause physical and psychological trauma to patients as well as a severe waste of economic resources [52]. Extensive data illustrate the pervasive impact of medical errors on global health outcomes. For example, multiple studies have found that nearly 1 in 10 hospitalized patients experiences adverse events, with approximately half of these events considered preventable [16]. Furthermore, medical errors are one of the leading causes of death in America, with only cancer and heart disease being more prevalent [28]. Finally, medical errors are expensive. One report found that the added claim costs due to 62,000 medical errors in Massachusetts over 1 year was $617 million ([7]). Therefore, improving patient safety is a critical point of leverage for improving global health and societal outcomes.

In Table 20.1, you will find definitions of key terms related to patient safety.

Health informatics pursues the effective uses of biomedical data, information, and knowledge for scientific inquiry, problem-solving, and decision-making, motivated by efforts to improve human health arising from revolutions in computational and communication technologies [5].

Table 20.1 Classification of patient safety events

Terms	Definitions
Safety	Freedom from accidental accidents
Error	The failure of planned action to be completed as intended (i.e., error of execution) or the use of a wrong plan to achieve an aim (i.e., error of planning). Errors may be errors of commission or omission and usually reflect deficiencies in the systems of care
Adverse event	An injury related to medical management, in contrast to complications of disease. Medical management includes all aspects of care, including diagnosis and treatment, failure to diagnose or treat, and the systems and equipment used to deliver care. Adverse events may be preventable or nonpreventable
Preventable adverse event	An adverse event caused by an error or other types of systems or equipment failure
"Near-miss" or "close call"	Serious error or mishap that has the potential to cause an adverse event but fails to do so because of chance or because it is intercepted. Also called potential adverse event
Adverse drug event	A medication-related adverse event
Hazard	Any threat to safety, e.g., unsafe practices, conduct, equipment, labels, names
System	A set of interdependent elements (people, processes, equipment) that interact to achieve a common aim
Event	Any deviation from usual medical care that causes an injury to the patient or poses a risk of harm. Includes errors, preventable adverse events, and hazards (see also "incident")
Incident (or adverse incident)	Any deviation from usual medical care that causes an injury to the patient or poses a risk of harm. Includes errors, preventable adverse events, and hazards
Potential adverse event	A serious error or mishap that has the potential to cause an adverse event but fails to do so because of chance or because it is intercepted (also called "near-miss" or "close call")
Latent error (or latent failure)	A defect in the design, organization, training, or maintenance in a system that leads to operator error and whose effects are typically delayed

Adapted from Sanchez et al. [41]

Examples of informatics applications in healthcare include electronic health records (EHRs) for digital patient records, clinical decision support systems (CDSS) aiding in diagnosis and decision-making, and telemedicine enabling remote patient care. These technologies can be both a challenge and an opportunity for patient safety. They are a challenge because they introduce new sources of medical error and complexity. They are an opportunity because they could help better address and prevent sources of medical error [44]. This chapter offers an overview of patient safety combined with examples of how evolving information technologies hold potential to change the field over the coming decades. We present the main decision frameworks and tools for improving patient safety that dominate the field and examine their applications in new lights and possible limitations in a rapidly evolving healthcare environment.

20.2 Brief History of Patient Safety

Patient safety is a relatively new field. While medical research can be traced to ancient times, patient safety only gained traction in the 1990s. One reason that Hippocrates was not concerned with patient safety is that physicians had little to offer for ailing patients and most died young and quickly in Ancient Greece. Healthcare systems became more complex over the course of the industrial revolution with new medical breakthroughs such as antibiotics and vaccines saving lives, but the health system itself created more opportunities for systemic failures that caused potential harm to patients.

A key milestone for patient safety was the 1999 publication of *To Err Is Human* by the Institute of Medicine, which estimated that as many as "44,000-98,000 Americans die each year due to preventable harm" and globally as many as 1 in 10 patients continues to be harmed from safety lapses during their care, resulting in well over three million deaths each year [18]. Unsafe care also has high financial and economic costs. In developed countries, the direct costs of treating patients who have been harmed during their care approaches 13% of health spending, amounting to US$606 billion a year [45, 46]. These reports sparked an increase in international awareness of iatrogenic harm and funding for patient safety research. The 2001 report *Making Health Care Safer* published by the Agency for Healthcare Research and Quality (AHRQ) called for a new research paradigm of applying evidence-based medicine principles and frameworks to the systematic reductions of patient harm [43]. The field of patient safety has developed to address an urgent public need, with abundant national funding, and an empirical approach to designing, implementing, and evaluating improvements. Governments, health systems, and providers are now seen to have a duty to protect patients and the public from harm.

The adoption of health information technology (HIT), particularly electronic health records (EHRs), was motivated in part by the patient safety movement and its growing attention following the *To Err Is Human* report. For example, EHR incumbent Epic Systems benefited from unprecedented EHR adoption following the regulatory tailwind of the 2009 HITECH act that aimed in part to address patient safety issues by requiring healthcare providers in the USA to adopt EHRs [50].

However, despite the aim of HIT to improve quality of care, reduce duplicate care, and reduce adverse health events, these systems may contribute to the patient safety problem. For example, poorly designed EHRs can lead to healthcare provider burnout, alarm fatigue, and unsafe workarounds that contribute to errors [26]. However, by contrast, alerts built into these systems can guard against prescribing a drug to which the patient may have an allergy or warn again drug interactions [1]. Similarly, telemedicine extends the hospital walls by increasing access to care and facilitating better monitoring of patients in their home [34]. However, telehealth solutions create new failure modes such as increased data privacy and security concerns, equitable access issues, and increased opportunities for health wearables device failures [8]. Further, given the limited robust outcomes data about EHRs, there is a need for greater transparency about the meaningful benefits of EHRs [48].

A key theme of this chapter is the growing realization that patient harm arises from systemic failures that are affected by every aspect of the health system that is highly coupled to its underlying informatics tools and platforms. The health informaticist needs to be aware that in the face of the conveniences and optimizations that health IT bring to healthcare, there may also be unintended risks. The risks of health IT to patient safety can be exacerbated by multiple human factors issues and the fact that technology-focused developers are often unaware of the risks inherent in complex systems and are not trained in patient safety principles.

20.3 Methods, Models, and Applications

20.3.1 Systems Thinking

Systems thinking is an approach to problem-solving that views problems as part of a wider dynamic system [55]. It recognizes and prioritizes the understanding of linkages, relationships, interactions, and interdependencies among the components of a system that give rise to the system‘s observed behavior. The principle that underlines all of patient safety is *systems thinking*. This principle stems from two insights. The first is that systems shape the behavior of individuals and create or mitigate the various ways things can go wrong, essential opposite sides of the same coin [2]. The second is that humans inherently make mistakes: "Human fallibility contributing to error causation is the result of intrinsic and unavoidable imperfections of human cognitive processes such as memory, vigilance, attention, concentration, and reasoning, as well as the tendency of human performance to degrade with fatigue, sleep-deprivation, distractions, excessive task demands, stress, and anxiety" [32]. Medicine has a long history of reviewing errors from the perspective of what individuals did wrong and overlooking or only giving tokenistic efforts to the underlying systemic causes of medical errors and harm. Studying the system at multiple levels and discovering what system-wide changes can be implemented are needed to reduce harm due to the inevitability of human errors [12].

20.3.2 The SEIPS Model: Conceptualizing Healthcare Systems

The Systems Engineering Initiative for Patient Safety (SEIPS) model is one of several models that endeavor to elicit the interrelationships between different aspects of the healthcare system [23]. The SEIPS model builds on the foundational Donabedian model for linking and evaluating healthcare quality, which conceptualizes a feedback loop from structure (i.e., work system), to processes, to outcomes. This framework could help improve the design and interpretation of informatics evaluative studies and represents the various subunits that make up a health system [27]. The patterns of behavior or processes in the system arise from the structure and inter-relationships of the work system. These processes create the ultimate outcomes of the system and outcomes shape the work system and processes in a series of interrelated feedback learning loops.

The SEIPS model's depiction of the health work system draws attention to the many interrelated elements that interact each day in a health system, such as the healthcare providers, organization, tools, and technologies, and the external regulatory and political environment. The SEIPS model underscores that healthcare is a *sociotechnical system*, that is, that technology does not exist in isolation, but rather healthcare staff interact with and use technology, and this interaction is shaped directly and indirectly by the physical and organizational environment, and circumstances. The SEIPS 2.0 authors observe, *"The deliberate placement of person(s) in the center of the sociotechnical system fits with the human factors approach... and emphasizes that design should support—not replace or compensate for—people"* [23].

The next key insight of the SEIPS model is that work processes and outcomes follow naturally from the work system. That is, when placed in a particular environment, people will tend to behave in certain ways afforded by the unique environment's structures and affordances. The model's holistic perspective accounts for the process of all the stakeholders: professionals, patients and their families, and the organizational leaders, and points out that the system's structure influences the processes and outcomes of each of the system's actors.

System thinkers like Jens Rasmussen remind us to think about healthcare systems at different scale levels [37], that is, microsystems, mesosystems, and macrosystems. Rasmussen, more than any other person, is credited with a renaissance in recent decades of interest in and appreciation for the fallibility of human behavior in high-risk systems (e.g., human reliability analysis as part of probabilistic risk analysis in the nuclear power and other process control industries, aviation, and medicine) [54]. Rasmussen's theories enriched our understanding of error and the nature of mental models and cognitive work and the application of these ideas to systems design [38]. At the top level of the macrosystem: are the environment, the architecture, the public policy, the population health, etc., represented by "work system" in Fig. 20.1. At the mesosystem level, you have a host of technologies, medium-scale internal environments, organizational culture, etc., and finally, when you drill down to individual units of care, the microsystems, represented in the diagram by "People." Patient safety research emphasizes the critical roles of studies and interventions at the microsystem level because "errors and failure occur within the microsystem, and ultimately it is the well-functioning microsystem that can prevent or mitigate errors and failure to avoid causing patient harm" [25]. Thinking about the healthcare system at different scale levels helps us to make sense of the interrelationships between subcomponents and study and implement changes in manageable units.

20.4 Culture of Safety

Medicine lags far behind other high-risk industries that share the characteristic of severe consequences for errors. There is an abundance of literature showing how the aviation and nuclear energy industries have progressed more rapidly than healthcare in terms of introducing and requiring a safety management system that includes error reduction, near-miss reporting, threat and error management, and a "safety culture" focused on reliability [40]. One of the core tenets of high-reliability organizations (HROs) is their active cultivation of a culture of safety. Creating a safety culture at the organizational level follows naturally the systems-thinking mindset because one of the foundational tools for shaping behavior at scale is through culture change. When high-reliability principles permeate an organization at the systemic and cultural levels, organizations build trust, engage employees fully, and, with time, gain the quality of a sys-

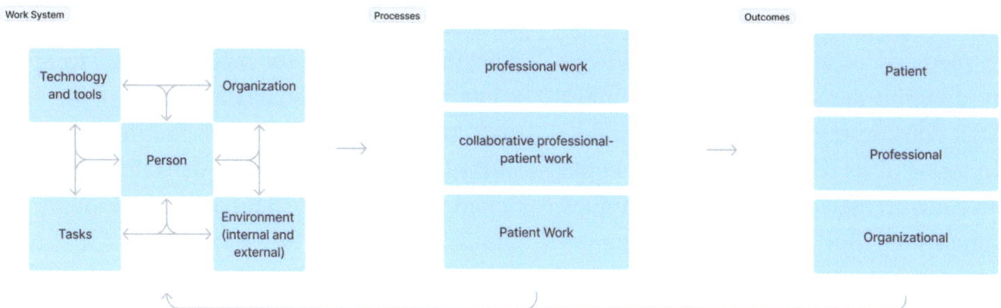

Fig. 20.1 Adapted from the SEIPS 2.0 model overview. [23]

tem's resilience. We define *Resilience* to mean that when humans make mistakes the organization has systems in place that can recover from a human error before harm occurs.

A culture of safety is defined as having the following attributes [25]:

1. A commitment of the leadership to discuss and learn from errors.
2. Communications founded on mutual trust and respect.
3. Shared perceptions of the importance of safety.
4. Encouragement and practice of teamwork.
5. Incorporation of nonpunitive systems for reporting and analyzing adverse events.

As noted above, a key tenet of a safety culture is psychological safety. Amy Edmonson defines this as the belief that one will not be punished or humiliated for speaking up with ideas, questions, concerns, or mistakes, and the team is safe for interpersonal risk-taking [19]. For management to get accurate information about near-misses and adverse events, care providers must feel comfortable and safe to speak up without work or other negative consequences. For interventions to be adopted by care providers, they must feel safe doing so. Psychological safety requires that an organization adopt a systems mindset to thinking about the causes of medical errors. In the absence of a systems' mindset, there is often a culture of individual blame, where individual care providers are assigned responsibility for an adverse event. This makes care providers less likely to report accurate information about mistakes and near-misses, and it means management is likely to miss the learnings about systemic factors that lead to patient harm [3].

Many of the models used to enhance patient safety are methods of analyzing the healthcare system by dividing the system into meaningful subunits and considering each subunit individually and in terms of its relationship to the whole. We present a few frameworks below as examples. These frameworks illustrate how choosing the right model can help to make sense of the complexity that comes with systems thinking. The examples also give a taste for the various conditions that lead to error and harm in health systems.

20.5 The Haddon Matrix

In the 1970s, Dr. William Haddon created a framework for reducing harm caused by car accidents [21]. The Haddon Matrix was a revolutionary injury prevention way of thinking about harm reduction because it deconstructed a harmful event into a matrix of the factors leading to the event and the phases of the event. This makes it possible to create harm reduction solutions for each component of the matrix. In the case of car accidents, the factors leading to harm can be the human, the vehicle, and the environment and the combinations of these three elements. The phases of harm are preinjury, injury, postinjury. For each cell in the grid, there are unique failure mode conditions that increase the risk and severity of injury. For example, the human-preinjury cell includes alcohol intoxication. The vehicle-injury cell includes sharp edges and surfaces.

We choose to adapt the Haddon Matrix to harm reduction in healthcare by delineating the causes of harm into factors like patient/family, healthcare provider, system, environment, and for each factor, consider harm-causing conditions at the pre-event, event, and postevent stages of error. We can use the Haddon Matrix to partition a complex web of factors leading to patient harm into subcategories, and then design interventions to prevent or mitigate the harm caused in each category. Furthermore, the Haddon Matrix offers a useful framework for mapping tools to appropriate parts of the healthcare process for better understanding the points of failure for patient safety (Barach & Johnson). An example of such a mapping of tools to their respective phase and human factors is as follows:

- Phase: pre-event.
  - Human factors: patient/family.
    - Tools: process mapping.
  - Human factors: healthcare professional.
    - Tools: probabilistic risk assessment, scenario building, hazard analysis, checklists.
  - Human factors: systems/environment.
    - Tools: FMEA, human factors engineering.
- Phase: event.
  - Human factors: patient/family.
    - Tools: interview.
  - Human factors: healthcare professional.
    - Tools: crew resource management, checklists.
  - Human factors: systems/environment.
    - Tools: root-cause analysis.
- Phase: post-event.
  - Human factors: patient/family.
    - Tools: interviews, focus groups.
  - Human factors: healthcare professional.
    - Tools: microsystem analysis, morbidity, and mortality conference.
  - Human factors: systems/environment.
    - Tools: root–cause analysis, artifact analysis.

20.6 The WHO Framework

Another framework for making sense of the diverse set of factors leading to errors in healthcare is the World Health Organization (WHO) framework [32]. The WHO framework focuses on advancing global health and considers all the conditions that make medical errors more likely and splits them into three categories: workplace conditions, human conditions, and organizational conditions. A significant challenge to learning from medical errors is that there is still no accepted taxonomy for categorizing different kinds of errors. The WHO framework offers a taxonomy of medical errors that can help to learn from healthcare errors in a more systematic way. The taxonomy is as follows:

- Work conditions (W)
  - Inadequate staffing, excessive patient–nurse ratio, excessive workloads
  - Undesirable shift patterns and work schedules that promote fatigue
  - Equipment poorly designed, not available, or poorly maintained
  - Poor ergonomic design of work area
  - Lack of administrative and managerial support
  - Protocols and standard procedures not available or hard to access
  - Use of unclear written communications and verbal communication methods that are prone to misinterpretation; unclear task design and lack of clarity of the organizational structure and about when and how to seek help
  - Inadequate supervision or backup
  - Poor team structure, functioning, and leadership
- Human conditions (H)
  - Mismatch between skills and healthcare worker and requirements of the job
  - Healthcare worker lacks knowledge, is in poor physical or mental health, is in a highly emotional state, is under stress, or does not consistently adhere to safety standards
  - Patient's condition is very complex or serious
  - Patient has language problems or hearing impairments that make effective communication more difficult
  - Patient personality and social factors make care more difficult
- Organizational conditions (O)
  - Financial constraints and economic pressures encourage production and efficiency over safety
  - Equipment, personnel, or other resources are either lacking or are not allocated to patient safety
  - Lack of policies, standards, goals, and regulations make it difficult to work safely
  - Excessively stringent regulations encourage violations

20.7 Failure Modes and Effects Analysis (FMEA)

An important part of informatics is assessing how new technologies can introduce added risks into the system and then mitigating that risk or using a data-driven approach to measure and this risk more transparent to the designers and users. Failure modes and effects analysis (FMEA) is a validated model of risk management that is used in a countless industries [17]. Failure modes and effects analysis (FMEA) is a structured risk management way to identify and address potential problems, or failures and their resulting effects on the system or process before a clinical adverse event occurs [33]. In comparison, root-cause analysis (RCA) is a structured way to address problems after they occur. FMEA involves identifying and eliminating process failures for the purpose of preventing an undesirable event. In short, for a given situation, a list is made of all the things that could go wrong, and for each thing that could go wrong, there is an assessment of its likelihood of occurrence and the severity of the consequences if it does occur [53]. In this way, failure modes are categorized into high, medium, and low likelihood, and high-, medium-, and low-impact risks. A completed FMEA matrix allows decision-makers to prioritize interventions and where best to allocate resources (see Table 20.2).

> Unnecessary noise, then, is the most cruel absence of care which can be inflicted either on sick or well.
> —Florence Nightingale, 1859

20.8 Case Study: Medical Device Alarm Fatigue

Medical device alarms are a ubiquitous feature of modern hospitals. Device alarms are used to alert nurses and physicians that there is a problem that needs to be addressed related to patient monitoring. Unfortunately, the poor design of medical alarms creates multiple adverse consequences for health outcomes. Firstly, noise created by medical alarms harms patient recovery because the noises interrupt sleep and create a stressful environment known to impede healing. Secondly, the overuse of sound-based medical alarms results in loud environments and the phenomenon known as alarm fatigue, whereby staff become desensitized to the alarms and when an urgent situation finally does arise they are less likely to respond to the alarm [47].

The problem is exacerbated by poor design decisions by the device manufacturers. For example, devices use alarm sounds that are difficult to interpret and difficult to differentiate from one another. In particular, the sound of a nonurgent alarm such as the need to replace a battery is, in many cases, difficult to distinguish from an urgent alarm such as a cardiac arrest. Furthermore, the over-prevalence of nonurgent alarms makes hospital staff less sensitive to the truly important alarms. Nurses will sometimes disable alarms because of frustration with the noise created by the devices [15]. Additionally, in many cases alarms will sound when the associated condition is not there. This is known as a false-positive alarm. Finally, the sounds of the alarms are often aesthetically unpleasing and tonally dissonant. While it may seem that aesthetics are a low-priority design constraint for a life-critical device, there is an abundance of evidence showing that the dissonant sonic landscape created by these bedside device alarms has a negative impact both on staff responsiveness, patient recovery, and on staff wellness [31].

Recent studies have shown success in using machine learning to reduce the frequency of false-positive alarms and withhold sounding of nonurgent alarms at inopportune times [13]. However, despite the successful use of machine learning in improving the alarm fatigue, the enthusiasm for these techniques reflects another theme of this chapter, which is the tendency to overly focus on technical solutions when a true solution requires a social-technical approach. While many scientists are developing algorithms for reducing the frequency of device alarms, there are comparatively few who are conducting qualitative interviews with stakeholders and co-designing more harmonious alarm sounds with staff and patients to asses how these solutions would align with real world clinical flow.

Table 20.2 Example: Failure modes and effects analysis (FMEA)—laboratory specimen collection and labeling process

Steps in the process	Failure mode	Failure causes	Failure effects	Likelihood of occurrence (1–10)	Likelihood of detection (1–10)	Severity (1–10)	Risk profile number (RPN)	Actions to reduce occurrence of failure
Electronic orders are entered for lab tests	Wrong patient is selected when entering the order	Similar patient names or medical record numbers Clinician is distracted during order entry Inadequate EHR alerts for same-name patients	A specimen is collected from the wrong patient, resulting in an error in treatment decisions	4	6	6	144	Implement hard-stop EHR alerts for same-name patients Display patient photo at order entry Educate staff on using two-identifier verification
Specimen is collected at the bedside	Specimen tube is mislabeled or unlabeled	Labels printed away from bedside Multiple patients drawn in rapid succession Poor lighting or space constraints	Results are reported for the wrong patient, resulting in misdiagnosis or delayed treatment	7	5	7	245	Require bedside label printing Limit phlebotomist workload to one patient at a time Conduct random audits of labeling compliance
Specimen is transported to the lab	Specimen leaks or is stored at the wrong temperature	Tube cap not fully sealed Cooler packs not replenished on night shift	Integrity of the sample is compromised, causing inaccurate or rejected test results and additional draws	5	4	3	60	Use leak-proof, temperature-monitored transport containers Post visual checklists for night-shift staff to verify cooler temperature

20

Lastly, regulatory challenges are another dimension often forgotten by the technologists. One of the key design problems with hospital alarms is that there is no required standardization of sounds and acoustic standards across machines and manufacturers. This lack of interoperability makes it even harder for staff to correctly interpret the multitude of heterogeneous sound alerts in the clinical environment. Thus, health informatics practitioners must be mindful not only of the technology aspects of their discipline, but also the other nontechnical interrelated factors that will ultimately determine whether their technology helps or harms staff and patients. That includes the social-technical, human factors elements, and regulatory elements. This case study emphasizes the underlying theme that adopting a systems mindset is essential to designing successful technology interventions in healthcare.

20.8.1 Challenges and Opportunities Ahead

The rapidly evolving technology landscape holds potential to disrupt healthcare and patient safety over the coming decades both for better and for worse. For example, HIT has the potential to reduce adverse drug evens and diagnostic errors, and improve transfusion safety and adherence with evidence-based care [22]. Additionally, artificial intelligence shows increasing promise as a tool to create meaningful improvements to patient safety by harnessing big data to develop early warning systems, improve patient monitoring, assist in diagnosis, improve access to care, and other novel applications [4, 11, 24] .

However, we are in the middle of a big hype cycle around machine learning and artificial intelligence. There is an abundance of academic literature and news coverage singing praises of the techno-optimism and the potential of these technologies to transform healthcare often obscuring or neglecting the risks and challenges of these powerful technologies. Indeed, health informatics technologies present remarkable opportunities for revolutionizing the reliability of patient care.

The first challenge is that adding more technology tends to make things more complicated, not less. And more complicated systems have more failure modes, create more error-inducing conditions, and are more difficult to navigate. Adding more devices, more user interfaces, more protocols, more data often creates more points of failure, increases staff mental workload, more staff burnout, and at least has failed to reliabily make a meaningful change in patient outcomes [9, 10, 29, 35].

Secondly, the hype around machine learning technologies and the lack of appreciation of the lived experience of staff, combined with the rapid onboarding of new technologies, means that frontline workers are at risk of putting too much trust in technologies they do not properly understand. For example, some of the most important use cases for predictive modeling are in computer-assisted diagnosis, but if healthcare professionals lack an understanding of the failure modes and limitations of deep learning models, they may fail to use the technology appropriately as a decision-making tool. Deep learning models are subject to multiple biases that occur when an algorithm produces results that are systemically prejudiced due to erroneous assumptions in the machine learning (ML) process. The results of the biased process can fail to generalize on data that is significantly different from the data they were trained and evaluated on [49].

Thirdly, technology-focused interventions tend to create problems when they do not respect the social systems they must inhabit. Human factors such as the culture, user interface, and the surrounding environment must be considered by technologists who want their solutions to be used in day-to-day encounters by healthcare professionals. The case study on medical device alarm fatigue points to what happens when technologists fail to consider the second- and third-order consequences of their designs and the unique needs of the people who must use them every day. Technologists should co-develop their informatics solutions in close concert with all the stakeholders in addressing these blind spots (often referred to as a user-centered design, which is discussed in Chaps. 8 and 9 in this book). This implies an abundance of informal interviews with end users and extensive consultations with people who understand the organization and culture of the end users. Failure to respect these design principles will likely lead in the best case to technologies that do not get adopted, have long prototypical gestational periods, and in the worst case, to technologies that do not get adopted due to more confusion, medical errors, and patient harm. In the latter case, machine learning and artificial intelligence can create unprecedented opportunities for disrupting care [6, 14] .

Finally, both an opportunity and challenge for health informatics as it relates to patient safety is the future of data acquisition and error detection. Patient safety improvement relies on gathering large amounts of accurate data on adverse events and near-misses and implementing solutions for systems change. Data acquisition and processing is one of technology's specialties, and improved remote patient monitoring also has the potential to be a life-saving evolution in the paradigm of remote care. But once again there are significant pitfalls to overcome. First, data acquisition is only useful if it enables meaningful action. There is historic precedent for health systems collecting lots of data that is either unusable (e.g., because its format is nonstandardized) or is never acted upon [20, 42].

In the absence of protocols for analyzing data and making data-enabled decisions, more data can just end up creating more confusion. Furthermore, as machine learning models become more powerful and impactful, the consequences and risks of biases in training data are magnified. A well-publicized early warning of this phenomenon is the case of racial bias in pulse oximetry monitors. A known design flaw of pulse oximetry is that patients with darker skin (compared to those with lighter skin) are more likely to experience occult hypoxemia—defined conceptually as substantial arterial hypoxemia (SaO_2) detected on blood gas but not noted on simultaneous pulse oximetry (SpO_2) [51]. If data pipelines and model deployments outpace the system's ability to ensure data integrity, health systems could end up with major blind spots due to statistical biases baked into models through problematic training data.

Finally, there are many examples of frontline workers failing to adopt new data collection technologies because of overwhelming working conditions and systemic distrust of healthcare management. Without a culture of psychological safety, attempts to monitor staff performance using health IT may be met with pushback, and attempts to analyze voluntary reporting of adverse events are only as good as the reports, which can be compromised if staff do not feel safe speaking up. Informatics experts and technologists must be mindful of the need to consider the social-technical challenges inherent in implementing new healthcare interventions and look beyond the narrow problem definitions of a technology-focused solution. If innovators in health informatics can skillfully integrate their technology expertise with careful consideration of the unique affordances of healthcare, then the next generation of health informatics technologies has the potential to take patient care to a new level of reliability while better managing the downside risks [30, 39] .

20.9 Conclusions and Recommendations

Healthcare is being disrupted by emerging technologies and health informatics. These new technologies offer many opportunities to streamline workflows, improve access to care, and augment data collection and patient monitoring. However, they also pose numerous organizational, professional, and patient challenges.

Medical errors are the third leading cause of death in America, and, thus, patient safety is critical to health outcomes. Patient safety is about delivering high-quality and reliable care by reducing the chances of causing patient harm due to medical errors. The first step in improving patient safety outcomes is adopting a systems mindset and learning to constantly reflect on the complex interrelationships between different elements of the healthcare system. High-reliability organizations in other industries have blazed a trail that healthcare can follow in establishing a culture of safety, which follows from a systems mindset because shaping culture is one of the most effective ways to create trust and staff engagement for systemic and lasting changes.

Systems thinking and culture of safety supports experts in informatics to apply various mental models for making sense of the failure modes in healthcare at every scale of the organization such as the Haddon Matrix and WHO frameworks. Interventions and studies can be designed for each failure mode. It is useful when planning organizational workflow change to assess the relative risks and impacts of the different failure modes using a risk management tool like failure modes and effects analysis.

Patient safety's core tenet of systems thinking implies that patient safety is shaped by every aspect of the health system and aspects of health informatics workflow. It is essential to ground a study of health informatics in the fundamental principles of the patient safety research and practice.

20.10 Epilogue

Your first day at your new job was rough, but after doing some feverish reading on patient safety in the context of health informatics you are ready to present an informed plan to your boss. The next day, you walk into your boss's office and explain how improving patient safety around EHRs is not an isolated initiative, but part of creating a new approach toward systemic changes in your organization. You present different frameworks for conceptualizing the interrelated processes within a healthcare system that lead to patient harm, and you explain how meaningful changes must start at a cultural level. You suggest analyzing the EHR problem using the Haddon Matrix and show your boss how you can assess the risks of your intervention using an FMEA. Armed with these principles of patient safety, you finally get to leverage your informatics toolkit to build a data pipeline for measuring patient process and outcome results. Your boss is so impressed that you are put in charge of your organization's first patient safety initiative. Good thing you learned about patient safety!

List of Learning Resources

- For an overview of national patient safety goals and standards, see The Joint Commission: https://www.jointcommission.org/
- For a series of short articles that give some background on different aspects of patient safety, see Patient Safety Network's Patient Safety 101: https://psnet.ahrq.gov/patient-safety-101
- For some useful statistics on patient safety, see WHO on Patient Safety: https://www.who.int/news-room/fact-sheets/detail/patient-safety
- For the 2001 report that brought international attention to the patient safety movement, see Donaldson, M. S., Corrigan, J. M., & Kohn, L. T. (Eds.). (2000). To err is human: building a safer health system.
- For a comprehensive standard textbook on patient safety, see Vincent, C. (2011). Patient safety. John Wiley & Sons.

Knowledge Check Questions

1. Why is a systems mindset critical to patient safety?
2. How would you use the tools described in the tools and methods section to design an improvement study for improving problems with medical device alarms as described in the case study?
3. Why are systems thinking and a culture of safety prerequisites for implementing successful health informatics interventions in health systems?
4. Select an area of health informatics from a different chapter in this book and list three opportunities and three challenges for this area as it relates to patient safety. You might use Google Scholar to search for recent articles on the subject.
5. Practice using a Haddon Matrix and FMEA matrix to analyze the failure modes for some-

thing you do regularly. For example, flying, bicycling, investing, starting a new job, and choosing to start a new degree program.

Answers

1. A systems mindset is critical to patient safety because the primary driver of patient harm is neither individual negligence nor isolated components of the healthcare system. Rather, patient harm results from the systemic challenges at the intersections between people, technologies, workflows, and organizational culture. The inherent fallibility of humans is amplified by the complexity and high-stress environment of healthcare organizations. A systems mindset enables practitioners to shift from a focus on blaming individuals to making sense of the underlying systemic failures that are contributing to patient harm.
2. Use systems thinking to analyze the interactions between medical device alarms and their interactions with different layers of the healthcare system. Start, for example, with the SEIPS model to examine how medical device alarms affect different parts of the system. Consider using the Haddon Matrix to investigate opportunities for interventions to reduce alarm-related harm. Using the Haddon Matrix, you can propose interventions at the pre-event, event, and post-event phases, and classified by patient, provider, system, and environmental factors. For example, a preevent intervention might consider machine learning algorithms for reducing false positive alarm signals. An event-level intervention might be to improve communication protocols for team members when alarms arise. Additionally, consider using a failure modes and effects analysis (FMEA) model to evaluate whether your interventions sufficiently address the various ways things can go wrong and the potential impact of insufficiently addressed failure modes. Finally, use qualitative methods like interviewing staff to help design interventions that will align with the team's practical needs and help to gain their buy-in.
3. Systems thinking is a prerequisite for implementing successful health informatics interventions because healthcare systems are complex socio-technical systems in which optimizing one isolated component without thinking about its systemic effects can result in unsafe and sub-optimal outcomes. A culture of safety is needed to learn from errors and near misses. If team members fear punishment for reporting errors then it is likely errors will remain unreported and the system will fail to learn from mistakes that harm patients. Additionally, health informatics tools are only effective to the extent that they are used by staff. A culture of safety is needed to create conditions in which it is natural for staff to use interventions and tools that support patient safety
4. Selected area: AI–based clinical decision support
   Opportunities:
   1. Early warning systems that alert staff to risk of patient deterioration.
   2. Reduce medication errors by checking prescription against historical data.
   3. Expand access to medical expertise in resource-constrained settings using AI-assisted support.

   Challenges:
   1. Model bias can exacerbate health outcomes disparities.
   2. Clinicians overly relying on AI recommendations without understanding model limitations.
   3. Increased system complexity, resulting in more cognitive load and new failure modes.
5. Example activity: Starting a new job
   Use a Haddon Matrix to analyze risk factors across phases (pre-event, event, post-event) and contributors (individual, organization, environment):

- Pre-event:
  - (Organization) inadequate onboarding
  - (Individual) insufficient training
  - (Environment) changing industry norms and tools
- Event:
  - (Organization, individual) miscommunication
  - (Individual) fatigue
  - (Environment) unfamiliar systems leading to errors
- Post-event:
  - (Individual) resistance to learning from mistakes
  - (Organization) lack of formal feedback mechanisms
  - (Environment) blame culture preventing learning

Using FMEA, the potential failure modes (e.g., misunderstanding critical procedures) would be rated by likelihood, detectability, and severity. High-risk failures could be mitigated through structured onboarding, mentorship, checklists, and feedback loops. This exercise mirrors patient safety analysis by proactively identifying risks and prioritizing interventions before harm occurs.

Identify multiples steps in the process for your chosen activity and for each step, identify:

Step in the process

Failure mode

Failure causes

Failure effects

Likelihood of occurrence (1–10)

Likelihood of detection (1–10)

Severity (1–10)

Risk profile number (= likelihood of occurrence × likelihood of detection × severity)

Actions to reduce occurrence of failure

As an example of one such row in the table, in the case of starting a new job:

Step in the process: day one onboarding

Failure mode: new employee deletes massive database

Failure causes: miscommunication, insufficient training, improper credential access management

Failure effects: loss of proprietary company data, loss of trust with customers

Likelihood of occurrence (1–10): 2

Likelihood of detection (1–10): 9

Severity (1–10): 9

Risk profile number (= likelihood of occurrence × likelihood of detection × severity): 162

Actions to reduce occurrence of failure: ensure that new employees do not have the ability to make destructive changes to databases.

References

1. Barach P, Arora VM. Hospital alarms and patient safety. JAMA. 2014;312(6):651. https://doi.org/10.1001/jama.2014.7648.
2. Barach P, Berwick DM. Patient safety and the reliability of health care systems. Ann Intern Med. 2003;138(12):997–8. https://doi.org/10.7326/0003-4819-138-12-200306170-00013. PMID: 12809458.
3. Barach P, Johnson JK. Assessing risk and preventing harm in the clinical microsystem. In: McLaughlin & Kaluzny's continuous quality improvement in health care. Burlington: Jones & Barlett Learning; 2020. p. 235–52.
4. Bates DW, Levine D, Syrowatka A, Kuznetsova M, Craig KJT, Rui A, Jackson GP, Rhee K. The potential of artificial intelligence to improve patient safety: a scoping review. Npj Digit Med. 2021;4(1):1–8. https://doi.org/10.1038/s41746-021-00423-6.
5. Bath PA. Health informatics: current issues and challenges. J Inf Sci. 2008;34(4):501–18. https://doi.org/10.1177/0165551508092267.
6. Baweja JA, Fallon CK, Jefferson BA. Opportunities for human factors in machine learning. Front Artif Intell. 2023;6:1130190.
7. Betsy Lehman Center for Patient Safety. The financial and human cost of medical error. Boston: Massachusetts; 2019.
8. Blandford A, Wesson J, Amalberti R, AlHazme R, Allwihan R. Opportunities and challenges for telehealth within, and beyond, a pandemic. Lancet Glob Health. 2020;8(11):e1364–5.
9. Bonabeau E. Understanding and managing complexity risk. MIT Sloan Manag Rev. 2007;48(4):62.
10. Borycki EM. Technology-induced errors: where do they come from and what can we do about them? In: Context sensitive health informatics: human and sociotechnical approaches. IOS Press; 2013. p. 20–6. https://ebooks.iospress.nl/doi/10.3233/978-1-61499-293-6-20.
11. Brodeur PG, Buckley TA, Kanjee Z, Goh E, Ling EB, Jain P, Cabral S, Abdulnour R-E, Haimovich A, Freed JA, Olson A, Morgan DJ, Hom J, Gallo R, Horvitz

E, Chen J, Manrai AK, Rodman A. Superhuman performance of a large language model on the reasoning tasks of a physician (No. arXiv:2412.10849). arXiv. 2024; https://doi.org/10.48550/arXiv.2412.10849.
12. Cassin BR, et al. Making sense of root cause analysis investigations of surgery-related adverse events. Surg Clin. 2012;92(1):101–15.
13. Chromik J, Klopfenstein SAI, Pfitzner B, Sinno Z-C, Arnrich B, Balzer F, Poncette A-S. Computational approaches to alleviate alarm fatigue in intensive care medicine: a systematic literature review. Front Digital Health. 2022;4:843747.
14. Cresswell K, Sheikh A. Organizational issues in the implementation and adoption of health information technology innovations: an interpretative review. Int J Med Inform. 2013;82(5):e73–86.
15. Cvach M. Monitor alarm fatigue: an integrative review. Biomed Instrum Technol. 2012;46(4):268–77. https://doi.org/10.2345/0899-8205-46.4.268.
16. de Vries EN, Ramrattan MA, Smorenburg SM, Gouma DJ, Boermeester MA. The incidence and nature of in-hospital adverse events: a systematic review. BMJ Qual Saf. 2008;17(3):216–23. https://doi.org/10.1136/qshc.2007.023622.
17. Dekker S. The field guide to human error investigations. Routledge; 2017. https://www.taylorfrancis.com/books/mono/10.4324/9781315202778/field-guide-human-error-investigations-sidney-dekker
18. Donaldson, M. S., Corrigan, J. M., & Kohn, L. T. (2000). To err is human: building a safer health system.. https://books.google.com/books?hl=en&lr=&id=Jj25GlLKXSgC&oi=fnd&pg=PT25&dq=Donaldson,+M.+S.,+Corrigan,+J.+M.,+%26+Kohn,+L.+T.+(Eds.).+(2000).+To+err+is+human:+building+a+safer+health+system.&ots=bKjgnsM37F&sig=CZac5vsWShAom8efsQXmxDlwJIE.
19. Edmondson AC, Bransby DP. Psychological safety comes of age: observed themes in an established literature. Annu Rev Organ Psych Organ Behav. 2023;10(1):55–78. https://doi.org/10.1146/annurev-orgpsych-120920-055217.
20. Foreman B. Neurocritical care: bench to bedside (eds. Claude Hemphill, Michael James) integrating and using big data in neurocritical care. Neurotherapeutics. 2020;17(2):593–605.
21. Haddon W. Energy damage and the ten countermeasure strategies. Hum Factors. 1973;15(4):355–66. https://doi.org/10.1177/001872087301500407.
22. Hall KK, Fitall E, Hettinger AZ. Updates in the role of health IT in patient safety. Updates in the Role of Health IT in Patient Safety. 2020. https://psnet.ahrq.gov/perspective/updates-role-health-it-patient-safety.
23. Holden RJ, Carayon P, Gurses AP, Hoonakker P, Hundt AS, Ozok AA, Rivera-Rodriguez AJ. SEIPS 2.0: A human factors framework for studying and improving the work of healthcare professionals and patients. Ergonomics. 2013;56(11):1669–86. https://doi.org/10.1080/00140139.2013.838643.
24. Howell MD. Generative artificial intelligence, patient safety and healthcare quality: a review. BMJ Qual Saf. 2024;33(11):748–54. https://doi.org/10.1136/bmjqs-2023-016690.
25. Johnson JK, Sollecito WA. McLaughlin & Kaluzny's continuous quality improvement in health care. Jones & Bartlett Learning; 2018. https://books.google.com/books?hl=en&lr=&id=JEBvDwAAQBAJ&oi=fnd&pg=PP1&dq=Johnson,+J.+K.,+%26+Sollecito,+W.+A.+(2018).+McLaughlin+%26+Kaluzny%27s+continuous+quality+improvement+in+health+care.+Jones+%26+Bartlett+Learning.&ots=C7imHJvy02&sig=IJj45RPsZ4GZ_hiig88Ui-kpbqY
26. Kroth PJ, Morioka-Douglas N, Veres S, Babbott S, Poplau S, Qeadan F, Parshall C, Corrigan K, Linzer M. Association of electronic health record design and use factors with clinician stress and burnout. JAMA Netw Open. 2019;2(8):–e199609.
27. Lilford RJ, Chilton PJ, Hemming K, Girling AJ, Taylor CA, Barach P. Evaluating policy and service interventions: framework to guide selection and interpretation of study end points. BMJ. 2010;341:c4413. https://www.bmj.com/content/341/bmj.c4413
28. Makary MA, Daniel M. Medical error—the third leading cause of death in the US. BMJ. 2016;353. https://www.bmj.com/content/353/bmj.i2139/
29. McBeth R. EPR implementation led to "catastrophic loss of confidence." Digit Health. 2016. https://www.digitalhealth.net/2016/02/epr-implementation-led-to-catastrophic-loss-of-confidence/.
30. McGinn CA, Grenier S, Duplantie J, Shaw N, Sicotte C, Mathieu L, Leduc Y, Légaré F, Gagnon M-P. Comparison of user groups' perspectives of barriers and facilitators to implementing electronic health records: a systematic review. BMC Med. 2011;9(1).46. https://doi.org/10.1186/1741-7015-9-46.
31. McNeer RR, Bohórquez J, Özdamar Ö, et al. A new paradigm for the Design of Audible Alarms that convey urgency information. J Clin Monit Comput. 2007;21:353–63. https://doi.org/10.1007/s10877-007-9096-6.
32. Nelson EC, Batalden PB, Godfrey MM. Quality by design: a clinical microsystems approach. Wiley; 2011. https://books.google.com/books?hl=en&lr=&id=ATA8gdpTfAUC&oi=fnd&pg=PR5&dq=Nelson,+E.+C.,+Batalden,+P.+B.,+%26+Godfrey,+M.+M.+(Eds.).+(2011).+Quality+by+design:+a+clinical+microsystems+approach.+John+Wiley+%26+Sons.&ots=ka-uQiF-dZ&sig=VMMDwBQTUpapTZJcBeWhibR_dkI
33. Parretti C, Tartaglia R, La Regina M, Venneri F, Sbrana G, Mandò M, Barach P. Improved FMEA methods for proactive health care risk assessment of the effectiveness and efficiency of COVID-19 remote patient telemonitoring. Am J Med Qual. 2022;37(6):535–44. https://doi.org/10.1097/JMQ.0000000000000089. Epub 2022 Oct 18. PMID: 36250651; PMCID: PMC9622365.
34. Parretti C, La Regina M, Tortu C, Candido G, Tartaglia R. Telemedicine in Italy, the starting point. Intern Emerg Med. 2023;18(3):949–51. https://doi.org/10.1007/s11739-022-03176-6. Epub 2022 Dec 21. PMID: 36539605; PMCID: PMC9767849.

35. Physician Burnout. n.d.. Retrieved January 7, 2025, from https://www.ahrq.gov/prevention/clinician/ahrq-works/burnout/index.html
36. PSNet Glossary. n.d.. Retrieved January 6, 2025, from https://psnet.ahrq.gov/glossary-0
37. Rasmussen J. Cognitive systems engineering. A Wiley-Interscience Publication. 1994. https://dl.acm.org/doi/abs/10.5555/179248.
38. Rasmussen J, et al. Tasks, errors and mental models: a festschrift to celebrate the 60th birthday of Professor Jens Rasmussen. In: Goodstein LP, Anderson HB, Olsen SE, editors. Tasks, errors and mental models. London: Taylor & Francis; 1988. p. 21–34. https://cir.nii.ac.jp/crid/1130282271197214336.
39. Safi S, Thiessen T, Schmailzl KJ. Acceptance and resistance of new digital technologies in medicine: qualitative study. JMIR Res Protoc. 2018;7(12):e11072.
40. Sanchez JA, Barach PR. High reliability organizations and surgical microsystems: re-engineering surgical care. Surg Clin North Am. 2012;92(1):1–14. https://doi.org/10.1016/j.suc.2011.12.005. Epub 2012 Jan 4. PMID: 22269256.
41. Sanchez JA, Barach P, Johnson JK, Jacobs JP. Surgical patient care: improving safety, quality and value. Cham: Springer; 2017. p. 683–94. https://doi.org/10.1007/978-3-319-44010-1.
42. Sedlakova J, Daniore P, Horn Wintsch A, Wolf M, Stanikic M, Haag C, Sieber C, Schneider G, Staub K, Alois Ettlin D. Challenges and best practices for digital unstructured data enrichment in health research: a systematic narrative review. PLoS Digit Health. 2023;2(10):e0000347.
43. Shojania KG, Duncan BW, McDonald KM, Wachter RM, Markowitz AJ. Making health care safer: a critical analysis of patient safety practices. Evid Rep Technol Assess (Summ). 2001;43:i–x, 1–668.
44. Sittig DF, Wright A, Coiera E, Magrabi F, Ratwani R, Bates DW, Singh H. Current challenges in health information technology–related patient safety. Health Informatics J. 2020;26(1):181–9. https://doi.org/10.1177/1460458218814893.
45. Slawomirski L, Klazinga N. The economics of patient safety: From analysis to action. 2022a. https://www.oecd-ilibrary.org/social-issues-migration-health/the-economics-of-patient-safety_761f2da8-en.
46. Slawomirski L, Klazinga N. The economics of patient safety: from analysis to action, OECD health working papers, no. 145. Paris: OECD Publishing; 2022b. https://doi.org/10.1787/761f2da8-en.
47. Solet JM, Barach PR. Managing alarm fatigue in cardiac care. Prog Pediatr Cardiol. 2012;33(1):85–90.
48. Subbe CP, Tellier G, Barach P. Impact of electronic health records on predefined safety outcomes in patients admitted to hospital: a scoping review. BMJ Open. 2021;11(1):e047446.
49. Sujan M, Pool R, Salmon P. Eight human factors and ergonomics principles for healthcare artificial intelligence. BMJ Health Care Inform. 2022;29(1) https://www.ncbi.nlm.nih.gov/pmc/articles/PMC8819549/
50. Trout KE, Chen L-W, Wilson FA, Tak HJ, Palm D. The impact of meaningful use and electronic health records on hospital patient safety. Int J Environ Res Public Health. 2022;19(19):12525.
51. Valbuena VSM, Merchant RM, Hough CL. Racial and ethnic bias in pulse oximetry and clinical outcomes. JAMA Intern Med. 2022;182(7):699–700. https://doi.org/10.1001/jamainternmed.2022.1903.
52. Vincent C. Patient safety. Wiley; 2011. https://books.google.com/books?hl=en&lr=&id=CbJwsamhVdoC&oi=fnd&pg=PR9&dq=impact+of+healthcare+patient+safety&ots=NGf4Rht8xe&sig=AAVoNum-m4poIcomU_MK0ms-BSk
53. Vohra PD, Johnson JK, Daugherty CK, Wen M, Barach P. Housestaff and medical student attitudes toward medical errors and adverse events. Jt Comm J Qual Patient Saf. 2007;33(8):493–501. https://doi.org/10.1016/s1553-7250(07)33053-5. PMID: 17724946.
54. Waterson P, Le Coze J-C, Andersen HB. Recurring themes in the legacy of Jens Rasmussen. Appl Ergon. 2017;59:471–82. https://doi.org/10.1016/j.apergo.2016.10.002.
55. York S, Lavi R, Dori YJ, Orgill M. Applications of systems thinking in STEM education. J Chem Educ. 2019;96(12):2742–51. https://doi.org/10.1021/acs.jchemed.9b00261.

Quality Improvement 21

Lindsay A. Adams and Katie A. McCarthy

Foundational Domains

This chapter addresses the following AMIA Foundational Domains: F1—Health, F3—Social and Behavioral Science, F4—Health Information Science and Technology.

Learning Objectives

After reading this chapter, you should be able to.

1. Define quality, quality improvement, patient safety, near-miss, error, adverse event, system, and process.
2. Explain the importance of systems thinking within a quality improvement project.
3. Identify and describe the phases within the Six Sigma DMAIC process.

21.1 Introduction and Case Study

To illustrate the concepts within this chapter, we will use a hypothetical case study that focuses on Tom, who is the director of Clinical Laboratories for a large healthcare system that includes ten hospitals and several hundred clinics. One of the hospitals is an academic medical center aligned with the region's largest research university.

In his role, Tom oversees all the laboratory departments that test patient samples and provide the results to clinicians, who treat patients, and help them manage their health. For example, a patient may report that they are very thirsty, have lost weight without changing their diet or physical activity, and are hungry all the time. A physician may order a blood test (such as an A1C laboratory test) to determine if a patient's blood sugar levels are high and may indicate that the patient has type 2 diabetes. A sample of the patient's blood is taken, and the sample and the physician's order for the A1C lab test are sent to one of the clinical laboratories that Tom leads. The sample is tested to get a result, and then a report with this result is sent back to the ordering provider so that they can diagnose the patient and work with the patient to determine the appropriate treatment.

While reviewing monthly reports for each of the laboratories, Tom discovers a problem—the results of one laboratory test are taking a long time to get to the clinicians who need them. He is concerned about this issue and decides to investigate further.

21.2 Overview of Quality

One department that Tom leads, the Complex Testing Laboratory (CTL), provides specialized testing to diagnose rare blood and genetic condi-

L. A. Adams
Clinic Manager, Froedtert & The Medical College of Wisconsin, Milwaukee, WI, USA

K. A. McCarthy (✉)
Sullivan School of Business, Engineering, and Technology, Carroll University, Waukesha, WI, USA
e-mail: kamccart@carrollu.edu

C. Eldredge et al. (eds.), *Introductory Textbook in Health Informatics*, Health Informatics,
https://doi.org/10.1007/978-3-032-16657-9_21

tions. While reviewing a monthly report for the CTL, Tom discovers a concerning trend in the turnaround time for one of the CTL's most popular tests, the Rare Blood Disease (RBD) panel. *Turnaround time (TAT)* is the amount of time between when the laboratory receives the patient sample and order to when the laboratory sends a test result back to the ordering provider.

According to CTL's website, the turnaround time for the RBD panel is 4–7 days. In the most recent TAT report, though, Tom discovers that the average TAT is 12 days. Tom knows that TATs longer than 7 days can negatively impact patient care.

Within the Clinical Laboratories, the Quality department helps laboratories improve the efficiency and effectiveness of their daily work. Tom decides to reach out to Mia, the manager of the Quality department, for assistance. Mia agrees to meet with Tom to discuss the issue and potential next steps.

21.2.1 What Is Quality?

During their meeting, Mia explains that *quality* is defined as the likelihood that healthcare services achieve desired outcomes and are consistent with professional standards [1]. In addition, the National Academy of Medicine (NAM) has identified six aims of quality healthcare (described in Table 21.1).

Table 21.1 Six aims of quality healthcare

Aim	Description
Safe	Avoiding injuries to patients [2]
Effective	Providing services based on scientific knowledge to those who will benefit [2]
Patient-centered	Providing care that respects and responds to patients' preferences, needs, and values [2]
Timely	Reducing wait times and harmful delays for both patients and providers [2]
Efficient	Avoiding waste of equipment, supplies, ideas, and energy [2]
Equitable	Providing consistent care, regardless of patients' personal factors [2]

Mia agrees with Tom that the definition of quality is not being met when the TAT for the RBD panel results is an average of 12 days, which could delay diagnosis and make treatment less timely and effective.

21.2.2 What Is Quality Improvement?

Next, Mia explains that the Quality department works with teams to complete quality improvement projects. *Quality improvement (*also known as *continuous improvement)* is an ongoing effort to improve processes, safety, and patient care [3].

A variety of frameworks (known as *quality methodologies*) exist for organizing quality improvement efforts. Table 21.2 describes some of the most common quality methodologies.

21.2.3 What Is Patient Safety?

Next, Tom asks, "How is quality improvement related to patient safety?" Mia explains that *patient safety* is the prevention of avoidable harm to a patient [7]. Within patient safety, the goal is to reduce near-misses, errors, and adverse events.

Table 21.2 Overview of quality methodologies

Quality methodology	Description
Baldrige Excellence Framework	Assesses a business's performance based on leadership, strategy, customer focus, workforce, operations, and results for long-term success [4]
Lean	Improves efficiency and effectiveness by eliminating waste [5]
Six Sigma	Improves business processes using statistical analysis and the DMAIC steps: Define, measure, analyze, improve, Control [6]. *Define*—What is important? *Measure*—How are we doing? *Analyze*—What is wrong? *Improve*—What needs to be done? *Control*—How do we guarantee performance?

- A *near-miss* is an error in medical care that is found and fixed before harming the patient [8].
- An *error* is incorrect planning or execution that leads or could lead to an unintended result [9].
- An *adverse event* is an event where care leads to a negative outcome, such as extended hospital stay, permanent harm, life-saving intervention, or death [10].

Mia explains that the RBD panel TAT could be considered an error because results are not being sent to providers according to the published turnaround time. This error may not be causing any adverse events right now, but a quality improvement team can identify what is causing the errors (the longer TATs) and try to reduce or stop them from occurring.

21.3 Defining a Quality Improvement Project

At the end of their discussion, Mia and Tom agree that a quality improvement team should be assigned to investigate the issues with the RBD panel TAT. To start this process, Tom first works with the Project Management Office (PMO) to submit a project request. Because the RBD panel TAT may be negatively impacting patient care, the request is approved and assigned a high priority. To learn more about project management and approval processes, refer to the project management chapter in this textbook.

21.3.1 Selecting a Quality Improvement Methodology

Once the project has been approved, Ahmad (a project manager) is assigned to lead the project. Ahmad, Tom, and Mia decide that the project will follow the Six Sigma DMAIC quality methodology (using the phases of define, measure, analyze, improve, control). Laboratory personnel have completed other Six Sigma projects, so they are familiar with this approach.

The first phase within the DMAIC methodology is the *Define* phase, during which the problem, areas for improvement, and project goals are identified [11].

21.3.2 Forming a Quality Improvement Team

Ahmad works with Tom and Mia to identify members of the quality improvement (QI) project team and define their roles and responsibilities within the project.

Tom and Mia will be the project champions and sponsors. They will help to address any resistance or barriers that the quality improvement team experiences. In addition, they will help to ensure that appropriate stakeholders are represented within the QI project team. A *stakeholder* is anyone affected by the outcome of a project [12]. For example, in this project, stakeholders may include laboratory personnel, quality personnel, and providers who order the laboratory tests and receive the results.

In addition to Ahmad, Mia explains that the team will also need a QI lead. Within her department, she has two types of staff who can serve in this role.

- A *quality engineer* ensures products and services meet specific quality standards [13].
- A *quality analyst* improves the quality of care by analyzing data, identifying issues, and recommending solutions to enhance patient outcomes [14].

Because this project focuses on the analysis and improvement of the testing process, Mia recommends one of the quality analysts, Elena, as the QI lead for this project.

Next, Ahmad, Tom, and Mia discuss the laboratory personnel who should be part of the QI project team. Tom recommends that the manager of the CTL, Ren, be included in the QI project, as he is responsible for overseeing the daily operations of the laboratory. In addition, Ada is the lead laboratory technologist who works on the RBD panel, so she will be included in the QI project team. A *laboratory technologist* collects tissue and fluid samples from patients and tests them to help doctors diagnose and treat diseases [15].

Finally, they decide to contact Keiran, a hematologist who often orders the RBD panel, and ask if he would be interested in joining the QI project team. A *hematologist* is a doctor specially trained to diagnose and treat blood disorders [16]. Keiran agrees to be part of the team.

21.3.3 Systems and Processes

With the QI project team members identified, Ahmad schedules the first team meeting. During the first team meeting, the QI lead Elena explains the importance of understanding the systems and processes involved in the RBD panel and its TAT.

21.3.3.1 What Is a System?

First, Elena explains that the RBD panel is more than test results and their TAT. The RBD panel is part of a larger system.

A *system* is a set of processes designed to achieve a specific goal or result [17]. Within a system, *inputs* enter that system and are *processed* to produce an *output*. To ensure that the outputs meet *standards*, the system will have *controls*, which are used to check that the process is performing as expected and the outputs meet standards. As the process runs and controls are used, *feedback* is provided to individuals within the process so they can identify issues immediately and correct them.

Finally, the system operates within an *environment*, which can include the individuals working within the system, the technology involved, and the physical layout of the facility. For example, the RBD panel testing uses an *assay analyzer*, which is an instrument used to find and measure the amount of specific substances in a sample [18]. A *laboratory information system (LIS)* is used to track lab orders, patient samples, test results, and result reports that are sent to providers.

To better understand the RBD panel system, the QI project team works together to describe each component of the system (a portion of which is shown in Table 21.3).

Table 21.3 Examples of components within the RBD panel system

Component	Description	RBD panel example(s)
Input	Resources put into a system[19]	RBD panel order for the patient. Patient blood sample.
Process	Activities or operations performed on the inputs [19]	Sample processing, which includes entering the RBD panel test order and labeling the blood sample. RBD panel testing, which includes preparing the sample for testing and completing the testing. Results review, which includes reviewing the results of the RBD panel testing, preparing a report of the results, and reviewing and approving the results report.
Output	Results and products of the system[19]	Test results from the RBD panel testing. RBD panel test results report.
Standard	Guidelines an organization follows to ensure consistent quality in processes [20]	The results review and reporting must be completed within 24 h from when the test results are available.
Control	Overseeing and guiding an activity to achieve the desired result [21]	At each step in the process, individuals must scan the label on the blood sample into the LIS. The LIS keeps track of when each step in the process occurs (such as when the CTL receives the sample from the Sample Processing Department).
Feedback	Information about how a process is performing, which is used to make changes and improvements [22]	Ada is paged if the assay analyzer indicates that RBD panel testing was unsuccessful. Ren is paged if a testing result has not been reviewed, corrected (if needed), and approved within 24 h.
Environment	The conditions, factors, and resources that impact how a process is carried out and its outcome [23]	The RBD panel is one of 35 tests that are done within the CTL. The primary technologies used in RBD panel testing are the LIS and the assay analyzer.

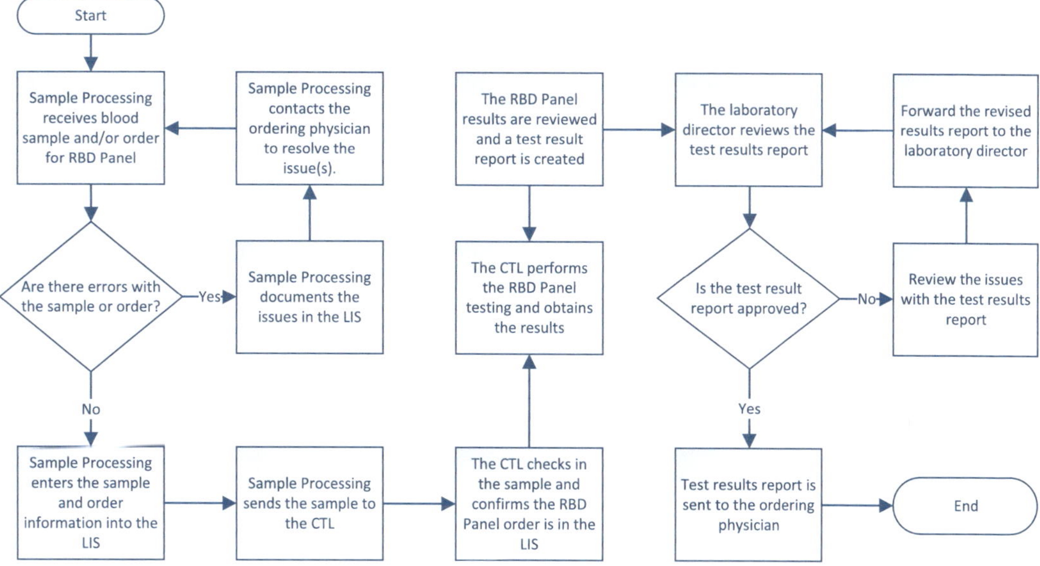

Fig. 21.1 Process map for RBD panel testing

21.3.3.2 What Is a Process?

Now that the team has a better understanding of the RBD panel system, Elena recommends that they map the three processes involved in the system: sample processing, RBD panel testing, and results review. A *process map* is a tool that visually displays a process's inputs, actions, and outputs in a clear, step-by-step map [24]. Process maps help the entire team visualize the steps within the process, as well as the roles that are responsible for each step, as shown in the process map for the RBD panel testing (Fig. 21.1).

21.3.4 Defining the Project Scope

With the RBD panel system and processes defined, Ahmad works with the team to define project goals, objectives, and scope.

Based on the information from Tom, the goal for the current project is to reduce the RBD panel TAT from an average of 12 days to a maximum of 7 days, in alignment with the CTL's published TAT for this test.

To achieve this goal, the project will have the following objectives:

- Identify processes and/or process steps that are the most significant contributors to the current TAT time (12 days on average).
- Based on these contributors, identify improvements to lower the overall TAT and implement these improvements within the CTL and RBD panel testing.
- Monitor these improvements to determine their effect on the RBD panel TAT.

Next, the team discusses the scope of the project. The project scope will include the three processes involved in the RBD panel system. This project will not include any research samples that are being completed by university researchers within the CTL.

21.4 Measuring the Process

With the Define phase of the project complete, the next phase is the *Measure* phase of the DMAIC methodology. In the Measure phase, data is gathered about the current process to find areas that need improvement [25].

Table 21.4 Example measurements for the RBD panel system

Measurement	Description	Reason
Sample processing time	The time from when the RBD order and sample are received by the Sample Processing Department until the labeled blood sample is sent to the CTL	Determine if the sample processing time is completed within 8 h (maximum)
Sample receipt errors	The number of RBD panel orders and/or samples received without the necessary information Errors include: RBD panel orders received within an associated blood sample RBD panel blood samples received without an associated order RBD panel orders received without the necessary information (full patient name, patient birthdate, provider name, and contact information) RBD blood samples received without the necessary information (full patient name, patient birthdate, name of the test, date/time the sample was taken from the patient)	Determine if errors are contributing to delays in the sample processing process

21.4.1 Identifying "Symptoms" of the Problem

During the next team meeting, Elena explains that the next step in the project is to identify "symptoms" of the TAT problem. A *symptom* is an indication that something is not working as expected within the RBD panel system. To identify these symptoms, the inputs, steps within the process, and the outputs need to be measured.

Using the standards, controls, and process maps from the Define phase, the team determines what measurements may be helpful. For each of the processes, they decide to measure the time to complete each process, as well as some key inputs and outputs. Examples of these measurements are shown in Table 21.4.

21.4.2 Creating a Measurement Plan

With the measurements identified, Elena works with the team to create a measurement plan. A *measurement plan* is a document that links goals to specific criteria to measure success [26]. Most measurement plans will have two primary components: operational definitions and a data specification.

Table 21.5 Examples of operational definitions for the RBD panel system

Term	Definition
CTL	Complex testing laboratory, which is one of the laboratories within the clinical laboratories
RBD panel	Rare blood disease panel, which is a laboratory test performed within the CTL
Sample processing time	The time from when the RBD order and sample are received by the Sample Processing Department until the labeled blood sample is sent to the CTL

An *operational definition* creates consistency by providing the entire team with the same definitions of key terms within the project [27]. Operational definitions can also include key acronyms used within the project, such as TAT, meaning "turnaround time." Examples of operational definitions are shown in Table 21.5.

A *data specification* is a guideline to ensure detailed and consistent data definitions and measurements [28]. In general, a data specification will include the name of the measurement; the source of the data for this measurement; and the steps for collecting the data, including the amount of data to collect. Table 21.6 shows a partial data specification for the measurements planned within the RBD panel system.

Table 21.6 Partial data specification for the RBD panel system

Measurement	Data source	Measurement process
Sample receipt errors	Spreadsheet that contains: RBD panel order ID (if available) Blood sample ID (if available) The error(s) identified for the order and/or associated blood sample	For 1 month, the staff within the Sample Processing Department will document each RBD panel order and associated blood sample within the spreadsheet For each order/sample, they will document any errors that occur such as RBD panel orders received within an associated blood sample RBD panel blood samples received without an associated order RBD panel orders received without the necessary information (full patient name, patient birthdate, provider name, and contact information) RBD blood samples received without the necessary information (full patient name, patient birthdate, name of the test, date/time the sample was taken from the patient)
Sample processing time	Report from the LIS that includes RBD panel order ID Blood sample ID Date/time the RBD panel order was received by the Sample Processing Department Date/time the RBD panel was received by the CTL	Ada will request LIS report from the Data reporting specialist (Ruth) Report should include RBD panel orders and samples from the past month (the month during which the sample receipt errors were documented) Report should not include any RBD panel orders or samples related to research Ada will review the report (to ensure the correct information was received) Ada will forward the report to Ahmad (so that the data is maintained with the rest of the project documentation)

21.4.3 Testing the Measurement Plan

As part of creating the measurement plan, Elena recommends that the QI project team "test" the measurement process they have defined. For one of the measurements, the team creates a spreadsheet to track the sample receipt errors.

Staff within the Sample Processing department try out this spreadsheet for 2 days. During that time, they discover that the spreadsheet is difficult to maintain, and they often forget to document the RBD panel samples they receive. Then, one of the Sample Processing staff members asks if the data from the LIS can be used, as the staff are required to enter any problems with the RBD panel order or associated blood sample that they are processing.

The QI project team was not aware that this data was entered into the LIS, so Ada works with Ruth to determine if this error information could be reported from the LIS. They determine that the LIS has all the information that the QI project team needs, so the team updates the data specification within the measurement plan to indicate that an LIS report will be used to collect this data.

Once all the measurements have been tested and the measurement plan has been updated, the QI project team finalizes the measurement plan.

21.4.4 Collecting Measurement Data

Following the measurement plan, the QI project team collects data for each of the measurements and provides the data to Ahmad for storage with the rest of the project documentation.

Ada asks Elena what would have happened if the measurement plan was not followed correctly, such as if the laboratory technologist who completed the RBD panel did not document the success indication from the assay analyzer. Elena explains that following the measurement plan is important for *data integrity*, which is ensuring data is accurate, complete, consistent, and valid [29].

To evaluate data integrity, the QI project team would need to work with the laboratory technologist and Ren to determine if the success indication information could be found elsewhere, such as in the log that the CTL maintains for all the testing they perform each day. If this information could be found in this log, then the team could document the indication from this log and, assuming the testing was successful, data integrity would no longer be a concern.

If the success indication information could not be found elsewhere, though, data integrity may be impacted. If the integrity of the data could not be assessed, then the data would need to be removed and not used for further work in the QI project.

21.5 Analyzing Data and Measurements

Next, the QI project team begins working on analyzing the data. In the *Analyze* phase of the DMAIC methodology, data from the Measure phase is used to identify the underlying cause of an issue [30].

21.5.1 Identifying Key Questions

The first step in analyzing the data is identifying the key questions that need to be answered during the analysis. The team works together to select the questions to use in the analysis. For example, one of the questions is "what is the average sample processing time?"

21.5.2 Selecting Analysis Techniques

Once the key questions are identified, the QI team determines the appropriate analysis technique for answering each question.

Descriptive statistics summarize the facts and proven outcomes of a data set [31]. They can be used to calculate basic information about the data such as counts, averages, minimum values, and maximum values. For example, the team calculates the minimum, maximum, and average values for the sample processing time, the RBD panel testing time, and the results review time.

Inferential statistics use sample data to draw conclusions about population data [31]. For example, the team determines if a statistical correlation (relationship) exists between the results review time and the overall turnaround time for the RBD panel. For example, when the sample processing time increases, does the overall TAT also increase?

21.5.3 Documenting the Results

After the QI project team completes their analysis, Elena helps the team document their findings using a template like shown in Table 21.7.

21.5.4 Summarizing the Results

Once the results for each measurement are documented, Elena works with the QI project team to summarize the findings from their analysis. These findings include

- The sample processing time average was 6.76 h. None of the samples reviewed in this analysis exceeded the maximum (8.0 h per laboratory policy).
- The CTL testing time average was 15.5 h. None of the samples reviewed in this analysis

Table 21.7 One measurement for the RBD panel system

Question	What is the average sample processing time?
Tool(s)	Statistical average, minimum value, maximum value (descriptive statistics)
Interpretation	The average sample processing time is 6.76 h with a minimum of 2.5 h and a maximum of 7.75 h The maximum value for this time is 8 h per laboratory policy Based on the calculations performed, we have confirmed that all samples used for this analysis were processed within the 8-h policy requirements

exceeded the maximum (24 h per laboratory policy).

- The result review time average was 7 days. Approximately 11% of the test results were completed within the 24-h maximum set by laboratory policy.
- The time from when the test results were available until the time the results report was created was an average of 5 days. This time was related to the laboratory technologist assigned to create the results report as well as the type of result. Abnormal results took the longest (on average, 6 days) while normal results took the least time (on average, 2 days).
- The time from when the results report was created until it was approved by the laboratory director was an average of 12 h.

21.6 Improving the Process

With the Analyze phase complete, the next phase in the DMAIC methodology is the *Improve* phase. In this phase, the team creates and implements solutions to the problems identified during the Analyze phase [32].

21.6.1 Identifying a Root Cause

The first step in the Improve phase is to identify the root cause. The *root cause* is the main cause of a problem or defect in a process [33].

In reviewing the analysis summary, the team identifies that the primary contributor to the increase in the RBD panel TAT is the results review, which is taking an average of 7 days. During the results review, the time from when the test results were available until the time the results report was created was an average of 5 days with the greatest delays occurring for abnormal results. In addition, one laboratory technologist (Sue) reviewed most of these abnormal results.

The team observes several days of the results review process and notes that two technologists (Ramon and Eva) are only reviewing normal results and, when asked, they state they are uncomfortable reviewing abnormal results. Sue is scheduled to review results 1 day per week. Based on this information, the root cause of the RBD panel TAT is how the technologists are reviewing the results (normal vs. abnormal).

21.6.2 Identifying and Selecting Improvements

Next, the QI project team brainstorms potential improvements. *Brainstorming* is a technique for generating new ideas and solving problems through creative thinking [34].

Some of the potential improvements include

- Additional training for Ramon and Eva.
- Changing Sue's schedule so she reviews results multiple times per week.
- Sending abnormal results directly to Sue for review.

To determine which improvement to implement, the QI project team assesses the total cost, the time to implement each change, and the likelihood the change will reduce the TAT. Based on these criteria, the team determines that sending abnormal results directly to Sue would be low cost and take a short time to implement. This improvement also has a high likelihood of reducing the TAT for the RBD panel, as Sue would be notified immediately when abnormal results were available for review. As a result, they select this improvement for implementation.

21.6.3 Developing an Implementation Plan

Once the improvement is selected, the QI project team identifies the key tasks to complete:

- The LIS team can set up the abnormal RBD panel results to be sent directly to Sue. This task will take 1 week.
- The change should be communicated to the CTL staff and the project sponsors and champions (Tom and Mia), as well as the hematologists who order the RBD panel.

Table 21.8 Partial implementation plan for selected improvement

Task	Deadline	Assigned to
Configure abnormal RBD panel results to be sent directly to sue	January 12	LIS analyst
Communicate change to RBD panel results to review to CTL laboratory staff	January 15	Ren

Based on this planning discussion, Ahmad creates an implementation plan (also known as a project plan) for this improvement. An *implementation plan* lists the tasks, timelines, and responsibilities for implementing the improvement. A portion of the implementation plan is shown in Table 21.8.

For more information about planning a project, refer to the project management chapter in this textbook.

21.7 Controlling and Monitoring Improvements

Once the Improve phase is complete, the final phase of the DMAIC methodology is the *Control* phase, during which the project's progress is tracked to ensure the improvements are sustained [35].

21.7.1 Identifying Monitoring Measurements

As part of the implementation planning, the QI project team identifies measurements they will use to determine if the improvement is working. During this monitoring, they decide to collect data for the following measurements:

- The results review time
- The overall TAT

For the first 2 weeks after this implementation, Ren will receive a daily report for the result review time and the overall TAT. After these 2 weeks, the QI project team, Ramon, Eva, and Sue, will meet to review all the measurement data and determine next steps, including if the improvement should continue.

21.7.2 Implementing the Improvement

With the monitoring plan determined, the QI project team implements the improvement. After 2 weeks, they find that the results review time decreases to an average of 27 h (with the maximum being 48 h). The average overall turnaround time is 6 days (with a maximum of 8 days). Based on this data, the team decides to allow the improvement to continue for another month.

After another month, the results review time decreases to an average of 20 h (with a maximum of 23 h). The average turnaround time is 4.5 days (with a maximum of 7 days). Based on these results, the improvement is maintained within the CTL. Tom and Ren continue to monitor the overall TAT using the regular monthly reports.

21.7.3 Identifying the Lessons Learned

As the project nears completion, Ahmad schedules a final meeting for the QI project team. During this meeting, Tom, Mia, and the QI project team reflect on the lessons they learned while working on this QI project. *Lessons learned* are the knowledge and skills gained during the project, which can be applied to future projects to avoid issues and improve project performance [36].

For example, the team recommends adding observation of the process as one of the measurements for future projects, as this observation was critical to identifying the issues with the results review. Ahmad documents these lessons learned in the project closeout report and stores this document as part of the project.

At the end of the meeting, Ahmad, Tom, and Mia surprise the team with handwritten thank you notes and gift cards to their favorite restaurants to celebrate the work they completed.

21.8 Summary

Elena, a quality analyst, provides leadership to quality improvement (QI) teams who work to improve the processes, safety, and patient care. Recently, she worked with stakeholders for the Complex Testing Laboratory (CTL) to reduce the turnaround time (TAT) for the Rare Blood Disease (RBD) panel.

With the support of CTL leadership, a QI project team worked through the Define, Measure, Analyze, Improve, and Control (DMAIC) phases of the Six Sigma methodology and completed key activities like defining the project goal; defining and collecting measurements; analyzing the measurement data; identifying improvements and planning their implementation; and monitoring the improvement to determine if it is having the intended effect on the RBD panel TAT.

By the end of the project, the RBD panel TAT has improved and meets the published standards. The team reflected on their work to identify lessons learned and celebrate this improvement, which will support more timely patient care.

21.9 Resources

See Table 21.9 for a list of process improvement resources.

Table 21.9 Process improvement resources

Resource	Website (link)
Professional organizations for process and quality improvement	American Society for Quality (ASQ) (https://asq.org/) The American Health Quality Association (AHQA) (https://www.ahqa.org/ahqa-member-organizations/) National Association for Healthcare Quality (NAHQ) (https://nahq.org/) International Association for Six Sigma Certification (IASSC) (https://iassc.org/)
Organizations for quality improvement in healthcare	Centers for Medicare & Medicaid Services (CMS) Quality Measurement and Quality Improvement (https://www.cms.gov/Medicare/Quality-Initiatives-Patient-Assessment-Instruments/MMS/Quality-Measure-and-Quality-Improvement-) Agency for Healthcare Research and Quality (AHRQ) (https://www.ahrq.gov/) Institute for Healthcare Improvement (https://www.ihi.org/) The Leapfrog Group (https://www.leapfroggroup.org/)
Information about careers in process and quality improvement	Quality analyst on Indeed (https://www.indeed.com/career/quality-analyst/salaries) Quality engineer on Indeed (https://www.indeed.com/career/quality-engineer/salaries) Six Sigma Black Belt salaries (https://www.indeed.com/career-advice/pay-salary/six-sigma-black-belt-salaries)

Quality Improvement - QUESTIONS

1. *Define quality and quality improvement.*
2. *Define patient safety, near miss, error, and adverse event.*
3. *Explain the importance of systems thinking within a quality improvement project.*
4. *Identify and describe the key activities within each phase of the Six Sigma DMAIC process.*

Quality Improvement - ANSWERS

1. Quality is the likelihood that healthcare services achieve desired outcomes and are consistent with professional standards.

   Quality improvement is an ongoing effort to improve processes, safety, and patient care.
2. A near miss is an error in medical care that is found and fixed before harming the patient.

   An error is incorrect planning or execution that leads or could lead to an unintended result.

   An adverse event is an event where care leads to negative outcomes, such as extended hospital stay, permanent harm, life-saving intervention, or death.
3. A system is a set of processes designed to achieve a specific goal or result. Systems consist of inputs, processes, outputs, standards, controls, feedback, and an environment. Therefore, when working within a quality improvement project, all of these components need to be reviewed and considered to avoid negative unintended consequences and increase the likelihood that improvements will have the intended effects.
4. In the Define phase, the problem, areas for improvement, and project goals are identified. As part of this work, the quality improvement methodology and team will be selected. Using the selected quality improvement methodology, the team will gather information about the system and processes involved.

   In the Measure phase, the team will gather data about the current process to find areas that need improvement. To complete this work, they will identify information about what is not working and create a plan to measure potential issues in the current process. The team will use this plan to collect data.
   In the Analyze phase, the team using the data they collected to identify the underlying cause of an issue in the current process. They identify the key questions that need to be answered and select analysis techniques that are appropriate for answering these questions. They complete their analysis and document the results.

   In the Improve phase, the team creates and implements solutions to the problems identified in the Analyze phase. Using their analysis, they identify a primary root cause and then identify and select improvements based on this cause. The team creates a plan to implement the improvements they have selected.

   In the Control phase, the team tracks the project's progress to ensure the improvements are having the intended effects. Before they implement the improvements, they will identify measurements that can be completed to determine if the improvement is working. Then, they implement the improvements and a process for gathering the measurements they identified. Finally, they will identify the lessons they learned from completing this process.

Glossary of Terms

Term	Definition
Adverse event	An event where care leads to a negative outcome, such as extended hospital stay, permanent harm, life-saving intervention, or death.
Analyze phase	A phase within the six sigma DMAIC methodology, during which data from the measure phase is used to identify the underlying cause of an issue.
Assay analyzer	An instrument used to find and measure the amount of specific substances in a sample.
Baldrige excellence framework	A quality improvement methodology that assesses a business's performance based on leadership, strategy, customer focus, workforce, operations, and results for lasting success.

Term	Definition
Brainstorming	A technique for generating new ideas and solving problems through creative thinking.
Continuous improvement	An ongoing effort to improve processes, safety, and patient care.
Control	Overseeing and guiding an activity to achieve the desired result.
Control phase	A phase in the six sigma DMAIC methodology, during which the project's progress is tracked to ensure the improvements are sustained.
Data integrity	Ensuring data is accurate, complete, consistent, and valid.
Data specification	A guideline to ensure detailed and consistent data definitions.
Define phase	A phase in the six sigma DMAIC methodology, during which the problem, areas for improvement, and project goals are identified.
Descriptive statistics	A type of statistics that summarizes the facts and proven outcomes of a data set.
Effective	Providing services based on scientific knowledge to those who will benefit.
Efficient	Avoiding waste of equipment, supplies, ideas, and energy.
Environment	The conditions, factors, and resources that impact how a process is carried out and its outcome.
Equitable	Providing consistent care, regardless of patients' personal factors.
Error	An error in planning or execution that leads or could lead to an unintended result.
Feedback	Information about how a process is performing, which can be used to make changes and improvements.
Hematologist	A doctor specially trained to diagnose and treat blood disorders.
Improve phase	A phase in the six sigma DMAIC methodology, during which solutions to the problems identified during the analyze phase are created and implemented.
Inferential statistics	A type of statistics that uses sample data to draw conclusions about population data.
Input	Resources put into a system.
Laboratory technologist	An individual who collects tissue and fluid samples from patients and tests them to help doctors diagnose and treat diseases.

Term	Definition
Lean	A quality methodology that focuses on improving efficiency and effectiveness by eliminating waste.
Measure phase	A phase in the six sigma DMAIC methodology, during which data is gathered about the current process to find areas that need improvement.
Measurement plan	A document that links goals to specific criteria to measure success.
Near-miss	Errors in medical care that are found and fixed before harming the patient.
Operational definition	Documentation that creates consistency by providing the entire team with the same definitions of key terms within the project.
Output	Results and products of the system.
Patient safety	The prevention of avoidable harm to a patient.
Patient-centered	Providing care that respects and responds to patients' preferences, needs, and values.
Process	Activities or operations performed on inputs and produces outputs.
Process map	A tool that visually displays a process's inputs, actions, and outputs in a clear, step-by-step graphic.
Quality analyst	An individual who focuses on improving the quality of patient care by analyzing data, identifying issues, and recommending solutions to enhance patient outcomes.
Quality engineer	An individual who ensures that products and services meet specific quality standards.
Root cause	The main cause of a problem or defect in a process.
Six sigma	A quality methodology that improves business processes using statistical analysis and the DMAIC steps: Define, measure, analyze, improve, control.
Stakeholder	Anyone affected by the outcome of a project.
Standard	Guidelines an organization follows to ensure consistent quality in processes.
System	A set of processes designed to achieve a specific goal or result.
Timely	Reducing wait times and harmful delays for both patients and providers.

References

1. Institute of Medicine (IOM). Medicare: a strategy for quality assurance, volume I. The National Academies Press; 1990.
2. Agency for Healthcare Research and Quality (AHRQ). Six domains of health care quality. https://www.ahrq.gov/talkingquality/measures/six-domains.html. Accessed 19 Mar 2025.
3. Rehkopf M. What is continuous improvement? https://www.atlassian.com/agile/project-management/continuous-improvement. Accessed 19 Mar 2025.
4. Louisiana Quality Foundation. Why you should consider the baldrige excellence framework for your business. 2021. https://louisianaquality.org/why-you-should-consider-the-baldrige-excellence-framework-for-your-business/. Accessed 19 Mar 2025.
5. Lean Enterprise Institute. What is lean? https://www.lean.org/explore-lean/what-is-lean/. Accessed 19 Mar 2025.
6. SixSigma. About Six Sigma. https://www.6sigma.us/six-sigma.php. Accessed 19 Mar 2025.
7. World Health Organization (WHO). Patient Safety. https://www.who.int/news-room/fact-sheets/detail/patient-safety. Accessed 19 Mar 2025.
8. Crane S, Sloane PD, Elder NC, Cohen LW, Laughtenschlager N, Zimmerman S. Implementing near-miss reporting and improvement tracking in primary care practices: lessons learned. https://www.ahrq.gov/patient-safety/reports/liability/crane.html. Accessed 19 Mar 2025.
9. Agency for Healthcare Research and Quality (AHRQ). Medical errors. https://www.ahrq.gov/topics/medical-errors.html. Accessed 19 Mar 2025.
10. U.S Department of Health and Human Services (HHS) Office of Inspector General. Adverse Events. 2023. https://oig.hhs.gov/reports/featured/adverse-events/. Accessed 19 Mar 2025.
11. 6signmastudy. Define Phase. 2021. https://www.6sigmastudy.com/article?title=define-phase. Accessed 4 Apr 2025.
12. Johnivan JR. Understanding different types of stakeholders and their roles. 2023. https://project-management.com/types-of-stakeholders/. Accessed 19 Mar 2025.
13. University of Massachusetts Amherst. What is a quality engineer? A comprehensive guide to the profession. 2024. https://bootcamp.umass.edu/blog/quality-management/what-is-a-quality-engineer. Accessed 4 Apr 2025.
14. ZenBit. Defining quality assurance in healthcare. https://zenbit.tech/blog/what-is-quality-assurance-in-healthcare/. Accessed 4 Apr 2025.
15. All Allied Health Schools. Learn how to become a clinical laboratory technologist. https://www.alalliedhealthschools.com/specialties/clinical-laboratory-scientist/. Accessed 4 Apr 2025.
16. National Cancer Institute (NCI). Hematologist. https://www.cancer.gov/publications/dictionaries/cancer-terms/def/hematologist. Accessed 4 Apr 2025.
17. MYOB. Business systems: what are they and how will they help your business? 2021. https://www.myob.com/au/blog/understanding-business-systems/. Accessed 4 Apr 2025.
18. News Medical Life Sciences. Immunoassay analyzers. https://www.news-medical.net/Clinical-and-Diagnostics/Immunoassay-Analyzers.
19. Jones K. The input-process-output model in project management. 2024. https://medium.com/@kyle-jones_47003/the-input-process-output-model-in-project-management-f8383873c33f. Accessed 4 Apr 2025.
20. Guevara P. A quick guide on quality standards. 2024. https://safetyculture.com/topics/quality-assurance-and-quality-control/quality-standards/. Accessed 4 Apr 2025.
21. ENERCORP Instruments LTD. What does process control mean? https://enercorp.com/what-does-process-control-mean/. Accessed 4 Apr 2025.
22. INTOO. Feedback mechanism. https://www.intoo.com/us/glossary/feedback-mechanism/. Accessed 4 Apr 2025.
23. IBM. System environment. 2024. https://www.ibm.com/docs/en/aix/7.2?topic=administration-system-environment. Accessed 4 Apr 2025.
24. Hessing T. Process mapping. https://sixsigmastudyguide.com/process-mapping/. Accessed 4 Apr 2025.
25. Six Sigma Online. How to collect data in the measure phase of the DMAIC process. https://www.sixsigma-online.org/dmaic-process-measure-phase/. Accessed 4 Apr 2025.
26. Flippo W. Creating measurement plans: what they are and why they are important. 2017. https://www.deptagency.com/insight/creating-measurement-plans-important/. Accessed 4 Apr 2025.
27. Harkhoe. Operational measure definition. https://www.dmaic.com/operational-measure-definition/. Accessed 4 Apr 2025.
28. Lightcast. Data definition specification. https://lightcast.io/open-skills/skills/KS122NV6KDQ72CYGSCK4/data-definition-specification. Accessed 4 Apr 2025.
29. Fortinet. What is data integrity? https://www.fortinet.com/resources/cyberglossary/data-integrity. Accessed 4 Apr 2025.
30. Management and Strategy Institute (MSI). Six Sigma DMAIC – Analyze stage. https://www.msicertified.com/blog/six-sigma-dmaic-analyze-stage/. Accessed 4 Apr 2025.
31. Kumar A. Comprehensive guide to descriptive vs inferential statistics. 2025. https://www.simplilearn.com/difference-between-descriptive-inferential-statistics-article. Accessed 4 Apr 2025.

32. SixSigma. DMAIC: approach to continuous improvement. https://www.6sigma.us/dmaic-process/. Accessed 4 Apr 2025.
33. Management and Strategy Institute (MSI). Define root cause. https://www.msicertified.com/define-root-cause/. Accessed 4 Apr 2025.
34. Miro. What is brainstorming? Accessed 4 Apr 2025. https://miro.com/brainstorming/what-is-brainstorming/.
35. Hessing T. Control phase (DMAIC). https://sixsigmastudyguide.com/control-phase/. Accessed 4 Apr 2025.
36. Project Management Institute (PMI), editor. A guide to the Project Management Body of Knowledge (PMBOK) Guide. 7th ed. Project Management Institute (PMI); 2021.

22 Interoperability

Christopher W. Lewis and Michael G. Leu

Foundational Domains [1]
This chapter addresses the following AMIA Foundational Domains: F2—Information Science and Technology, F4—Health Information Science and Technology.

Learning Objectives
After reading this chapter, you should be able to

1. Define the terms commonly used to describe health information interoperability and interoperability levels in healthcare.
2. Describe the different types of data standards required for health data exchange.
3. List and explain different frameworks for health data interoperability.
4. Discuss the current state of interoperability in healthcare and interoperability challenges.

22.1 Vignette

Interoperability supports the practice of medicine by ensuring that a patient's medical records are available when needed to support continuity of care. Prior to digital records, patients carried their physical medical records between their physician visits or health records were requested to be mailed or faxed between facilities. Even with the advances of digital health records, interoperability capabilities are not uniform. One example of one of these legacy inconsistencies is in the recording of immunizations. While numerous immunization registries exist, participation by providers in registries is not always mandatory. Further complicating this is the ability to get immunizations at the drug store, supermarket, or community centers. Noncompulsory reporting and diverse locations result in inconsistent, incomplete, and stale immunization records forcing people to carry "Immunization cards" with them for medical appointments, school, travel, and other requirements. Without immunization cards and reliable records, people may receive unneeded extra vaccine doses, or if going from potentially inaccurate verbal history, may receive incomplete vaccine series.

C. W. Lewis (✉)
Department of Rehabilitation Medicine, University of Washington, Seattle, WA, USA
e-mail: clewis56@uw.edu

M. G. Leu
Department of Pediatrics, of Biomedical Informatics and Medical Education, and of Family Medicine, University of Washington, Seattle, WA, USA

C. Eldredge et al. (eds.), *Introductory Textbook in Health Informatics*, Health Informatics,
https://doi.org/10.1007/978-3-032-16657-9_22

22.2 Definitions

As defined by the Institute of Electrical and Electronics Engineers [2], *interoperability* is "the ability of two or more systems or their components to exchange information and to use the information that has been exchanged."

An *electronic medical record (EMR)* is a digital version of a patient medical record that contains the medical and treatment history of the patient at a single institution or practice. This includes patient demographics, medical history, diagnoses, treatments, and test results. This system may also include log administrative data such as who accessed the records and what time various actions took place [3, 4].

An *electronic health record (EHR)* is an EMR that can share medical records with other EMR systems through interoperability. This means that the information collected at a single institution can be shared beyond that institution as well as data can be brought in from outside the institution [3, 4].

Health information exchange (HIE) has two meanings. When used to describe an action, it describes the electronic movement of health-related information among organizations according to nationally recognized standards. HIE facilitates the secure exchange of patient data across different healthcare entities [5]. This term can also be used to describe companies that specialize in coordinating record exchange so that patient information can be accessed, often from all the health systems in a geographical region.

22.3 A Brief History of Interoperability

Moving patient data together with patients as they are being seen across different healthcare teams and geography has always been a challenge. When patients are seen for the first time at a hospital, they would often need to repeat their entire medical history unless they brought copies of their records. Despite advancements in EHR interoperability, there is a continued reliance on faxed copies as the ubiquitous method of transferring patient medical records between medical institutions. While it is a method for transferring paper records, faxing provides information that must be manually reviewed and can lead to delays and inefficiencies in care delivery. Even when these records are available, providers might not digest them completely due to their length (sometimes tens to hundreds of pages), complexity, and sometimes lack of organization.

The increasing reliance on specialty care has further fragmented the healthcare system, often resulting in gaps in patient-centered care. As patients move between multiple specialists, key details of their medical history may be lost or inconsistently communicated, leading to incomplete care plans. This lack of continuity can cause repetitive diagnostic tests, unnecessary treatments, and increased costs, ultimately impacting the quality of care. Without a centralized and accessible record of the patient's health information, opportunities for comprehensive, coordinated care may be missed and vital medical management may be overlooked.

In 2009, the US Congress passed the Health Information Technology for Economic and Clinical Health (HITECH) Act that established the EHR Program [2]. The HITECH Act was part of the broader American Recovery and Reinvestment Act (ARRA) of 2009 introduced by the Obama administration. ARRA aimed to stimulate economic growth while promoting the adoption and meaningful use of health information technology to improve healthcare delivery [6]. Given the new requirements for protecting patient information through the Health Insurance Portability and Accountability Act (HIPAA) and the incentives from HITECH, the adoption rate of EHR in hospitals increased from 9% in 2008 to 97% in 2014 [7, 8]. This rapid adoption involved hospital systems adopting multiple vendor-supplied EHRs as well as "home-grown" EMRs developed in-house. At the time, HITECH had no requirements for interoperability [7].

The customization of EHRs by hospitals and vendors has created significant challenges to interoperability. Each system may use proprietary formats, unique data structures, or customized interfaces. While each medical system has its own idiosyncrasies that need to be incorporated into the design of the EHR, these changes can make it difficult for different platforms to communicate effectively. This lack of standardization further exacerbates the problem of information blocking, where entities knowingly interfere with the exchange or access of electronic health information. This practice not only limits care coordination but also contradicts the goals of patient-centered care. To address these barriers, the Office of the National Coordinator for Health Information Technology has implemented rules to prohibit information blocking and promote data exchange, marking a critical step toward improved interoperability [9].

In April 2018, the Centers for Medicare and Medicaid Services (CMS) changed the EHR Incentive Programs to the Medicare and Medicaid Promoting Interoperability Programs, which rewarded institutions that met certain interoperability standards and required that patients have access to their health data [10]. See Fig. 22.1 for the timeline of federal legislation and policies for interoperability over the past couple decades [11–13].

22.4 Stakeholder Perspectives

Patients may expect their medical records to be available to all their providers when needed at the point of care; however, when patients move between healthcare institutions or geographical locations, there may be gaps in health information as not all health systems (as of this writing) provide the interoperability needed so that these records can be available to any other practice. Furthermore, doctors and other healthcare providers value having a complete medical history of their patients as it reduces redundant work/testing, streamlines patient communications, and helps build the contextual knowledge necessary to provide high-quality care.

Payers also believe that giving providers access to the complete health record will reduce the costs of providing healthcare services by reducing redundant testing and medical errors [8]. However, while it is technically possible to exchange clinical notes and other health data between HIT systems, there are several challenges to doing so. For example, there is a large burden to keep these IT systems up to date with evolving standards that help enable health data exchange. Future development will require the coordinated adoption of interoperability standards among all healthcare systems, which is challenging.

Interoperability also had an impact on public health surveillance. While standardized data collection formats have been used in the past, the need for real-time information exchange has become increasingly critical, especially in responding to public health emergencies. For example, early surveillance systems did identify

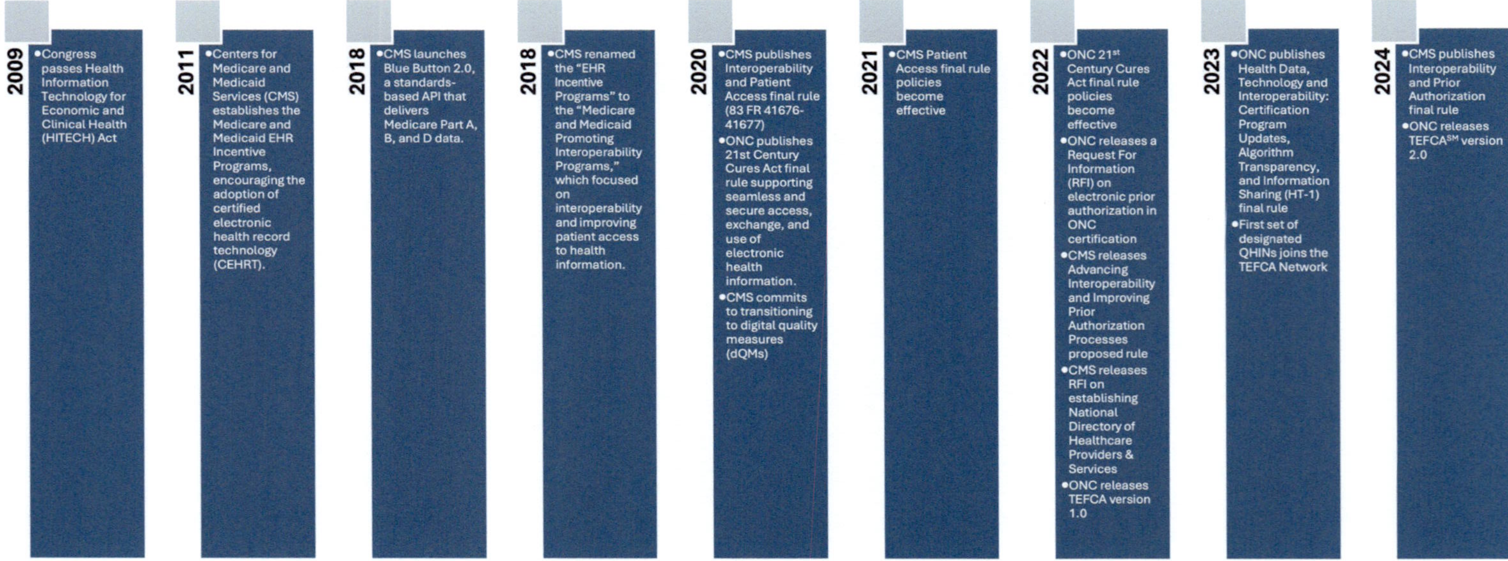

Fig. 22.1 A summary of the timeline of federal interoperability efforts

early cases of COVID-19 in Washington State [14, 15]. However, the benefit of these data across institutions benefits from interoperability as they can be shared and integrated with other datasets in real time. A more interoperable system would allow for the rapid flow of data and a quicker aggregation and analysis of that data. This would allow policymakers to make data-driven policy decisions regarding resource allocation and intervention strategies [16, 17].

22.4.1 Application of Interoperability in Informatics Disciplines

Interoperability is a critical concept throughout all areas of practice in informatics. The exchange of information between systems requires not only the ability to move data from one system to another securely but also requires standards to ensure the data can be interpreted correctly by the receiving organization. This can be particularly challenging in healthcare as there are many vendor-supplied EHR systems with differing adherence to data exchange and interoperability standards. This has led to heterogeneity in the data exchange capabilities of health systems. Additionally, new technologies continue to be developed (i.e., consumer devices and activity trackers) that can generate clinically useful data. However, these devices may not inherently exchange information with existing EHR systems, thereby limiting the ability of the healthcare team to use that data for clinical decision-making. Finding efficient and secure ways to exchange data between these systems will allow patients to have a more streamlined healthcare experience and providers have a larger wealth of data to make sound clinical decisions.

Interoperability is also important in clinical research, as this research may rely on retrospective review of data generated routinely in the care of patients. If clinical research systems and EHRs are interoperable, then patient data can be efficiently extracted and used for many purposes. For example, data can be collected and collated between multiple healthcare systems to perform multicenter research. Using data collected for one purpose (e.g., patient care) for another (e.g., research) is referred to as "secondary use."

Clinical informatics is the operational management of how data are acquired, structured, stored, processed, retrieved, analyzed, and communicated to support clinical operations. The day-to-day technology needs of the hospital require continuous evaluation, updating, and maintenance. Interoperability is a cornerstone for the seamless utilization of the disparate technologies and systems that are required to optimize a modern healthcare system.

22.5 Standards

Standards are established guidelines and specifications that define how data are formatted, transmitted, secured, and interpreted. In healthcare, standards ensure consistency and compatibility between different systems. There are over 40 standards development organizations (SDOs) in health information technology (HIT), who both create standards as well as provide guidance on how to implement those standards [18, 19]. Examples include the Health Level Seven (HL7) [20] Messaging Standard and HL7 Fast Healthcare Interoperability Resources (FHIR) [21]. HL7 is an international organization that helps to set standards for the exchange, integration, sharing, and retrieval of electronic health information. HL7 Messaging Standard is widely used in healthcare to enable interoperability between different systems. FHIR is a modern standard for exchanging healthcare information electronically. FHIR is designed to be easy to implement and support the exchange of data in a web-friendly format and allows apps to be written that are integrated with EHRs [21, 22].

Notably, standards may change and evolve over time. Therefore, SDOs should communicate if there are changes to these standards so that the new versions can be used. Individual standards may have weaknesses. Refer to Table 22.1 for a selection of standards relevant to the interoperability of medical records.

Table 22.1 Selection of standard development organizations (SDOs), standard types, and applications as related to HIT interoperability

Standards development organization	Standards	Practical application
American National Standards Institute (ANSI); X12	Electronic Data Interchange (EDI)	Guidelines and protocols defining data formatting between devices and health systems
Digital Imaging and Communications in Medicine (DICOM) Standards Committee (DSC)	DICOM	Images from studies such as radiographs and computed tomography (CT) scans
Health Level Seven (HL7) international	HL7 messaging standard, Fast Healthcare Interoperability Resources (FHIRs)	Information is organized and exchanged between EHRs as well as third-party applications
International Health Terminology Standards Development Organization (IHTSDO)	Systematized Nomenclature of Medicine Clinical Terms (SNOMED CT)	List of problems and diagnoses that a provider makes
National Library of Medicine	Unified Medical Language System (UMLS), RxNorm	Standard health and biomedical vocabulary, and standard terminology for medications, respectively
National Council for Prescription Drug Programs (NCPDP)	Billing unit standard	Used in medication claims processing for how pharmaceuticals are billed
Regenstrief institute	Logical Observation Identifiers Names and Codes (LOINC)	Defining laboratory and clinical observations
OpenID foundation	OpenID Connect Core 1.0	Allows client applications to verify the identity of an end user and obtain basic profile information
World Health Organization (WHO)	International Classification of Diseases (ICD)	The ontology of medical diagnoses is often used for defining the patient's problem list[a] and billing codes

[a]Problem list: a list of active medical conditions relevant to a patient's clinical visit that can be relevant for history documentation and billing

22.6 Data Warehouses

A *clinical data repository (CDR)* or *data warehouse (DW)* is a centralized database that consolidates health data from different sources within a healthcare organization or can also include data from outside the organization. It facilitates the storage and retrieval of clinical information [23]. The advantage of a data warehouse is to create a collective of data from multiple and often disparate systems, atop which analytics and visualizations can be built. With current technology, it would be nearly impossible to create and maintain reports or visualizations atop many disparate individual data sources.

CDRs are typically organized as relational databases. Typical database architecture has a patient key associated with each patient. This helps track patient medical care over time and link all the appropriate updates to the correct patient. This can have challenges due to situations where patient information is added in an emergency when there isn't time to check if the patient already exists or the patient's identity isn't known. There has been consideration to create a national patient identifier, but this hasn't been accomplished. The challenge is that patients can have multiple patient identifiers across multiple medical EHR systems.

Patient matching is the process of accurately linking and matching patient records across different healthcare systems to ensure that information about a particular patient is correctly identified and aggregated. One way to address this issue is by creating a *master patient index (MPI)*. HIEs may use MPIs in the process of patient record reconciliation and deduplication between and within healthcare systems, mapping multiple local patient IDs to a single entry in the MPI.

Patient matching is a significant interoperability challenge as accurately reconciling patient records requires more than just a matching name and birth date between institutions. For example, a patient may arrive at the emergency department unable to identify themselves and without any identifying documentation. In this case, a new patient record number may be assigned even though the patient already has an existing record. When the patient is identified, the disparate records should be linked so that they refer to the same patient. However, merely fixing this at the level of the health system is insufficient if there is also an HIE involved. For these types of reasons, HIE MPIs may require significant effort to maintain, with maintenance often requiring a combination of automated matching and manual confirmation with patients.

There are a variety of types of patients matching and several considerations regarding patient matching. Deterministic matching includes the comparison of specific fields (name, date of birth, etc.) for exact matches. For example, Robert Brown and Bob Brown with a date of birth variation would not return a match. Probabilistic matching, on the other hand, looks at probable matches based on the likelihood of certain data elements occurring together. For example, Robert Brown born on 2/3/2000 and Bob Brown born on 3/2/2000 might return a match with probabilistic matching. Algorithms are used to learn these combinations and therefore the accuracy can improve over time. Hybrid matching combines both deterministic and probabilistic matching together, and contextual matching adds contextual information, such as medical history, to increase the accuracy of the matching schemes. Regardless of the matching scheme, reliable and standardized data increases matching accuracy.

There as some key considerations regarding patient matching that cannot be overlooked. Privacy and security are essential. HIPAA requires that patient data that is going to be aggregated and analyzed must be deidentified.

22.7 Frameworks and Technical Requirements for Interoperability

In this section, we will explore different frameworks that are considered when providing interoperability from the lowest level to the highest level.

- The Open System Interconnection (OSI) model is used to describe the specific technical capabilities connecting systems and users when data is being transmitted from one site to another.
- The Four Levels of Interoperability describe the capabilities for the data to be interpreted correctly after transmission.
- The Office of the National Coordinator for Health Information Technology (ONC) and the Interoperability Standards Advisory (ISA) initiative describe how to store information to support the highest level of interoperability in healthcare.

22.7.1 The Open System Interconnection (OSI) Model

The OSI model [24–27] is divided into seven different technology layers when exchanging information. This model was introduced in Chap. 5. The purpose of this model is help visualize the technical solutions used to move data from one system to another. This model can be reviewed when troubleshooting transmission problems. The Seven Layers (Health Level 7, HL7) is a common set of standards to ensure information systems can communicate effectively. The information being communicated must pass through these seven layers (from the physical hardware to the application you see on your screen) [28]. The details of HL7 are discussed in Chap. 5.

There are multiple designs that are commonly used when developing a network. Examples of network architectures [29]:

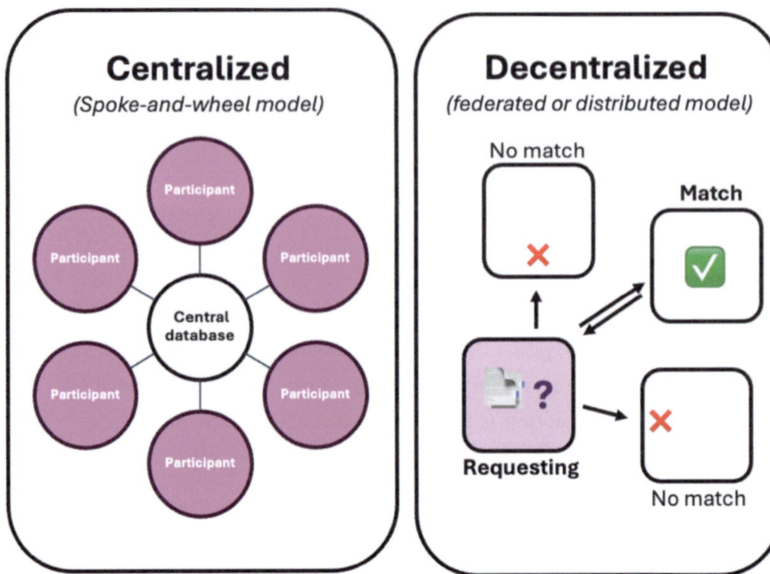

Fig. 22.2 Network architecture examples

- *Centralized (spoke-and-wheel)*: In a centralized model, all participants contribute information to a central database that can then be accessed by all participants. Users report centrally and do not exchange data directly with each other. The data must follow the specific formatting criteria of the central database (i.e., public health surveillance data). The "hub" can sometimes also reach out to have data pulled from the "spokes." In HIEs, this architecture is common but expensive to maintain because it requires significant effort to match data with standardized formatting to report it centrally. It also requires resources to continually maintain, update, and send reports.
- *Decentralized (federated or distributed model)*: All participants are registered in a peer network. Effectively, a data federation allows multiple systems to function as one—an information request made by one site is made to all and typically one system will respond and then they will exchange data as a pair. A common example of this network architecture is the banking system, where data is requested and exchanged regarding account balances. All banks are responsible for the accounts they represent and track the transfer of funds in and out of those accounts. Given the large amount of data exchanged in HIEs, a full federated model is deemed to be impractical at this time.
- *Hybrid models:* There are multiple types of hybrid models that take advantage of both the strong security and control that is available in the distributed model and the accessibility of the centralized model. One method for creating a hybrid federated model utilizes a record locator service that can identify the institutions at which the data is located [29] (Fig. 22.2).

22.7.2 The Four Levels of Interoperability

Assuming that data can be exchanged as described in the OSI model, healthcare data has additional requirements for interoperability. Even if characters (i.e., letters, numbers, symbols) can be exchanged using a network, the meaning of what the clinician is entering into their EHR (i.e., medical diagnoses) still needs a shared key to code and decode the information. The Four Levels of Interoperability [30, 31] (Fig. 22.3) represents a continuum of the capabilities of data exchange in healthcare. This model establishes the requirements for one system or application to securely exchange data with another. The Four Levels are

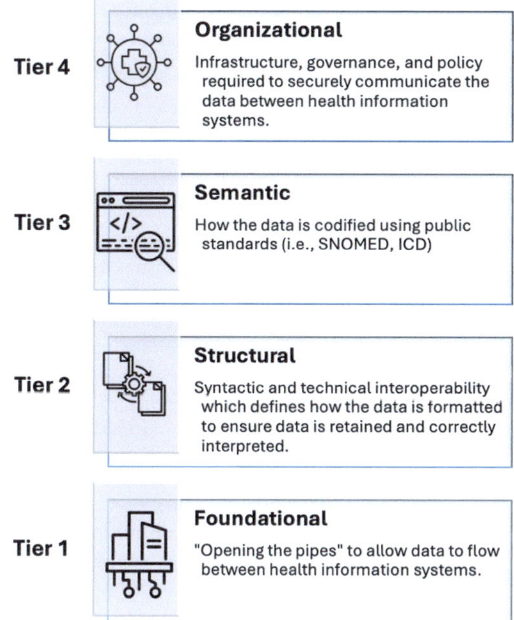

Fig. 22.3 The Four Levels of Interoperability. Icons open source from The Noun Project [32–35]

defined by the Healthcare Information and Management Systems Society as.

1. *Foundational*: The "opening of the pipes" for the data to flow from one HIT system to another. Associated with Stage 1 of Meaningful Use. At this level, information can be successfully moved from point A to point B but how to interpret the information by the receiving party may be unclear.
2. *Structural*: Also known as syntactic or technical interoperability, defines how the data is formatted when it is exchanged between HIT systems. At this level, the data types are known so that the information can be exchanged in a way that the underlying structure of the data can be interpreted (such as the string of characters represents a "text string" vs. "an integer number"), so that it can be stored appropriately. However, the receiver receiving the string "shortness" or number 157 may not know how to interpret the information sent.
3. *Semantic*: Defines how the data is codified, often drawing from standardized definitions that are shared publicly (i.e., SNOMED, ICD). At this level, the two parties have a shared understanding of the meaning of the data that was exchanged.
4. *Organizational*: The infrastructure required to securely use and communicate data between organizations and individuals. This is accomplished when all the previous levels are completed and internal governance, policy, and legal considerations are addressed.

22.7.3 Office of the National Coordinator for Health Information Technology (ASTP/ONC) and the Interoperability Standards Advisory (ISA)

The ISA process represents the model by which the ONC (now ASTP/ONC) will coordinate the identification, assessment, and determination of "recognized" interoperability standards and implementation specifications for industry use to fulfill specific clinical health information technology interoperability needs.

The ISA is structured into four sections [36]:

1. *Vocabulary/Code Sets/Terminology*: Standards and Implementation Specifications (i.e., "semantics").
2. *Content/Structure*: Standards and Implementation Specifications (i.e., "syntax").
3. *Standards and Implementation*: Specifications for Services and Exchange (i.e., the infrastructure components deployed and used to address specific interoperability needs).
4. *Administrative*: Standards and Implementation Specifications (i.e., payment, operations, and other "nonclinical" interoperability needs).

Through ISA, ONC recommended the standards and specifications that the country should follow when creating interoperable systems for healthcare.

22.8 Current State of Interoperability in Healthcare

Interoperability has the potential to make healthcare more cost-effective. As an example, if a provider sees in the patient record that their patient had a recent CT scan, they may decide to not order another scan. However, if the scan was done at a different healthcare system that doesn't provide interoperable records, then even if the patient remembered that the scan was done (which is not a given), the provider would not have the results. In the end, the patient may be subjected to repeat scanning that costs time, money, and resources, as well as exposes the patient to unnecessary testing (and radiation in this case).

In practice, the day-to-day benefits of interoperability are more nebulous. The best examples are in individual EHRs where instances of EHR at different institutions can share information in real time. As many patients see providers from multiple specialties (i.e., primary care, surgery, physical therapy, occupational therapy, social work), the members of their team may be scattered between multiple organizations. Care is more coordinated when highly interoperable systems allow transparency of what has occurred and the medical decision-making, and providers can more easily work together to create a comprehensive care plan.

22.9 Summary and Vignette Resolution

Considering everything covered in this chapter, we can return to the immunization vignette from Sect. 22.1. In a future of highly interoperable systems, every time a patient receives a vaccine (e.g. at a school, pharmacy or clinic), the EHR would automatically update patient's immunization history. Just as a travel website automatically updates with the most recent flight prices, the EHR would automatically update with the most recent immunizations. Although the standards and technology exist today to support this potential future, the challenge now is ensuring they are applied consistently to achieve seamless health information exchange.

References

1. Khairat S, Feldman SS, Rana A, et al. Foundational domains and competencies for baccalaureate health informatics education. J Am Med Inform Assoc. 2023;30(10):1599–607. https://doi.org/10.1093/jamia/ocad147.
2. IEEE Standard Computer Dictionary. A compilation of IEEE standard computer glossaries. IEEE Std. 1991;610:1–217. https://doi.org/10.1109/IEEESTD.1991.106963.
3. Singh A, Jadhav S, Roopashree MR. Factors to overcoming barriers affecting electronic medical record usage by physicians. Indian J Community Med. 2020;45(2):168–71. https://doi.org/10.4103/ijcm.IJCM_478_19.
4. Garrett P, Seidman J. EMR vs EHR—What is the Difference? Webpage. Accessed 17 Mar 2024. https://www.healthit.gov/buzz-blog/electronic-health-and-medical-records/emr-vs-ehr-difference.
5. Hersh W, Totten A, Eden K, et al. Health information exchange. Evid Rep Technol Assess (Full Rep). 2015;220:1–465. https://doi.org/10.23970/AHRQEPCERTA220.
6. Alder S. What is the HITECH act? Webpage The HIPAA J Updated, 2025. Accessed 21 Jan 2025. https://www.hipaajournal.com/what-is-the-hitech-act/.
7. Adler-Milstein J, Jha AK. HITECH act drove large gains in hospital electronic health record adoption. Health Aff Millwood. 2017;36(8):1416–22. https://doi.org/10.1377/hlthaff.2016.1651.
8. National Trends in Hospital and Physician Adoption of Electronic Health Records, Health IT Quick-Stat #61. The Office of the National Coordinator for Health information Technology (ONC). Updated October 4, 2022. Accessed 28 Mar 2024. https://www.healthit.gov/data/quickstats/national-trends-hospital-and-physician-adoption-electronic-health-records.
9. Information Blocking. Webpage. Assistant secretary for technology policy. Update 2024. Accessed 21 Jan 2025. https://www.healthit.gov/topic/information-blocking.
10. Promoting Interoperability Programs. Centers for medicare & medicaid services. Updated 2024. Accessed 28 Mar 2024. https://www.cms.gov/medicare/regulations-guidance/promoting-interoperability-programs.
11. TEFCA. Assistant Secretary for Technology Policy. Updated 2024. Accessed 11 Feb 2025. https://www.healthit.gov/topic/interoperability/policy/trusted-exchange-framework-and-common-agreement-tefca.

12. Turbow S, Hollberg JR, Ali MK. Electronic health record interoperability: how did we get here and how do we move forward? JAMA Health Forum. 2021;2(3):e210253. https://doi.org/10.1001/jamahealthforum.2021.0253.
13. A Brief History of Federal Interoperability Efforts. Portable document format. Centers for Medicare & Medicaid Services. Accessed 11 Feb 2025. https://www.cms.gov/files/document/hiig-federal-interoperability-timeline-brief-history-federal-interoperability-efforts.pdf.
14. Chu HY, Englund JA, Starita LM, et al. Early detection of Covid-19 through a citywide pandemic surveillance platform. N Engl J Med. 2020;383(2):185–7. https://doi.org/10.1056/NEJMc2008646.
15. McLaughlin HP, Hiatt BC, Russell D, et al. COVID-19 response efforts of Washington state public health laboratory: lessons learned. Am J Public Health. 2021;111(5):867–75. https://doi.org/10.2105/AJPH.2021.306212.
16. Burkhardt HA, Brandt PS, Lee JR, et al. StayHome: a FHIR-native Mobile COVID-19 symptom tracker and public health reporting tool. Online J Public Health Inform. 2021;13(1):e2. https://doi.org/10.5210/ojphi.v13i1.11462.
17. Greene DN, McClintock DS, Durant TJS. Interoperability: COVID-19 as an Impetus for Change. Clin Chem. 2021;67(4):592–5. https://doi.org/10.1093/clinchem/hvab006.
18. Resources: Standards Developing Organizations (SDOs). American National Standards Institute. Accessed 30 Mar 2024. https://www.standardsportal.org/usa_en/resources/sdo.aspx.
19. Standard-Setting and Related Organizations. Centers for medicare & medicaid services. Update 2024. Accessed 30 Mar 2024. https://www.cms.gov/priorities/key-initiatives/burden-reduction/administrative-simplification/hipaa/standard-setting-related-organizations.
20. Dolin RH, Alschuler L, Beebe C, et al. The HL7 clinical document architecture. J Am Med Inform Assoc. 2001;8(6):552–69. https://doi.org/10.1136/jamia.2001.0080552.
21. Ayaz M, Pasha MF, Alzahrani MY, Budiarto R, Stiawan D. The fast health interoperability resources (FHIR) standard: systematic literature review of implementations, applications, challenges and opportunities. JMIR Med Inform. 2021;9(7):e21929. https://doi.org/10.2196/21929.
22. Enabling health interoperability through FHIR: Application Registry. HL7 FHIR Foundation. Accessed 03 Feb 2025. https://fhir.org/implementations/registry/.
23. Cimino JJ, Ayres EJ. The clinical research data repository of the US National Institutes of Health. Stud Health Technol Inform. 2010;160(Pt 2):1299–303.
24. Amin MS, Rahman S. An introduction of open system interconnection (OSI) model and its architecture. Preprints.org; 2023.
25. Windows network architecture and the OSI model. Microsoft. Updated 2023. Accessed 25 Mar 2024. https://learn.microsoft.com/en-us/windows-hardware/drivers/network/windows-network-architecture-and-the-osi-model.
26. Interoperability: Physical Layer. Federal communications commission. Updated 2016. Accessed 02 Apr 2024. https://www.fcc.gov/general/interoperability-physical-layer.
27. Data processing — open systems interconnection — basic reference model. Computer Netw (Amsterdam, Netherlands: 1976). 1981;5(2):81–118. https://doi.org/10.1016/0376-5075(81)90066-0.
28. What is HL7? Health level seven defined. Webpage. Surety systems. Updated 2024. Accessed 03 Feb 2025. https://www.suretysystems.com/insights/what-is-hl7-health-level-seven-defined/.
29. McCarthy DB, Propp K, Cohen A, Sabharwal R, Schachter AA, Rein AL. Learning from health information exchange technical architecture and implementation in seven beacon communities. EGEMS (Wash DC). 2014;2(1):1060. https://doi.org/10.13063/2327-9214.1060.
30. Lee AR, Kim IK, Lee E. Developing a transnational health record framework with level-specific interoperability guidelines based on a related literature review. Healthcare (Basel). 2021;9(1) https://doi.org/10.3390/healthcare9010067.
31. Interoperability in Healthcare. Webpage. Healthcare Information and Management Systems Society (HIMSS). Update 2021. Accessed 17 Mar 2024. https://www.himss.org/resources/interoperability-healthcare.
32. Elvariani AR. Data interoperability (Image#6467387). PNG file The Noun Project Updated 2023. Accessed 15 Mar 2024. https://thenounproject.com/icon/data-interoperability-6467387/.
33. Mahira C. Meta description (Image#5659568). PNG file. The Noun Project Updated 2023. Accessed 15 Mar 2024, https://thenounproject.com/icon/meta-description-5659568/.
34. Aditia S. Versioning (Image#6618009). PNG file The Noun Project Updated 2024. Accessed 15 Mar 2024. https://thenounproject.com/icon/versioning-6618009/.
35. Edwin P. Business technology (Image#5267415). PNG file The Noun Project Updated 2022. Accessed 15 Mar 2024. https://thenounproject.com/icon/business-technology-5267415/.
36. Interoperability Standards Advisory (ISA). Office of the National Coordinator for Health Information Technology. Updated 2023. Accessed 30 Mar 2024. https://www.healthit.gov/isa/.

Health Informatics Standards and Standard Development Organizations

23

Christina Eldredge and Melissa Hood

Foundational Domains
This chapter addresses the following AMIA Foundational Domains: F4—Health Information Science & Technology, F8—Professionalism, F9—Interprofessional Collaborative Practice.

Learning Objectives
After reading this chapter, you should be able to

1. List and describe key standard development organizations in health informatics.
2. Distinguish between standard development methods and standard development stages.
3. Compare and contrast the common types of standards in health informatics.
4. Using the case study provided, describe the benefits and challenges of applying health informatics standards in practice.

23.1 Introduction to Standards

In this chapter, we will cover the need for standards in health informatics and the common types of standards used in the field. Secondly, the chapter will cover the organizations that develop and maintain these standards. Furthermore, we will discuss the common types of methods used to develop standards and the various stages a standard will progress through as it moves toward adoption in the field. Finally, the chapter will explain the benefits and challenges posed by the implementation of these standards and illustrate some of these in a case study.

23.1.1 Definitions

A *Standard* is an agreed-upon "set of rules and definitions that specify how to carry out a process or produce a product" [1] (p. 211).

Standard development organizations (SDOs) are organizations that bring stakeholders together in a field or domain to develop, maintain, publish, and disseminate standards in that area. In the context of health informatics, SDOs create standards that guide the collection, creation, use, security, application, and exchange of health data.

Standard development methods are the methods or processes used by an organization, members, stakeholders, and volunteers to create, implement, and maintain standards.

SDO Accreditation is a formal process in which SDOs are reviewed by an organization that accredits health informatics SDOs to determine if their standard development processes meet predetermined standards. Once accredited, the SDOs are continually reviewed on a regular basis [2].

C. Eldredge (✉) · M. Hood
School of Information, University of South Florida, Tampa, FL, USA
e-mail: celdredge2@usf.edu

C. Eldredge et al. (eds.), *Introductory Textbook in Health Informatics*, Health Informatics,
https://doi.org/10.1007/978-3-032-16657-9_23

23.1.2 What Are Standards?

Standards are used in various fields to establish common definitions, guidelines, rules, requirements, or processes that allow different entities (or parts) to work together to achieve a common goal [2]. At its most basic level, a *standard* is an *agreed-upon* way of doing things. Typically, standards in health informatics are developed to minimize variation or "excessive diversity" for more efficiency through improved collaboration, consistency, quality, and security in the context of health data and health information systems [1] (212).

23.1.3 Brief History of Standards

Standards have been used for centuries. The Egyptians used a cubit rod as a unit of measurement for length that was determined by the distance from the elbow to the tip of the middle finger of the Pharaoh at the time [3]. In more recent times, standard spacing of railroad ties and standards for lamps enabled interchangeability of railroad cars and lightbulbs [4 (248), 5], In these examples, there is a common theme of using standards to improve the consistency of a process so it is more reliable/dependable and can be communicated with relatively similar results between groups of people or during a building process.

In a similar way, standards in health informatics have evolved over the years to improve data quality, security, and exchange. Historically, among the first attempts at health data standards were early efforts in the late 1800s to classify causes of death using the Bertillon Classification of Causes of Death. This method later evolved into the International Classification of Diseases (ICD) that we use today [6]. In 1972, identifier standards for medications in the form of a unique National Drug Code (NDC) for commercially available drugs [7]. Later in the 1980s, standards such as Health Level Seven International (HL7) were created for health data exchange and Digital Imaging and Communications in Medicine (DICOM) standards for medical imaging data [8, 9].

23.1.4 Why are Standards Needed in Health Informatics?

In health informatics, standards are designed to ensure health information quality, privacy, and security while promoting data exchange and access. Generally, this is achieved through a consensus process and the creation of terms, methods, or processes that are important to achieve the goals of the community that the standard will serve, for example, the stakeholders [10]. Additionally, standards aid in the implementation of health information technology that is safe, secure, and easy to use, while meeting its intended purpose. In other words, health informatics standards are used to establish a common way of doing things so health information systems can securely share data to provide better care for patients, support research, and improve public health.

23.2 AMIA Specialty Areas

Standards and SDOs apply to all AMIA specialty areas. The specific type of standards used in the specialty area of health informatics will vary depending on the requirements of that field. For example, imaging informatics uses standards specific to the exchange of imaging data such as Digital Imaging and Communications in Medicine (DICOM) standards to store and exchange medical images and relevant information.

23.3 Standards and Interoperability

Standards play a key role in the *interoperability* of health systems. The use of standards aids in facilitating the exchange of health information and the development of quality, secure health IT systems that support this exchange. In health informatics, standards are needed to enable *interoperability* of data to support healthcare, biomedical research, and public health. *Interoperability* is defined as the ability of one health information system (HIS) to transfer health data/information to another HIS and, importantly, the receiving HIS is able to understand and act on the exchanged data/information. Facilitating interoperable HIS may reduce healthcare costs, improve healthcare quality, and reduce adverse events (improving patient safety) [11].

In clinical medicine, without data interoperability, an incomplete picture of the patient history can lead to duplicate care, inaccurate diagnoses, treatment delays, and adverse events. For example, a clinician treating a patient transferred from another medical facility with a penicillin allergy may not trigger an allergy-related clinical decision support system alert in the pharmacy information system if the data regarding the patient's drug allergy was not received from the transferring facility's clinical information system [e.g., their electronic medical record system (EMR)]. In biomedical research, silos of data may lead to information bias toward specific study populations. Furthermore, the lack of the ability to consolidate community public health data to regional, state, and national dashboards can hinder public health responses in emergencies such as the COVID-19 pandemic [12].

In addition to facilitating the transport of data from one facility to another, standards aid in ensuring the content of the data transferred is private and secure. Government regulation has determined what types of health information require patient consent for release. In addition, regulation under the *Health Information Portability and Accountability Act (HIPAA)* determines the types of healthcare organizations covered under this regulation and which types of health data need to be private and secure [13]. This information will also be covered in a later chapters of this book.

Finally, standards aid in patient identification. Having a single, standardized patient identifier provides value in terms of interoperability, it facilitates the linking of multiple medical/health records from different healthcare facilities for the same patient, and therefore, the exchange of health information. This standardization can lead to reduced errors and costs associated with duplicate records and mismatching of records. An example of errors associated with duplicate health records is missed abnormal lab results, that is, a clinician is not able to review abnormal lab results and provide the appropriate healthcare service to the patient because the clinician did not receive the lab results from one of the versions of the health record [14].

23.4 Standards Development

There are several different types of methods for the development of standards in the field of health informatics.

The methods used in health informatics are described by Dr. Hammond et al. and include four distinct methods:

1. Ad hoc method
2. De facto method
3. Governmental mandate method
4. Consensus method [1] (215)

The *ad hoc method* is an informal method of developing standards in health informatics by a group of experts or stakeholders interested in the topic area. It may not be supported by a standard development organization (SDO) as this method does not require rigorous methodology. In this method, a group of stakeholders agree on a standard without using a formal development process [15].

The *de facto method* occurs "by default" due to a single stakeholder having enough influence in the domain to dictate the standards for that field or area. A frequently used example of this would be how Microsoft 365 is used in the business and educational domains.

The definition of the *government mandate* method is reflected in its title. In this method, the government determines the standards required for an industry, product, process, etc.

In comparison, the *consensus method* is typically a volunteer-led effort that consists of stakeholders across the field coming together to determine standards for a particular topic. For example, *HL7 standards* such as *FHIR* would be considered a consensus effort in health informatics [16]. We will discuss more on this standard below. Standards development in health informatics generally uses the consensus method;

however, with multiple stakeholders across several fields, this can be challenging at times. Considering most participants in this effort are volunteers, coordinating meetings and moving the process forward can be time consuming. Furthermore, standards must be consistently supported and updated. This is where SDOs come into the picture.

23.5 Standards Development Organizations (SDOs)

Standard development organizations develop, support, and maintain standards. SDOs generally support the consensus method of developing standards using open forums and promoting transparency. At the end of the development process, the SDOs will disseminate the standard by publishing the final version and maintain the standard through updates and revisions as necessary. Several national and international organizations are dedicated to the development of health informatic standards. Other organizations have workgroups or committees that are specific to the context of health informatics. HIMSS notes on their website that there are over 40 different SDOs in the health information technology area alone [17]. Furthermore, these SDOs vary in their organization, membership, and their standard development processes.

Functions of SDOs

- Provide transparency
- Support open forums
- Set milestones in health informatics standards development
- Disseminate (publish)
- Maintain standards (and revise if necessary)

Important SDOs in Health Informatics

In this section, we will highlight some of the most prevalent SDOs in health informatics today. The majority of these organizations are volunteer supported and many use the consensus method of standard development.

Health Level Seven International (HL7)—Founded in 1987

HL7 is named after the Open Systems Interconnection (OSI) application level and represents over 50 countries with over 1600 members. The mission of this organization is "to provide standards that empower global health data interoperability" [8] The standards developed and maintained by HL7 are grouped into reference categories, one of which is the *Fast Healthcare Interoperability Resources (FHIR®)*. This standard is used to exchange health information between healthcare organizations and consists of two parts:

1. Content model (resources)
2. Specifications for health information exchange (RESTful interfaces, messaging, and documents) [8]

Clinical Data Interchange Standards Consortium (CDISC)—Founded in 1997 [18]

CDISC is a global nonprofit organization that creates and supports data standards for clinical research. Its aim is for research data to be "accessible, interoperable, and re-useable." CDISC is comprised of over 500 global organizational members from multiple industries, including, but not limited to, academia, government, pharmaceutical, BioTech, medical device companies, and technology service providers [19].

Digital Imaging and Communications in Medicine (DICOM)—First Published in 1993

DICOM is an international standard for the formatting of medical imaging data in fields such as cardiology, radiology, ophthalmology, and dentistry. This organization is recognized by the ISO and the DICOM standard is managed by the Medical Imaging & Technology Alliance, a division of the National Electrical Manufacturers Association [20]. For more on DICOM, please refer to the chapter on Imaging Informatics.

CEN/TC 251 Health Informatics—Founded in 1990 [21]

The aim of this SDO is to develop, deliver, and maintain health informatics standards for Europe.

CEN/TC 251 coordinates with other global SDOs in developing standards, emphasizing cooperation [22].

ISO Technical Committee 215—Health Informatics—Founded in 1998
This committee is a part of the International Organization for Standardization that has 171 member countries and 834 technical committees and subcommittees [23]. Health Informatics is represented by the Technical Committee 215. This committee works on standards in the health domain to promote standard capture, use, and exchange of data in health information systems [24].

SNOMED International—Founded in 1965
SNOMED International is responsible for SNOMED-CT, the Systemized Nomenclature of Medicine—Clinical Terms. This nomenclature provides a core set of clinical terminology [25]. See the chapter in this textbook on controlled vocabularies and terminologies for additional information on SNOMED-CT.

Observational Health Data Sciences and Informatics (OHDSI)—Founded in 2014
OHDSI supports an open data standard called the Observational Medical Outcomes Partnership (OMOP) Common Data Model (CDM). The organization's mission is to support the use of data to generate evidence to improve health outcomes [26].

Office of the National Coordinator for Health Information Technology—Founded in 2004 [27]
While the ONC, now referred to as the Assistant Secretary for Technology Policy (ASTP)/ONC [27], is not necessarily an SDO, this government office has a "process" for developing standard models in health informatics called the *Interoperability Standards Advisory (ISA).* The ISA process is how the ASTP/ONC "will coordinate the identification, assessment, and public awareness of interoperability standards and implementation specifications that can be used by the United States healthcare industry to address specific interoperability needs including, but not limited to, interoperability for clinical, public health, and research purposes" [28].

One standard supported by the ASTP/ONC is the United States Core Data for Interoperability (USCDI). This standard is a part of the *Cures Act Final Rule,* which defines health data classes and data elements to promote health data exchange and health IT system interoperability [29]. This is discussed further in the textbook chapter on interoperability.

23.6 Standard Development Process

The standard development process will entirely depend on the method used. As noted in the section above, there are several different methods of developing standards, some of which may be more informal than others. If the ad hoc method is used, a few meetings between stakeholders may be all that is required. Also, the de facto method may not require a formal process.

However, the government mandate and consensus methods are formal processes that undergo stages of standards development. In these processes, the idea for the standard will move through stages in a process that takes the idea/concept to a formal published standard. An example of a formal process for standards development can be found on the International Standards Organization (ISO) website. The ISO process has several stages from the initial proposal stage, the preparatory stage, committee stage, enquiry stage, approval stage, and, finally, the publication stage [30]. Within each stage, important steps will be performed by the SDO such as the recruitment of volunteers for workgroups/committees, initial proposal writing, public comment, and so forth. For an illustration of common steps included in these stages, see Fig. 23.1.

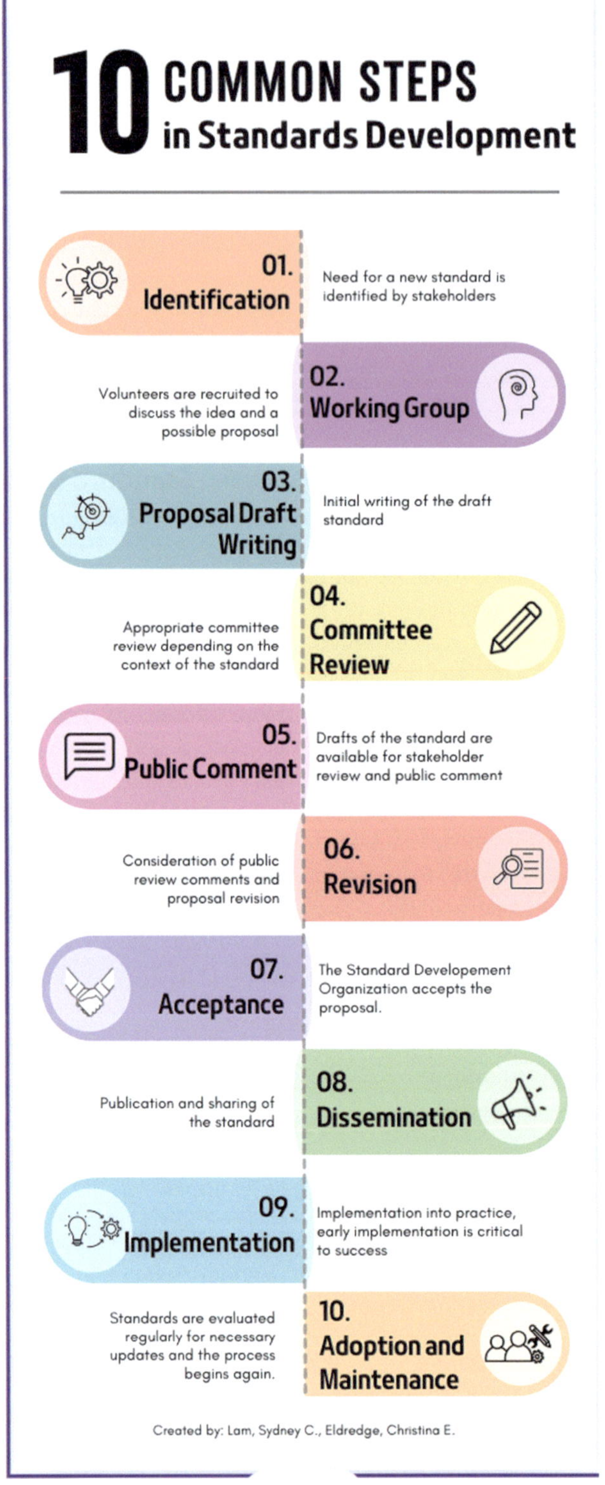

Fig. 23.1 Ten common steps in standards development

23.6.1 Standards Development Stages

In health informatics, standards are typically developed using the consensus method discussed above. Developing a standard using this method involves a process where the idea must go through various stages that take the identification of the need for the standard to its final form. SDOs typically take the lead in this process and aid in dissemination, publication, and maintenance of the standard. Each SDO may have a different process; however, there are generally commonalities in their processes [33]. Hammond et al. define various stages of standard development below, while emphasizing the implementation of the standard, conformance, and certification as important aspects in the process:

- Identification
- Conceptualization
- Discussion
- Specification
- Early implementation
- Conformance
- Certification

It is important to note that if the standard that is developed is not "implementable" or not "adopted" by the stakeholders, it will not achieve its purpose or goals [4]. Therefore, the last stages of the standards development should include methods or process for implementation and maintenance as noted above in order for the standard to continue to be relevant in the dynamic healthcare environment [1] (217).

23.7 Types of Standards

Most standards can be classified into different types. However, as the field of health informatics evolves, it is important to note that new standards will need to be created to support new challenges and innovations, especially in the setting of the increasing use of artificial intelligence (AI).

In this chapter, we will use the Health Information Management Systems Society (HIMSS) categorization of health information technology standards. HIMSS is one of the largest health information professional organizations. HIMSS identifies five different types of health data standards:

- Identifier standards
- Content standards
- Transport standards
- Vocabulary/terminology standards
- Privacy and security standards [17]

Below we will discuss identifier, content, and transport standards in more depth. Vocabulary and terminology standards are discussed in depth in the Health Informatics Controlled Vocabularies chapter of this textbook and privacy and security standards are discussed in depth in the Privacy and Security chapter.

Identifier Standards

Identifier standards provide methods for the identification of unique patient records and unique healthcare providers. This type of standard plays an important role in health information exchange. Without these standards, there is a risk of mismatching data, for example, the clinical results from patient A may be placed in the record of patient B. ASTP/ONC notes the importance of identification in providing a "comprehensive view" of the patient's records that will aid in providing quality healthcare and supporting interoperability [31].

Care must be taken in what can be considered a patient identifier as it should meet several characteristics to be used effectively. Those characteristics include the following: (1) must belong to only one person, (2) must be permanent, (3) must not disclose personal information, (4) everyone must have one and only one, and (5) it must not change over time. There is no single health identifier that is universal, and none nationally in the United States. For US citizens, the Social Security Number is the closest we have to a national identifier [17]. In some countries, there is the use of one identifier per patient/person. However, in the United States, with multiple healthcare providers, each may have their own method of identification, often referred to as the *"medical record number" (MRN)*. HIMSS defines the MRN as an "organization-specific code" [17]. Similarly, healthcare providers may have codes for identification such as the *National Provider ID (NPI)* or the *National Council of State Nursing ID (NCSBN ID)* [17].

Content Standards

Content standards define the contents and structure or "syntax" of the message or document contents to be exchanged [32]. That is, these standards describe what data and metadata are to be included in the contents of the message and how that is structured within the data package during an exchange from one health system to another health system, from a healthcare provider to a patient health record/portal, from a healthcare provider to a health insurance company, etc. Some specific examples of content standards are HL7 Version 2.x (a messaging standard) and C-CDA (template standard) [32].

Vocabulary and Terminology Standards

Vocabulary or terminology standards focus on the "semantics," that is, how humans would define and classify the data so that is consistently understood across health information systems. These standards focus on the consistent use of terms to define concepts such as diseases, symptoms, drug names, and procedures. One example of terminology variation is the use of "hair loss" versus "alopecia." If one system uses a numeric code for "hair loss" and the receiving system only recognizes the code for "alopecia," important patient information may be lost in the data exchange. For one system to understand, analyze, and use the data that another health information technology system is sending, it is important to use consistent terminology. For more details on these standards, please refer to the Health Informatics Controlled Vocabularies chapter in this textbook.

Transport Standards

Transport standards establish the format of data as it moves from one health IT system to another. The ASTP/ONC describes these standards as ways to "package" data for transport or the standards that describe "how" the data is moved securely and reliably from one system to the other in the health setting [32].

Privacy and Security Standards

Given the sensitive nature of health-related data, privacy and security standards exist to guide healthcare organizations in securing patient data while maintaining patient confidentiality. These standards and associated regulations are discussed in depth in the privacy and security chapter in this textbook.

Interoperability and Standards

In the previous chapter on interoperability, the levels of interoperability were discussed. HIMSS defines these levels as

1. Foundational
2. Structural
3. Semantic
4. Organizational [17]

Each level may be supported by a different type of standards (see Fig. 23.2). For example,

SDO	ABBREVIATION	STANDARD SUPPORTED	STANDARD TYPE
HEALTH LEVEL 7	HL7	CLINICAL DATA ARCHITECTURE (CDA)	CONTENT
DEPARTMENT OF HEALTH AND HUMAN SERVICES	HHS	HIPAA PRIVACY RULE	PRIVACY
DIGITAL IMAGING AND COMMUNICATIONS IN MEDICINE	DICOM	DICOM	TRANSPORT
DEPARTMENT OF HEALTH AND HUMAN SERVICES	HHS	HIPAA NATIONAL PROVIDER IDENTIFICATION (NPI)	IDENTIFIER
INTERNATIONAL HEALTH TERMINOLOGY STANDARDS DEVELOPMENT ORGANIZATION	IHTSDO	SYSTEMIZED NOMENCLATURE OF MEDICINE - CLINICAL TERMS (SNOMED-CT)	TERMINOLOGY

Fig. 23.2 Examples of health informatics SDOS and standard types

the structural level of interoperability defines the data fields and format of the data that will be exchanged, while the semantic level uses terminology or vocabulary standards to prevent loss of meaning during the data exchanged. Therefore, the structural level of interoperability is supported by messaging and format standards while the semantic level is supported by terminology and vocabulary standards. Recall from the data, information, and knowledge pyramid from Chap. 4. Unorganized data does not convey information, so the data must be organized and coded to be understood on the other side of the exchange. If the data is organized by data fields (structured) and consistently coded (semantic level), it will be better understood on the receiving end of the exchange. The organizational level of interoperability encompasses the entire exchange process, bringing all levels of interoperability together and is supported by standards that address privacy, security, and transport.

23.8 Standards Accreditation

Founded in 1918, the *American National Standards Institute* (ANSI) is a private, nonprofit organization dedicated to facilitating the creation of quality standards in multiple industries and areas, including health. According to their website, ANSI "administers and coordinates the U.S. voluntary standards and conformity assessment system" [34]. In other words, ANSI helps with the process of standards development across industry, government, and public sectors through stakeholder involvement and standardized processes. It is important to note that ANSI is not a standard development organization; rather, ANSI oversees the development of standards by other SDOs. This is a large organization that has millions of professional members and over 250,000 organizational partnerships [34].

23.9 Opportunities and Challenges

What Opportunities/Benefits Exist for the Use of Standards?

The use of standards can improve the ability of healthcare organizations, including government-based and private organizations, to exchange health information in a meaningful way. That is, the data exchanged from organization A to organization B can be understood and used for improving health outcomes. Further, as discussed in this chapter, standards can facilitate data exchange and minimize "silos" of data that can facilitate clinical research and continuity of care. Standards can also aid in maintaining privacy and security of health information. For example, the *Health Insurance Portability and Accountability Act of 1996 (HIPAA)* required the U.S. Department of Health and Human Services (HHS) to develop rules and regulations for the minimum privacy and security requirements for healthcare organizations who maintain, use, or exchange healthcare data [35].

What Are the Key Challenges of Developing Standards?

One of the most challenging aspects of standards development is *adoption* of the standards into practice. In order for adoption to take place, there must be willingness to change and a positive "return on investment" for the community who will adopt the standard [35, 36]. One method of addressing this challenge is involving stakeholders (users) in the standard development process. As discussed in the consensus method above, steps in the standard development process include the recruitment of working group members and the release of drafts for public comment. These steps can encourage stakeholder engagement. However, as the consensus process relies on coordination of volunteers (often from different time zones), coordination during the process can be challenging. Another challenge often mentioned in the health informatics space is the existence of too many standards. In other words, if too many SDOs publish similar standards, then there is essentially no consensus "standard" that can be shared amongst the organizations.

23.10 Case Study

To illustrate how all of this works together and the roles of people, organizations, and accrediting agencies in the process, let us consider HL7 and the newer FHIR standard. Refer to Fig. 23.3 as we describe the process. The SDO involved in developing this standard would be HL7 and its accreditor ANSI. The stakeholders include both the people (e.g., volunteers such as clinicians, information technologists, data analysts) and participating organizations such as government agencies, healthcare organizations, and mobile application developers (e.g., those who volunteer to participate in the standard development). The method for developing FHIR standards is the consensus method and process is defined by HL7 on its website. Stakeholders may elect to begin a project by submitting an FHIR Implementation Guide proposal, creating content, testing, submitting content for balloting (voting), revisions if required (reconciliation), and publication [37].

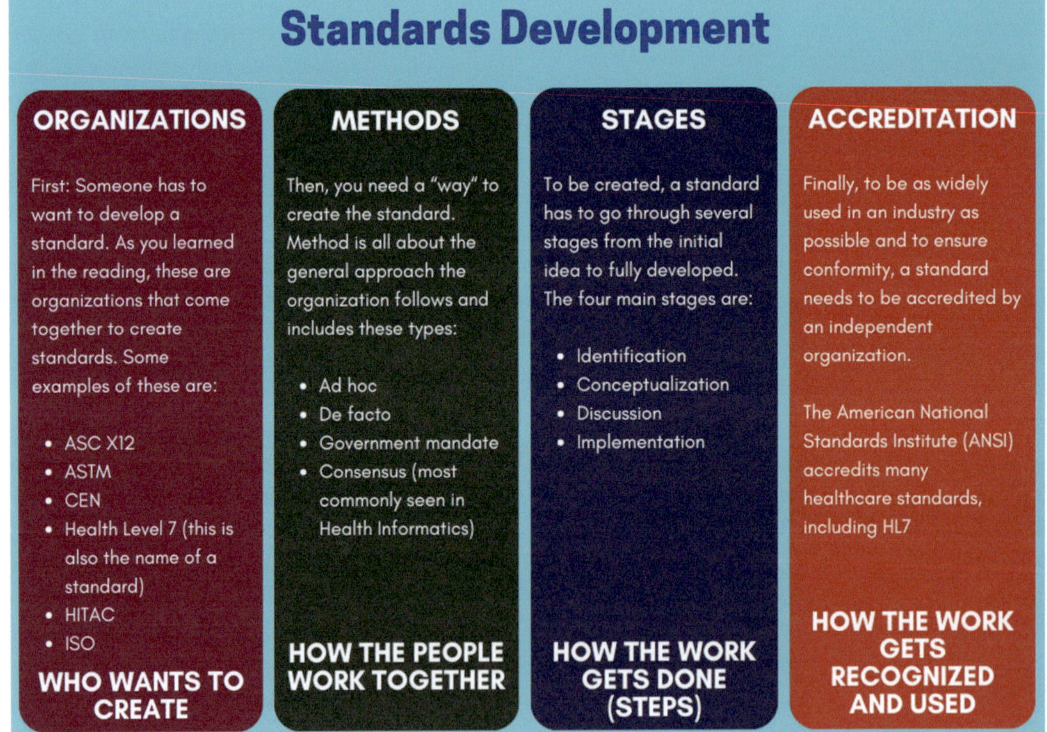

Fig. 23.3 Standards development

23.11 Additional Student Resources

Free resources that will help the reader understand the topic.

- HL7 website: https://www.hl7.org/
- HealthIT.gov: https://www.healthit.gov/topic/interoperability/standards-and-technology
- OHDSI website: https://www.ohdsi.org/
- ONC Standards Bulletin: https://www.healthit.gov/topic/standards-technology/onc-standards-bulletin

Knowledge Check Questions

1. Which of the following are standards development organizations in health informatics? (select all that apply)
   (a) HL7
   (b) FDA
   (c) ISO Technical Committee 215
   (d) SNOMED International
   (e) OHSDI
2. Which of the following is the most commonly used method of standards development in health informatics?
   (a) De facto
   (b) Ad hoc
   (c) Government mandate
   (d) Consensus
   (e) All of the above
3. Adoption of the standard by health organizations can be challenging, which of the following are ways to aid in improving early implementation and maintenance? (select all that apply)
   (a) Stakeholder involvement in the development process
   (b) Avoiding the public comment step
   (c) Limiting publication of the standard to within the SDO
   (d) Consensus building during discussion and proposal writing
   (e) None of the above

Answers

1. (a), (c), (d), (e)
2. (d)
3. (a) and (d)

Glossary of Terms

Term	Definition
HIMSS	Health Information Management Systems Society
HIPAA	Health Information Portability and Accountability Act

References

1. Hammond WE, Jaffe C, Cimino JJ, Huff SM. Standards in biomedical informatics. In: Shortliffe EH, Cimino JJ, editors. Biomedical informatics: computer applications in health care and biomedicine. 4th ed. London: Springer; 2014. p. 211–53.
2. ANSI. American national standards (ANS) process [Internet]. Washington: American National Standards Institute; 2024 [cited 2024 June 1]. Available from: https://www.ansi.org/american-national-standards/info-for-standards-developers/accreditation.
3. Kaaronen RO, Manninen MA, Erronen JT. Body-based units of measure in cultural evolution. Science. 2023;380(6648):948–54.
4. Russell AL. Standardization in history: a review essay with an eye to the future. In: Bolin S, editor. The standards edge: future generations. Ann Arbor: Sheridan Press; 2005. p. 247–60.
5. USDOE. The history of the light bulb [internet]. Washington: US Department of Energy; 2013 [cited 2025 March 13]. Available from: https://www.energy.gov/articles/history-light-bulb.
6. Raminani SR. International classification of diseases [Internet]. Britannica; Date unknown [cited 2025 March 13]. Available from: https://www.britannica.com/topic/International-Classification-of-Diseases.
7. Brion G, Bunkers L. Expiration Dating and National Drug Code Rules [Internet]. Treasure Island: StatPearls Publishing; 2023 [cited 2025 March 13]. Available from: https://pubmed.ncbi.nlm.nih.gov/34033382/#:~:text=In%201972%2C%20the%20United%20States,National%20Drug%20Code%20(NDC).
8. HL7. HL7 Standards - Section 1c: FHIR® [Internet]. Ann Arbor: Health Level Seven International; 2026 [cited 2026 Mar 26]. Available from: https://www.hl7.org/implement/standards/product_section.cfm?section=12.

9. DICOM. History [Internet]. Arlington: Digital Imaging and Communications in Medicine; Date unknown [cited 2024 May 24]. Available from: https://www.dicomstandard.org/history.
10. McKenzie L. Understanding the standards process [Internet]. Ann Arbor: Health Level Seven International; 2022 [cited 2024 May 24]. Available from: https://confluence.hl7.org/display/HL7/Understanding+the+Standards+Process.
11. Li E, Clarke J, Ashrafian H, Darzi A, Neves AL. The impact of electronic health record interoperability on safety and quality of care in high-income countries: a systematic review. J Med Internet Res. 2022;24(9):e38144.
12. Liaw ST, Kuziemsky C, Schreiber R, Jonnagaddala J, Liyanage H, Chittalia A, Bahniwal R, He JW, Ryan BL, Lizotte DJ, Kueper JK, Terry AL, de Lusignan S. Primary care informatics response to covid-19 pandemic: adaptation, progress, and lessons from four countries with high ICT development. Yearb Med Inform. 2021;30(1):44–55.
13. HHS. Health information privacy [Internet]. Washington: US Department of Health and Human Services; Date unknown [cited 2024 June 1]. Available from: https://www.hhs.gov/hipaa/index.html.
14. Joffe E, Bearden C, Byrne M, Bernstam E. Duplicate patient records—implication for missed laboratory results. Paper presented at AMIA Annual Symposium Proceedings 2009. 2009; San Francisco.
15. AMIHM. Healthcare information systems standards [Internet]. Marlborough: American Institute for Healthcare Management; 2021 [cited 2024 May 24]. Available from: https://www.amihm.org/healthcare-information-system-standards/.
16. FHIR. Welcome to the HL7 FHIR foundation [Internet]. Health Level Seven International; Date unknown [cited 2024 June 1]. Available from: https://fhir.org/.
17. HIMSS. Interoperability in healthcare [Internet]. Chicago: Health Information and Management Systems Society; 2024 [cited 2024 May 02]. Available from: https://www.himss.org/resources/interoperability-healthcare.
18. CDISC. Founder and president emeritus [Internet]. Austin: Clinical Data Interchange Standards Consortium; 2024 [cited 2024 May 24]. Available from: https://www.cdisc.org/about/president-emeritus.
19. CDISC. New to CDISC – Academic Researcher [Internet]. Ann Arbor: Clinical Data Interchange Standards Consortium; 2024 [cited 2024 May 24]. Available from: https://www.cdisc.org/new-to-cdisc/academic.
20. DICOM. About DICOM: Overview [Internet]. Arlington: Digital Imaging and Communications in Medicine; Date unknown [cited 2024 May 24]. Available from: https://www.dicomstandard.org/about-home.
21. IPS. CEN/TC 251 [Internet]. The International Patient Summary; 2024 [cited 2024 May 24]. Available from: https://international-patient-summary.net/cen-tc-251/.
22. eHealth Standards. CEN/TC 251 Health Informatics [Internet]. eHealth Standards; Date unknown [cited 2024 May 24]. Available from: https://www.ehealth-standards.eu/about/.
23. ISO. About ISO [Internet]. Geneva: International Organization of Standardization; Date unknown [cited 2024 May 24]. Available from: https://www.iso.org/about-us.html.
24. ISO. ISO/TC 215 Health informatics [Internet]. Washington: International Organization of Standardization; Date unknown [cited 2024 May 24]. Available from: https://www.iso.org/committee/54960.html.
25. SNOMED. 5-step briefing [Internet]. London: SNOMED International; 2024 [cited 2024 Apr 27]. Available from: https://www.snomed.org/five-step-briefing.
26. OHDSI. Who we are [Internet]. Observational Health Data Sciences and Informatics; 2024 [cited 2024 May 24]. Available from: https://ohdsi.org/who-we-are/.
27. ASTP. The birth of ONC [Internet]. Washington: The Office of the National Coordinator for Health Information Technology; 2024 [cited 2024 May 24]. Available from: https://www.healthit.gov/20years/#:~:text=The%20Office%20of%20the%20National%20Coordinator%20for%20Health%20IT%20was,Bush%20in%20April%202004.
28. ISA. About the ISA [Internet]. Washington: Interoperability Standards Advisory; Date unknown [cited 2024 May 24]. Available from: https://www.healthit.gov/isa/about-isa.
29. ASTP. Cures act final rule: United States core data for interoperability [Internet]. Washington: The Office of the National Coordinator for Health Information Technology; Date unknown [cited 2024 May 24]. Available from: https://www.healthit.gov/sites/default/files/page2/2020-03/USCDI.pdf.
30. ISO. Stages and resources for standards development [Internet]. Geneva: The International Organization of Standardization; Date unknown [cited 2024 May 24]. Available from: https://www.iso.org/stages-and-resources-for-standards-development.html.
31. ASTP. Patient identity and patient record matching [Internet]. Washington: The Office of the National Coordinator for Health Information Technology; 2024 [cited 2024 May 02]. Available from: https://www.healthit.gov/topic/interoperability/standards-and-technology/patient-identity-and-patient-record-matching.
32. ASTP. The ONC health IT playbook: 3.5 follow health IT standards [Internet]. Washington: The Office of the National Coordinator for Health Information Technology; 2022 [cited 2024 May 24]. Available from: https://www.healthit.gov/playbook/health-information-exchange/#section-3-5.

33. ASTP. Standards development organizations [Internet]. Washington: The Office of the National Coordinator for Health Information Technology; Date unknown [cited 2024 June 1]. Available from: https://www.healthit.gov/playbook/sdo-education/chapter-2/.
34. ANSI. About ANSI [Internet]. Washington: American National Standards Institute; 2024 [cited 2024 May 24]. Available from: https://www.ansi.org/about/introduction.
35. HHS. HIPAA for professionals [Internet]. Washington: Department of Health and Human Services; 2021 [cited 2024 May 24]. Available from: https://www.hhs.gov/hipaa/for-professionals/index.html.
36. van de Kaa G. Standards adoption: a comprehensive multidisciplinary review. Heliyon. 2023;9(8):e19203. https://doi.org/10.1016/j.heliyon.2023.e19203. PMID: 37664752; PMCID: PMC10468385.
37. HL7. G-ballot specification and reconciliation [Internet]. Ann Arbor: Health Level Seven International; 2024 [cited 2024 June 1]. Available from: https://confluence.hl7.org/display/HE/G%2B-%2BBallot%2BSpecification%2Band%2BReconciliation.

Health Informatics Controlled Vocabularies, Terminologies, and Nomenclatures

24

Melissa Hood and Christina Eldredge

Foundational Domains

This chapter addresses the following AMIA Foundational Domains: F4—Health Information Science and Technology, F9—Interprofessional Collaborative Practice.

Learning Objectives

After reading this chapter, you should be able to

1. Identify the key controlled vocabularies and terminologies used in health informatics.
2. Explain how controlled vocabularies and terminologies support interoperability.
3. Describe the common use cases for controlled vocabularies and terminologies in health informatics.

24.1 Definitions

There are many definitions of controlled terminologies and their related terms in health informatics. For the purposes of this chapter, we will follow the definitions below that are in line with the International Organization of Standardization's (ISO) Standard 1087. Also, for the purposes of this chapter, we will use "terminology" as an umbrella term to represent the topic.

Controlled vocabularies are organized arrangements of terms, words, and phrases used to index content and/or to retrieve content through browsing or searching.

Nomenclature is essentially the term or terms applied to something that follow "pre-established naming rules." In healthcare, nomenclature provides a common language for consistent indexing, storing, and retrieving clinical data [2] (225).

Ontologies are the concepts that show relationships between medical terminologies.

Taxonomies use a hierarchical method to classify terms where there is a "parent" or broader term and "child" or narrow terms beneath the parent.

Term is defined by ISO as a "general concept by linguistic means" [2]. In other words, a term is similar to a single idea. The term described a discrete concept within a standard terminology.

Terminologies are "a set of terms representing the system of concepts of a particular subject field" [3] (1083). In healthcare, these can simply refer to the words that are used in one context of health and healthcare. These terminologies are meant to be comprehensive sets of terms (standardized) that allow disparate systems to speak the same language.

Vocabularies are described by ISO as dictionaries "containing the terminology of a subject field" [2].

M. Hood (✉) · C. Eldredge
School of Information, University of South Florida, Tampa, FL, USA

C. Eldredge et al. (eds.), *Introductory Textbook in Health Informatics*, Health Informatics, https://doi.org/10.1007/978-3-032-16657-9_24

24.2 Introduction

In the previous two chapters, both the concepts of interoperability and standards were introduced. In this chapter, the focus will shift to terminologies and controlled vocabularies, which are essential components of standardization and are required for interoperability to be most effective, especially when connecting disparate health information systems (HIS). In other words, terminologies and controlled vocabularies enable clear and consistent communication between two or more HIS.

According to the National Library of Medicine (NLM), the functions of controlled terminologies include [1] providing a standardized way of "expressing a concept" [4], creating a method for cross-referencing these terms, and [2] providing a structure to the term relationships such as broader and narrower terms or parent and child terms [5]. In the healthcare system, controlled terminologies are used to code diagnoses, treatments, and procedures for administrative and billing purposes. These codes are required by payers such as insurance companies and Medicare. In the public health setting, the World Health Organization (WHO) requires the United Nations' member nations to report mortality statistics using International Classification of Diseases (ICD) codes [6]. This example illustrates how the use of one standardized method of coding disease terms can be understood and shared around the world today.

Terminologies have been in use in healthcare since at least the late nineteenth century when causes of death were first categorized. At that time, the first iteration of the ICD (discussed above) was born. In the years since, ICD has grown to encompass a larger set of terminologies. Additionally, many other terminologies have been released to address other areas of healthcare. Some well-known examples of healthcare terminologies include CPT, LOINC, SNOMED, UMLS, and more. In this chapter, we will dive deeper into these standardized terminologies.

24.3 AMIA Specialty Areas

Controlled vocabularies and terminologies apply to all American Medical Informatics Association (AMIA) areas of practice and can be used to support a single area of practice or multiple areas, depending on the needs of a specific setting. The type of vocabulary or terminologies applied to the area of practice will depend on the context of that area, e.g. type of data collected, users of data, and intended purpose. Across all domains, the use of controlled vocabularies and terminologies may improve data quality and interoperability, in the practices of clinical, consumer health, research, translational, and public health informatics.

24.4 Types of Controlled Vocabularies and Terminologies Used in Health Informatics

Table 24.1 provides a high-level overview of some of the more common terminologies used in health informatics.

24.4.1 ICD

Our deeper dive into these common terminologies will start with the *International Classification of Disease (ICD)* codes overseen by the World Health Organization (WHO). ICD codes are the most widely known terminologies in use today. The ICD system is used internationally to track diseases in populations using a coding structure made up of both letters and numbers (alphanumeric). The first versions of what would become ICD date back to the late 1700s. In 1948, the WHO took over ownership of ICD when it was in its sixth revision. In its early revisions, this system was known as the International List of Causes of Death. It was originally designed to be a way to classify "causes of mortality that could be used across borders and languages" [7]. When

Table 24.1 Common terminologies used in health informatics

Common name/ acronym of the terminology	Full name	Owner	Year created	Primary use
CPT	Current procedural terminology	AMA	1966	National coding system using evidence-based codes for use in coding medical services and procedures
HCPCS	Healthcare common procedure coding system	CMS	2000	Two-tier coding system for health insurance claims
ICD	International statistical classification of diseases and related health problems	WHO	1948[a]	International, systematic coding for classifying diseases, injuries, and causes of death
LOINC	Logical observation identifiers names and codes	Regenstrief Institute	1994	Common language for identifying health measurements, observations, and documents
McSH®	Medical subject headings	NLM	1963	Controlled specialized vocabulary used for PubMed citations
NDC	National Drug Code Directory	FDA	1972	This directory provides data submitted for all finished drugs, including over-the-counter drugs
RxNORM	RxNORM	NLM	2001	Provides normalized names for clinical drugs
SNOMED-CT	Systemized nomenclature of medicine—Clinical terms	SNOMED	1965	Standardized, multilingual core set of clinical terminology

[a]This is for the sixth revision of the standard when the WHO took over ownership of the classification. The first iterations of what would become ICD date back to the late 1700s

the WHO took ownership of the system in 1948, causes of diseases (morbidity) were added and the name was changed to the current International Classification of Disease [7].

Commonly referred to by its most recent revision, this terminology is now known as ICD-11, which became effective January 1, 2022, but was actually adopted in 2019 [6]. Over time, the years between revisions have grown. Figure 24.1 shows the versions under the WHO, the year adopted, and the number of years between updates.

Once the WHO has published a new ICD revision, the National Center for Health Statistics in the United States develops a clinical modification of the classification. For ICD-10, most commonly in use today, this modification is called ICD-10-CM [6]. Originally, the ICD coding system was designed to enable morbidity and mortality tracking at a disease-specific level. As the revisions have improved the coding, the ICD system is used for much more now, including broader public health tracking, patient care efforts like disease management, and tracking of outcomes for research purposes [8]. More information about how the CM version of ICD is used is discussed in the Case Study further in the chapter.

Table 24.2 shows the differences between ICD-9-CM and ICD-10-CM. As you can see, there were significant changes, which require time for organizations to update their systems and implement the new version.

The biggest difference between ICD-9-CM and ICD-10-CM, as demonstrated in Table 24.2, is the addition of further modifiers that increases the level of detail in the coding significantly.

Examples of ICD-10-CM codes include

- G44.85: Primary stabbing headache
- S06.OX1A: Concussion with loss of consciousness of 30 min or less, initial encounter
- Z12.31: Encounter for screening mammogram for malignant neoplasm of breast

24.4.2 CPT

CPT®, or *Current Procedural Terminology*, was created by the American Medical Association. It

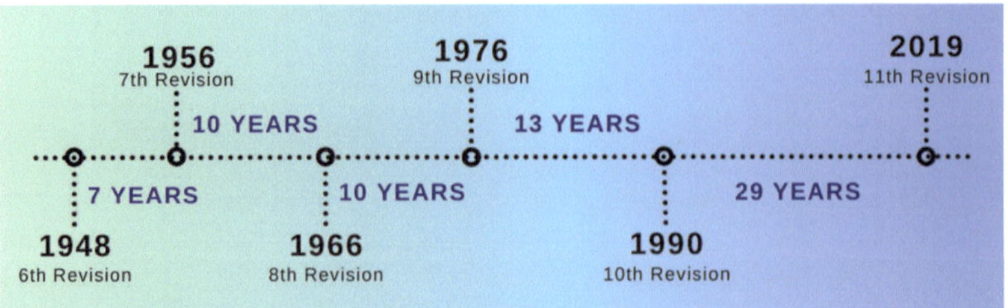

Fig. 24.1 ICD revision timeline

Table 24.2 ICD-9 and ICD-10 comparison [9]

ICD-9-CM and ICD-10-CM structure comparison	
ICD-9-CM	ICD-10-CM
3–5 characters	3–7 characters
First character is numeric or alpha (E or V)	First character is alpha (all letters except U used)
Characters 2–5 are numeric	Character 2 is numeric
Always at least 3 characters	Characters 3–7 are alpha or numeric
Use of decimal after 3 characters	Use of decimal after 3 characters
	Use of dummy placeholder "x"
	Alpha characters are *not* case-sensitive

is one of the oldest terminologies still in use in health informatics. This terminology was established more than 50 years ago and offers healthcare professionals a common/uniform language in which to code medical services and procedures.

The CPT was designated by the U.S. Department of Health and Human Services under the Health Insurance Portability and Accountability Act (HIPAA) as a national coding set. CPT uses evidence-based codes and is divided into four types of codes shown below [10].

- Category I: Descriptors that correspond to a procedure or service. This category is the primary set of CPT codes in use in standard procedures and services
- Category II: Optional, supplemental coding used for performance measurements
- Category III: Temporary codes for new and developing procedures, services, or technology
- PLA: "Proprietary Laboratory Analyses" codes that can be provided by a single lab or licensed and marketed to multiple providing laboratories

Some examples of the Category I primary set of codes include

- 99214 for an office visit
- 90658 for the administration of a flu shot
- 87635 for a COVID-19 test

24.4.3 HCPCS

Otherwise known as the *Healthcare Common Procedure Coding System*, it is produced by the Centers for Medicare and Medicaid Services (CMS). This coding system is used in health insurance claims, those by Medicare and other insurers.

HCPCS is split into two levels. The first level is made up of those codes that are in Current Procedural Terminology (CPT) described above. These codes are 5-digit numerical codes known as HCPT. The second level is codes that identify products, supplies, and services that are not in the CPT. These are also 5-digit codes, though the first digit is a letter, and the four remaining are numerical. These are known as HCDT [11].

24.4.4 LOINC

Logical Observation Identifiers Names and Codes was created in 1994 through the Regenstrief Institute to standardize health measurements and observations. At the time of creation, there was a trend toward the electronic submission of clinical data between laboratories, data producers, hospitals, and medical centers that was growing [12]. Without the coding values, the disparate systems would not be able to understand the data that was being sent and/or received.

24.4.5 MeSH®

The *Medical Subject Headings* (MeSH®) were created by the National Library of Medicine (NLM) in 1963. MeSH® is a controlled, hierarchical vocabulary that is used for indexing, cataloging, and searching health-related information. MeSH® is updated annually. The 2024 version is currently in use, and at the time of writing this chapter, the 2025 version is in progress. For 2024, there were new MeSH® descriptors created, some descriptors changed, and new terms related to psychological stress were added. The 2025 version in progress will have new terms related to Artificial Intelligence and Machine Learning [13].

MeSH® descriptors are organized into categories like anatomic terms or diseases, and then by subcategories [14]. Below is an example of how this organization works for Migraine, using the MeSH® Subject Headings 2023 browser [15].

Nervous System Diseases [C10]

Central Nervous System Diseases [C10.228]

Brain Diseases [C10.228.140]

Headache Disorders [C10.228.140.546]

Headache Disorders, Primary [C10.228.140.546.399]

Migraine Disorders [C10.228.140.546.399.750]

24.4.6 NDC

NDC is the FDA's *National Drug Code Directory*. This directory provides data submitted for all finished drugs, including over-the-counter drugs. It is important to know that listings in this directory do not mean that the drug is FDA approved or that the information has even been verified; unapproved drugs are also listed. The FDA owns the NDC, but the entries belong to the labeler who submits the file [16].

In addition to the finished drug products, the NDC also has an unfinished drugs database that is also required for drug establishments producing active pharmaceutical ingredients. The unfinished drug database includes active pharmaceutical ingredients, drugs for further processing, and bulk drug substances for compounding [16].

24.4.7 RxNORM

Created by the National Library of Medicine (NLM), *RxNorm* consists of two linked parts. The first part is the normalized naming system for generic and branded drugs, and the second part is a tool that helps interaction between drug terminologies and pharmacy knowledge base systems [17].

The purpose of RxNorm ties back to interoperability. It provides a way for various hospitals, pharmacy, and other organizations to communicate with one another. Many systems use different sets of drug names, so RxNorm gives a way to interpret and link those between systems efficiently and reduce errors. RxNorm's scope is focused on both prescription and over-the-counter drugs in the United States. Food or dietary supplements and homeopathic pharmaceuticals are not included in the scope [17].

RxNorm is available to users through the UMLS Metathesaurus (see later entry for UMLS) or through a UMLS account. Additionally, there is an API page, a navigation application, and files can be directly downloaded. Where many of the other terminologies we have discussed have annual or longer release schedules for new revisions, the entire RxNorm dataset is released monthly. There are also some weekly updates [17].

24.4.8 SNOMED-CT

SNOMED CT, started in 1965 as Systemized Nomenclature of Pathology (SNOP). In 1975, it was expanded to meet the growing needs of medicine and renamed *Systemized Nomenclature of Medicine (SNOMED)*. A partnership between the College of American Pathologists and the National Health Service in the United Kingdom led to the creation of SNOMED CT (CT stands for Clinical Terms). The first version of SNOMED CT was released in 2002 [26].

SNOMED-CT is multilingual and mapped to other international standards and in use in more than 80 countries. It is a comprehensive terminology that is released monthly. It is divided into concepts, descriptions, and relationships. The use of SNOMED-CT in electronic health records can make those records much more effective in the processing of clinical information [18].

Health records that implement SNOMED-CT enable linking between clinical guidelines and clinical records, enhancing quality care, and potentially reducing costs. The opportunities presented with using SNOMED-CT include improvement in clinical decision support and more accurate reporting for billing purposes and research [18].

24.4.9 UMLS

While not a controlled terminology of its own, the National Library of Medicine (NLM) also maintains the *Unified Medical Language System* (UMLS) in addition to MeSH® and RxNorm. A major component of the UMLS is the Metathesaurus, a makeup of many of the terms from biomedical vocabularies we have discussed here, including ICD-10-CM, SNOMED-CT, LOINC, MeSH®, RxNorm, and others [19].

The UMLS is a set of files and software. It can be accessed in several ways: web browsers, local installation, and through web services APIs. To use the UMLS, a user should request a license from NLM. There is no charge for the license. With licensing, UMLS is a great tool for interoperability, allowing the user to link terms between providers, map between terminologies, and even create their own local terminology [19].

24.5 Use Cases for Terminology Standardization

In Fig. 24.2, you can see the different use cases for incorporating standardized terminology in healthcare information technology, including information capture, communication, knowledge organization, information retrieval, and decision support [20].

24.5.1 Information Capture

Terminologies provide a common way for providers to capture patient information in an electronic health record. This can include documenting clinical findings, conditions, and outcomes. Having standardized terminology allows for more structured data within the electronic health record that can then be used for purposes such as reporting, quality improvement, and population-level research. Healthcare system processes in the United States that depend on terminologies such as ICD include public health policy development, patient quality and safety initiatives, insurance claims processing, and outcome reporting for use in research. Coding systems such as ICD or CPT can also be utilized for billing and reimbursement [7].

To put this in perspective, Poterack and Ramakrishna looked at the anesthetic record of a patient through the lens of electronic health records (EHRs). According to the authors, the purpose of the anesthetic record has always been to capture data about the patient's "anesthetic experience" [21]. Capturing data using standardized terminology allows for the ability to communicate, organize, and retrieve information across health information systems.

24.5.2 Communication

As has been discussed previously, communication is an important use for standardized terminology. Terminology standardization facilitates health information exchange between disparate health IT systems while maintaining data quality and security. Furthermore, maintaining data quality and meaning is important for patient safety.

24.5.3 Knowledge Organization

The use of controlled terminologies aids in organizing information within an electronic health record system to create valuable knowledge for providers. These terminologies provide ways to organize by classification of conditions, treatments, outcomes, diagnoses, etc.. Having the

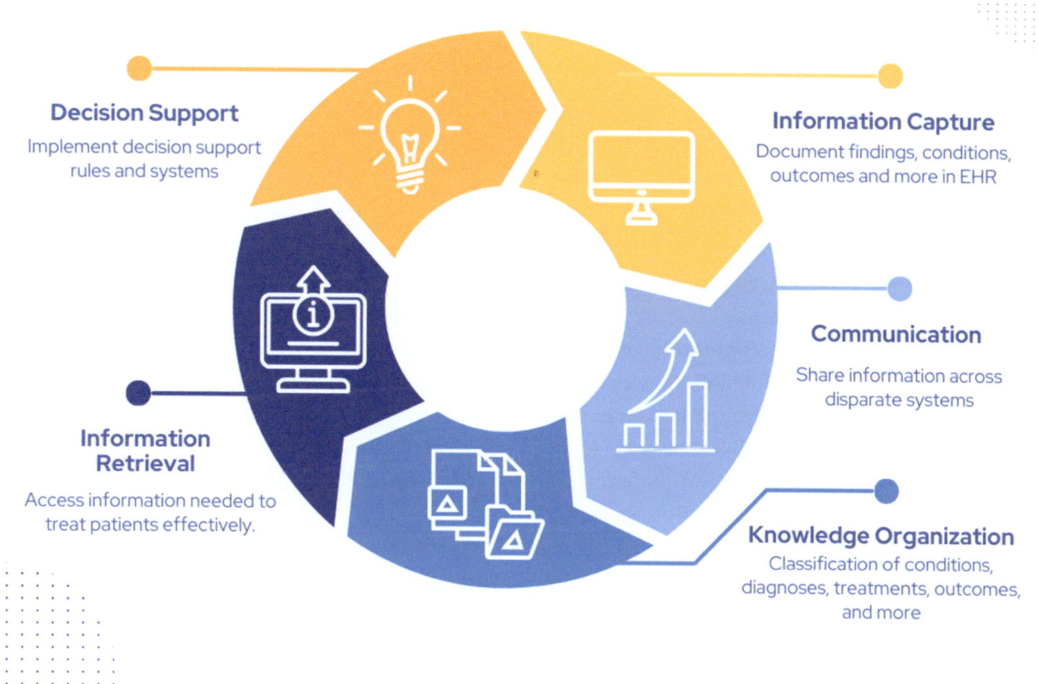

Fig. 24.2 Standardized terminology use cases

knowledge organized under these classifications can aid in the identification of disease, management strategies to improve health outcomes by recognizing similar characteristics or trends in health records.

Returning to our anesthetic record example, when controlled terminologies have been used, data can be compared across health information systems to create "patterns of interactions" that produce information that can be observed and researched creating "knowledge" for evidence-based practice [21].

24.5.4 Information Retrieval

An important part of using standardized terminologies is the ability for providers to easily retrieve critical information about their patients to help inform their treatment. The use of standard terms improves precision and recall when searching for medical information within a health information system. Precision is the percentage of information that is relevant from all information retrieved in a search, while recall is the percentage of information that is relevant from all information in the system [22].

24.5.5 Decision Support

The previous use cases discussed above support the ability of a health information system to incorporate decision support rules that aid the provider at the time of care with effective recommendations. This integration improves the knowledge and information needed by the provider, lowers the risk of errors, and reduces duplication of tests and services.

Cimino notes that decision support tools "will be easier to create and maintain when they can rely on the classification of terms in the terminology to make their inferences" [23]. This means that the tools that support providers in making appropriate clinical decisions will work better with controlled terminologies in place.

24.6 Opportunities

There are several benefits that emerge from the use of controlled vocabularies and terminologies. As discussed in the above use cases, having controlled vocabularies and terminologies in place allows for disparate systems to communicate with one another (see the chapter on interoperability for more information on this process). Additionally, even within the same system, the use of standardized terminologies improves communication between healthcare providers and hospital systems (e.g., departments), Again, these terminologies allow for consistent and secure exchange of health data to support patient transfers between departments for facilities, quality improvement efforts, biomedical research, and medical billing.

24.7 Challenges

While the use of terminologies does help facilitate interoperability, scaling of use from a local to a regional or global setting can be challenging as different organizations may have competing terminology standards. Furthermore, electronic health records systems within the same organization may not be interoperable with one another due to site variations in use or customizations of terminologies. Numerical coding of terminologies may be easier to implement and maintain in many cases as it may bridge a global divide. Additionally, as Cimino points out, when terminologies are updated and new "versions" created, historical data and descriptions of prior versions are important as "changes may be hard to detect when a user of historical data has only the codes for the data and the most recent version of the terminology" [23].

24.8 Case Study

As mentioned above, implementation of a new version of ICD can take years for healthcare systems. ICD is currently in its 11th revision, and yet, within the past decade, the US healthcare system has only updated its use of ICD from version 9 to version 10. In preparation for this, the Department of Health and Human Services offered courses and educational material to help institutions transition from one version of this terminology to another (see version explanation above). This transition offered some opportunities for improvement in the coding of diagnoses; however, there were several challenges.

First, let us look at some of the benefits of transitioning to ICD-10-CM. The overall benefit of using the newer classification system is to provide better data for the facility, which allows for

- Measuring the quality, safety, and efficacy of care
- Designing payment systems and processing claims for reimbursement
- Monitoring resource utilization
- Improving clinical, financial, and administrative performance
- Preventing and detecting healthcare fraud and abuse

There are also benefits to the broader healthcare community:

- Conducting research, epidemiological studies, and clinical trials
- Setting health policy
- Tracking public health and risks [9]

As mentioned, transitions like this are not without challenges. These challenges derive from the differences in the coding when moving from one to another, such as ICD-9-CM to ICD-10-CM, and the ability to "map" terms from one version to the next. The version modifications are key to achieving the benefits listed above but are still a challenge during the transition process. Below is a list of the differences.

- All codes are alphanumeric in ICD-10-CM. The first character is always alpha, but alpha characters may appear throughout the code.
- The codes can be longer at up to seven characters in length.

- Code titles are more complete that eliminates the need to refer to a category or subcategory.
- The side of the body affected (laterality) has been added to the code.
- There is expanded use of combination codes, such as poisonings and associated external causes.
- The ICD-10-CM codes reflect updated medical terminology [9].

As the lists above show, ICD-10-CM provides further detail for coding and reflects updated terminology and changes in medicine. But transitions are not without their challenges. The complexity of code changes can impact every part of a hospital's operations, from technical support to workflow and billing. Krive et al. observe that "although CMS provides forward and backward mappings between *ICD-9-CM* and *ICD-10-CM*, many codes share complex reciprocal relationships that may lead to confusion and incorrect coding" [24]. Essentially this means that with the increased detail in ICD-10-CM, some codes from ICD-9-CM may not directly map to the updated version or may not map at all. Care must be taken to identify the appropriate code as providers begin to use ICD-10-CM and a process must be established to address those codes without matches. The authors conducted a study to look at the accuracy of Emergency Department codes billed to Illinois Medicaid. They found that nearly 10% were clinically inaccurate. These types of errors can impact the clinical workflow and the financial stability of the hospital. The study demonstrates how changes in coding are difficult and must be handled appropriately for accuracy [24].

In this chapter, our focus for the ICD system has been ICD-10-CM and the transition from ICD-9-CM. But as you can see from Fig. 24.1, the current revision is ICD-11-CM. While the 11th revision was adopted in 2019, its effective date was January 1, 2022. Countries implement updated ICD revisions on their own schedules as the WHO does not set requirements for implementation. As of February 14, 2023, 64 WHO member states (countries) were in various stages of ICD-11 implementation [25].

As Feinstein et al. discuss, there are challenges to adopting ICD-11, including the in-depth mapping from ICD-10-CM codes to ICD-11 codes. With more than 70,000 codes and ICD-11's improved the level of detail, the authors point out that this mapping is "not a straightforward 1-to-1 process" [7]. Processes and activities that will require updates include billing, data processing algorithms, and statistical programs. Additionally, because the code structure for ICD-11 is different, "electronic health record systems and databases will need to be modified" [7].

24.9 Summary and Future Trends

As this chapter has demonstrated, the use of terminology standards in healthcare is important for multiple reasons, including data interoperability, information retrieval, decision support, communication, research, healthcare administration, and knowledge organization. Standardization is key to establishing interoperability between HIS for the secure exchange of quality health information. Using the most up-to-date versions of terminology standards is important because having multiple versions of terminologies can create challenges with data interoperability across health information systems. Also, as we also saw in the previous chapter, the use of standards, including terminologies and controlled vocabularies, is valuable in reducing medical errors.

Moving into the coming years, we are likely to see increases in the types of health informatics-related terminologies to support the use of artificial intelligence and machine learning in biomedical research and healthcare delivery. Mentioned above, MeSH® is already growing the inclusion of descriptors for AI use in the 2025 release version. It will be critical to keep a watch on new developments and guidelines from government healthcare agencies, such as the World Health Organization and the Centers for Disease Control and Prevention, in regard to the impact of artificial intelligence to key healthcare terminologies.

24.10 Additional Resources

Resource name	Website name	URL
Medical Subject Headings	National Library of Medicine	https://www.nlm.nih.gov/mesh/meshhome.html
Unified Medical Language System (UMLS)	National Library of Medicine	https://www.nlm.nih.gov/research/umls/index.html
SNOMED in Action	SNOMED International	https://www.snomed.org/snomed-in-action
International Statistical Classification of Diseases and Health Related Problems (ICD)	World Health Organization (WHO)	https://www.who.int/standards/classifications/classification-of-diseases
ICD-10-CM	Centers for Disease Control and Prevention (CDC)	https://www.cdc.gov/nchs/icd/icd-10-cm/index.html

Questions

1. What are five of the common controlled vocabularies or terminologies used in health informatics?
2. In what ways does the use of controlled vocabularies or terminologies support interoperability of electronic health record systems?
3. What are the five common use cases for controlled vocabularies and terminologies?

Answers

1. Possible answers include: CPT, HCPCS, ICD, LOINC, MeSH, NDC, RxNorm, SNOMED-CT.
2. Using controlled terminologies supports interoperability by providing a common set of terms which can be used to connect disparate HIS systems and allow HIS systems to communicate effectively with one another and effectively use the health information exchanged.
3. Possible answers include: Decision support, information capture, communication, knowledge organization, and information retrieval.

References

1. Khairat S, Feldman SS, Rana A, Faysel M, Purkayastha S, Scotch M, Eldredge C. Foundational domains and competencies for baccalaureate health informatics education. J Am Med Inform. 2023;30(10):1599–607.
2. ISO. ISO 13119:2022(en), Health informatics-clinical knowledge resources-metadata [Internet]. Geneva: International Organization of Standardization; 2022 [cited 2024 May 16]. Available from: https://www.iso.org/obp/ui/en/#iso:std:iso:13119:ed-2:v1:en https://www.iso.org/obp/ui/.
3. Shortliffe E, Cimino JJ. Glossary. In: Chiang M, editor. Biomedical informatics: computer applications in health care and biomedicine. 5th ed. New York: Springer; 2021. p. 1083.
4. Hammond WE, Jaffe C, Cimino JJ, Huff SM. Standards in biomedical informatics. In: Shortliffe E, Cimino JJ, editors. Biomedical informatics: computer applications in health care and biomedicine. 4th ed. New York: Springer; 2014. p. 211–53.
5. NLM. DB/metadata management program (MMP): using medical subject headings (MeSH®) in cataloging [Internet]. Bethesda: National Library of Medicine; 2017 July 17 [cited 2024 March 28]. Available from: https://www.nlm.nih.gov/tsd/cataloging/trainingcourses/mesh/mod1_050.html.
6. WHO. International statistical classifications of diseases and related health problems (ICD) [Internet]. Geneva: World Health Organization; 2024 [cited 2024 Apr 4]. Available from: https://www.who.int/standards/classifications/classification-of-diseases.
7. Feinstein JA, Gill PJ, Anderson BR. Preparing for the international classification of diseases, 11th revision (ICD-11) in the US health care system. JAMA Health Forum. 2023;4(7):e232253.
8. Hirsh JA, Nicola G, McGinty C, Liu RW, Barr RM, Chittle MD, Manchikanti L. ICD-10: history and context. AJNR Am J Neuroradiol. 2016;37(4):596–9.
9. CDC. International classification of diseases, 10th revision, clinical modification (ICD-10-CM) [Internet]. Atlanta: Centers for Disease Control and Prevention; 2023 [cited 2024 Apr 24]. Available from: https://www.cms.gov/medicare/coding/icd10/downloads/032310_icd10_slides.pdf.
10. AMA. CPT overview and code approval [Internet]. Chicago: American Medical Association; 2024 [cited 2024 Mar 28]. Available from: https://www.ama-assn.org/practice-management/cpt/cpt-overview-and-code-approval.

11. CMS. Healthcare common procedure coding system (HCPCS) [Internet]. Baltimore: Centers for Medicare and Medicaid Services; 2024 [cited 2024 Apr 24]. Available from: https://www.cms.gov/medicare/coding-billing/healthcare-common-procedure-system.
12. LOINC. About LOINC [Internet]. Indianapolis: Regenstrief Institute; 2024 [cited 2024 Apr 16]. Available from: https://loinc.org/about/.
13. NLM. What's new in MeSH [Internet]. Bethesda: National Library of Medicine; 2024 [cited 2024 Apr 27]. Available from: https://www.nlm.nih.gov/mesh/whatsnew.html.
14. NLM. MeSH tree structures [Internet]. Bethesda: National Library of Medicine; 2023 [cited 2024 May 28]. Available from: https://www.nlm.nih.gov/mesh/intro_trees.html.
15. NLM. MeSH subject headings 2023 [Internet]. Bethesda: National Library of Medicine; 2024 [cited 2024 May 28]. Available from: https://meshb-prev.nlm.nih.gov/search.
16. FDA. National drug code directory [Internet]. Washington: Federal Drug Administration; 2022 [cited 2024 May 02]. Available from: https://www.fda.gov/drugs/drug-approvals-and-databases/national-drug-code-directory.
17. NLM. RxNorm overview [Internet]. Bethesda: National Library of Medicine; 2024 [cited 2024 Apr 24]. Available from: https://www.nlm.nih.gov/research/umls/rxnorm/overview.html.
18. SNOMED. 5-step briefing [Internet]. London: SNOMED International; 2024 [cited 2024 Apr 27]. Available from: https://www.snomed.org/five-step-briefing.
19. NLM. Unified medical language system (UMLS) [Internet]. Bethesda: National Library of Medicine; 2021 [cited 2024 May 08]. Available from: https://www.nlm.nih.gov/research/umls/index.html.
20. Chute C. Medical concept representation. In: Chen H, Fuller S, Hersh W, Friedman C, editors. Medical informatics: advances in knowledge management and data mining in biomedicine. New York: Springer-Verlag; 2005. p. 162–82.
21. Poterack KA, Ramakrishna H. Converting data into information and knowledge: the promise and reality of electronic medical records. Ann Card Anaesth. 2015;18(3):290–2.
22. Ting KM. Precision and recall. In: Sammut C, Webb GI, editors. Encyclopedia of machine learning. Boston: Springer; 2011. Available from: https://doi.org/10.1007/978-0-387-30164-8_652.
23. Cimino JJ. High-quality, standard, controlled healthcare terminologies come of age. Methods Inf Med. 2011;50(2):101–4.
24. Krive J, Patel M, Gehm L, Mackey M, Kulstad E, Li J, Lussier YA, Boyd AD. The complexity and challenges of the international classification of diseases, ninth revision, clinical modification to international classification of diseases, tenth revision, clinical modification transition in EDs. Am J Emerg Med. 2015;33(5):713–8.
25. WHO. ICD-11 2023 release is here [Internet]. Geneva: World Health Organization; 2023 [cited 2024 May 28]. Available from: https://www.who.int/news/item/14-02-2023-icd-11-2023-release-is-here.
26. Bird L. Where does SNOMED CT® come from?. In: The essential guide to SNOMED CT®. Health information technology standards. Cham: Springer; 2025. https://doi.org/10.1007/978-3-031-97788-6_5.

25 Health Information Privacy and Security

Gary Schwebach and R. N. Josette Jones

Foundational Domains
This chapter addresses the following AMIA Foundational Domains: F4—Health Information Science and Technology, F6—Social and Behavioral Aspects of Health, F8—Professionalism.

Learning Objectives
After reading this chapter, you should be able to

1. Understand the US regulatory environment governing the use of health records.
2. Recognize protected health information in documents and information exchange.
3. Gain knowledge of individual rights to the privacy of their health information.
4. Understand the requirements for protecting the security of those rights.
5. Become aware of the consequences of failing to secure individual health information.

G. Schwebach (✉)
Luddy School of Informatics, Computing and Engineering, Indiana University- Indianapolis, Indianapolis, IN, USA
e-mail: gschweba@iu.edu

R. N. Josette Jones
Luddy School of Informatics, Computing and Engineering, Indiana University- Indianapolis, Indianapolis, IN, USA

Regenstrief Institute - Biomedical Informatics, Indianapolis, IN, USA
e-mail: jofjones@iu.edu

25.1 Introduction

Imagine that you are on vacation and not feeling well. You decide to go see a nurse practitioner at a local retail urgent care clinic. She takes your medical history, discusses what's going on in your life, diagnoses your most pressing health issues, and provides you with a prescription. You fill your prescription, pay with your credit card, and go on with your life. Over the next several months, you get a WhatsApp message from someone you don't know that asks you if you are better and would like to connect to talk about your conditions. This is followed by someone publishing a TikTok post that discusses your health conditions in detail. Then you receive a text message that someone has used your card to purchase gift cards from the drugstore chain.

25.1.1 What Is Going On?

Personal health information is some of the most valuable information for cybercriminals because it contains information about the person's identity, health conditions, personal situations, and financial circumstances and means [1]. This information can be exploited in many ways by the entity that acquired it and sold it to other cybercriminals via the dark web. The other aspect of health information that makes it a target is that it is stored electronically in electronic health

C. Eldredge et al. (eds.), *Introductory Textbook in Health Informatics*, Health Informatics,
https://doi.org/10.1007/978-3-032-16657-9_25

records (EHR). This makes it easier to obtain for those who can access the system. This relatively easy availability makes it a prime target for people to use and misuse.

This chapter will discuss the laws and regulations governing how individually identifiable health information, which is called protected health information (PHI), is protected from potential loss or theft. You will learn about the ways health data is protected and what can happen to those who access this data without authorization. We will start with a description of the environment in which these data live and some of threats that exist to the data. We will then explore the laws and regulations that have been put in place to protect the privacy of the person and the security of the person's information. Next the ways organizations should protect this information will be discussed. Then we'll explore what happens if the privacy and security of healthcare information is not protected by the organization [2]. Finally, we will let you apply these to your situation to cement how you can keep personal health information from being misused or abused.

25.2 The Health Information Environment

The health information environment is very complex. The majority of health information is collected, stored, and used in EHR systems that are maintained by multiple providers. If everyone were on the same system, protecting that information would be much easier since these systems could communicate with all the relevant organizations. That is not the case, however, which adds to the difficulty in keeping health data protected. What leads to this difficulty?

There are many different sources of health data. Within a provider's organization, multiple departments generate and maintain health-related information. This includes diagnostic and treatment details, information about the person's identity, location and social conditions, and the financial resources available for paying for the care [3]. This information is collected and transmitted in multiple ways, including administrative and admission notes collected in person, diagnostic and treatment notes entered in the EHR by hand or transmitted by wireless networks from various sensors, financial information transmitted electronically from the person's bank, and data collected and sent from smart phones and watches. All these data flowing along multiple channels must be protected within a healthcare organization.

If that weren't enough complexity, this information is then shared across multiple organizations. The provider must share this information with the insurance companies to be compensated for their services. They also need to share the patient information with pharmacists, labs, and diagnostic centers to provide the full range of care. Finally, in certain cases the information must be shared with local, state, and national governmental agencies, especially in cases of health surveillance.

Every time this information is transferred from one place or organization to another, there is a risk that the security of the information will be threatened. This can be accidental by people authorized to access the information or intentional by cybercriminals who are trying to obtain the information for their own purposes. In 2022, health information was improperly exposed by or obtained from over 590 organizations who legitimately obtained or used the data [4]. This impacted 48,600,000 individuals whose records were contained in those organizations. The costs associated with this were substantial; the average cost of a successful cyberattack to the healthcare system was $10,100,000 [4]. These mistakes, attacks, and costs continue to increase.

So, what can be done to protect some of the most private information that our society has? That is the topic for the remainder of this chapter.

25.3 Foundations for Protecting Health Information

Let's get started with the foundational underpinnings for protecting health information. We will address two concepts, *privacy* and *security*, which are two aspects of protecting the health information of individuals. Privacy is the right of every person to control access to their personal health information [5]. Every individual owns their health information and has a right to make decisions about who can access it unless there is a need for that information that serves the public interest. Security is how the personal health information is protected and controlled by the people who have a right to access, use, or disclose this information. Security is the method used to protect the individual's health data privacy. Both privacy and security are the responsibility of those who are authorized to work with personal health information [6].

There are two US federal laws that govern how privacy and security are applied to health information. These will be the topic for the remainder of this chapter. The first is the *Health Insurance Portability and Accountability Act of 1996 (HIPAA),* which sets the rules for protecting all personal health information. The second is the *Health Information Technology for Economic and Clinical Health Act 2009 (HITECH),* which protects personal health information in its electronic form. How do these two different laws protect health information?

HIPAA and HITECH are different in the scope of what they cover. HIPAA sets the foundational rules for protecting all health information. This includes what needs to be done, how it should be done, and what happens if it isn't done. HITECH promotes the use of health information technology (HIT) and EHR while guaranteeing the privacy and security of health information used in these systems. This covers how HIT and EHRs are to be used, how they are to be protected, and the mechanisms for increasing the meaningful use of this information. Regulations have been developed to govern the application of both HIPAA and HITECH. These regulations are regularly amended to address new situations dealing with privacy and security [7]. Now that we have a general background, we will delve into both HIPAA and HITECH to learn more about how each of these laws work.

25.4 The Health Insurance Portability and Accountability Act (HIPAA)

HIPAA, as the name implies, goes well beyond regulation privacy and security for health information. Its broader scope is to improve the portability and continuity of health insurance coverage while holding those providing the coverage accountable for doing so. The privacy and security provisions fall under the accountability sections of the law. These provisions establish the legal and regulatory regimen for protecting health information. It establishes the right of consumers to control the access and use of their personal health information. The law then creates restrictions and boundaries to using this information while holding the users accountable for its use. HIPAA also specifies that the privacy protection for consumers is to be balanced with the public good when determining whether and how the health information can be used. Finally, HIPAA publishes two rules, the Privacy Rule and the Security Rule, which govern the protection of health information as it is used [8].

Protected Information: There is a very specific type of information that HIPAA protects from unauthorized use or disclosure called PHI. PHI is defined as individually identifiable health information held or transmitted by a covered entity or its business associate, in any form or media, whether electronic, paper, or oral. PHI is information that can be used to identify the person to whom it refers. This information is protected in its use, storage, or transmission by specific entities. It also does not matter how the information is stored or shared. PHI is protected under every circumstance [5].

Applicable Organizations: HIPAA only applies to three specific organizations that the law defines. The first of these are *Covered Entities (CEs).* There are four categories of CEs who are authorized users of PHI.

1. Healthcare providers who are defined as any individual or organization that provides healthcare services in any form to individuals.

   - Company health plans, which are defined as organizations that provide health insurance to their employees through a sponsored plan
   - Healthcare insurance companies that sell or provide health insurance to organizations or individuals
   - Healthcare clearinghouses, which are organizations that process reimbursement claims from providers for submission to employer plans or insurance companies [9]

The second type of individual or organization to which HIPAA applies are *Business Associates (BAs)*. BAs must be [1] a person or organization that is not employed by the CE that [2] provides certain services, activities, or functions, which [3] require access to the PHI controlled by the CE. CEs contract with these external BAs to provide specialized services, such as accounting, legal, financial, administrative, or managerial services, that require access to PHI in order to complete those services. This relationship is governed by a business associate agreement, a contract that is specified by HIPAA and must be signed before access to PHI can be provided [9].

The third type of organization or people covered by HIPAA are *Business Associate Subcontractors*. These are individuals or organizations with whom a BA contracts to provide services to business involving access to or use of PHI. This relationship is governed by the same type of requirements as the CE and BA relationship in which the BA assumes the role of the CE.

Enforcement Responsibility: HIPAA assigned the responsibility for establishing regulations and rules to the Department of Health and Human Services (HHS). These rules and regulations provide guidance for how CEs provide the privacy and security of PHI. HIPAA then assigned the Office of Civil Rights (OCR) within the HHS to enforce these rules and regulations. The OCR investigates violations and can levy civil fines and/or refer to the Department of Justice (DOJ) for criminal penalties. It also has the authority to waive enforcement of regulations during public health emergencies, as occurred with the recent COVID-19 pandemic [10].

25.4.1 HIPAA Special Provisions

Now that you understand HIPAA's basic provisions, we will now go into more depth on the specific provisions of HIPAA. We will start with the Privacy Rule.

25.5 The HIPAA Privacy Rule: Standards for Privacy of PHI

The HIPAA Privacy Rule establishes the rights of individuals to control their PHI. While not absolute, it is substantial and protects PHI from being used in inappropriate ways. The Privacy Rule has two purposes. It defines and limits the circumstances in which an individual's PHI may be used or disclosed by CEs and BAs. It also works to protect privacy in the context of promoting high-quality care and protecting the public's health and well-being. This rule balances individual privacy with the public interest in better population health [11].

Categories of PHI: The Privacy Rule addresses three different situations related to health information by splitting it into three different categories:

1. Regulated data consists of PHI held or transmitted by a covered entity or its business associate, in any form or media, whether electronic, paper, or oral. Regulated data is subject to all provisions of HIPAA.
2. De-Identified data is health information that neither identifies nor provides a reasonable basis to identify an individual. This data is not subject to HIPAA rules and regulations. The primary means of converting PHI to de-identified data is to remove the 18 direct identifiers (Table 25.1) [12]. It can also be de-identified by receiving a certification from a qualified statistician that it is impossible to identify any specific person from the data.

Table 25.1 Complete listing of direct identifiers of protected health information for exclusion in de-identified or limited datasets

Patient name	Medical record number
Geographic subdivision smaller than a state: street address, city, county, precinct, and ZIP codes beyond the first three digits	Certificate/license number
All elements of dates (except year) for birth date, admission date, discharge date, and death or exact age of a patient older than 89	Vehicle identifier and license plate number
Telephone number	Device identifiers and serial number
Fax number	Web Universal Resource Locators (URLs)
Email address	Internet Protocol (IP) address
Social Security Number	Biometric identifier, including finger and voiceprint
Health plan beneficiary number	Full-face photograph and any comparable image
Account number	Any other unique identifying number, characteristics, or codes

3. Limited data is a PHI data set used for specific purposes that excludes any direct identifiers that are unrelated to the purpose. Limited data can only be used and disclosed for research, healthcare operations, and public health purposes. These data are subject to HIPAA regulations that require a separate data use agreement that requires specified safeguards for the included protected health information [13].

25.6 The Minimum Necessary Rule: Restrictions on the Volume of PHI

The Privacy Rule limits the amount of PHI that can be used or disclosed. It does this with the minimum necessary rule. This rule limits the use, disclosure, and any requests for PHI is to the minimum necessary amount of data needed to accomplish the intended purpose. CEs make their own assessment of the minimum necessary for a particular purpose and need to document how that was determined [14].

25.7 Authorized Uses or Disclosures of Health Information

The Privacy Rule also defines and limits the circumstances in which an individual's PHI may be used or disclosed by CEs and BAs. There are multiple circumstances in which PHI is authorized to be used or disclosed without the individual's permission. PHI must be protected from use or disclosure unless it falls into one of these categories [15].

1. Individual authorization is where an individual authorizes the use or disclosure of their PHI in a specific written format that is specified by the Privacy Rule. The minimum necessary rule does not apply to this circumstance since the individual owns their own data without restriction.
2. Uses and disclosures related to providing healthcare services specify that PHI can be used to ensure that healthcare will be effectively provided to patients. There are three areas that are covered by this provision [1]. PHI related to the treatment of the individual can be used for providing, coordinating, or managing healthcare and related services [2]. PHI can also be used to ensure that providers receive payment for reimbursable services and that the health plans receive premium payments to provide the reimbursement [3]. PHI can be used to support healthcare operations to ensure that healthcare can be efficiently provided to the population.
3. Uses and disclosure when the individual has the opportunity to agree or object, whether they are able to or not, covers emergent situations where healthcare is needed. The first is where an individual needs care and the provider informally obtains permission

either verbal or by signing a non-HIPAA authorized waiver, either by asking for permission or being in circumstances that clearly give the individual the opportunity to agree, acquiesce, or object. The second is circumstance where the individual is incapacitated, in an emergency situation or not available. CEs in this situation may make use of PHI in the best interest of the individual for treatment purposes.

4. Disclosure incident to an otherwise permitted use and disclosure occurs when an unauthorized person is exposed to PHI while engaged in an otherwise authorized activity. This requires an assessment of the risk that the PHI can be used or disclosed by that person. For example, when a member of the maintenance staff is working around people using electronic health records is exposed to PHI, this does not rose to the level of a breach due to the remote possibility that the data would be misused.
5. Use and disclosure for public interest and benefit activities permits PHI to be utilized without an individual's authorization or permission (U.S. Department of Health and Human Services, Summary of the HIPAA privacy rule, 2022). These activities must satisfy national priority purposes to qualify for this exemption. The use must be done in a way that balances individual privacy interests with the public need. There are multiple categories under this circumstance (Table 25.2) [5].

So how are these rights under HIPAA protected?

Table 25.2 Public interest and benefit categories for which use and disclosure is permitted under the HIPAA privacy rule

Required by law	Victims of abuse, neglect, or domestic violence
Public health activities	Health oversight activities
Judicial and administrative proceedings	Law enforcement purposes
Research	Essential government functions
Serious threat to health or safety	Workers' compensation

25.8 The HIPAA Security Rule: Security Standards for the Protection of Electronic PHI (ePHI)

The HIPAA Security Rule establishes the rules and methods for protecting privacy of ePHI while allowing the adoption of new technologies to improve the quality and efficiency of patient care (U.S. Department of Health & Human Services, Summary of the HIPAA Security Rule, 2022). It is a subset of the Privacy Rule that specifically addresses PHI that is collected, stored, or transmitted by electronic means, including tape and disc [6]. It goes beyond HIPAA to require far more comprehensive security measures and provides a greater level of detail about how to achieve these requirements. The Security Rule does not apply to PHI that is transmitted or stored on paper or provided orally; however, most organizations apply these same methods to all PHI (U.S. Department of Health & Human Services, Summary of the HIPAA Security Rule, 2022).

25.9 Required Outcomes of the Security Rule

The Security Rule applies to the same three organizations or persons as the Privacy Rule—CEs, BAs, and BA subcontractors. The CE is responsible for developing the means for complying with the Security Rule and ensuring that BAs and BA subcontractors follow them [9]. It requires the CE to achieve three specific outcomes to ensure the workable protection of ePHI. *Confidentiality* protects the ePHI by ensuring that is not available or disclosed to unauthorized persons. *Integrity* ensures that the ePHI is accurate and is not altered or destroyed in an unauthorized manner. *Availability* makes sure that ePHI is accessible and usable on demand by an authorized person for an appropriate use or disclosure. These three outcomes are collectively known as CIA or the security triad [6].

25.10 Responsibilities Under the Security Rule

Four proactive responsibilities are required under the Security Rule for CEs.

1. They are required to "ensure the Confidentiality, Integrity and Availability (CIA) of all ePHI they create, receive, maintain or transmit.
2. They must identify and protect against reasonably anticipated threats to the security or integrity of the information" (U.S. Department of Health & Human Services, Summary of the HIPAA Security Rule, General Rules, 2022).
3. The next responsibility is that each CE protects against reasonably anticipated, impermissible uses and disclosures.
4. Finally, they must ensure compliance by their workforce, which is often the most difficult aspect of the Security Rule (U.S. Department of Health & Human Services, Summary of the HIPAA Security Rule, General Rules, 2022).

25.11 The Flexibility of the Security Rule

The Security Rule acknowledges that CEs are very different from each other in their uses of ePHI. It states that there is need for each CE to adopt security measures that are appropriate for their individual situations. It is meant to be flexible and scalable to allow CEs to analyze their needs and implement appropriate solutions. CEs can implement policies, procedures, and technologies that are appropriate and reasonable for their size, organizational structure, and risks to ePHI [6].

25.12 The Three Steps to Implement the Security Rule

The Security Rule provides specific guidance to CEs on how to achieve these protections. The first step to protecting ePHI is for the CE to determine the risk to their ePHI. This is done through a process known as *risk analysis*. Risk analysis requires that the CE conduct an accurate and thorough assessment of the potential vulnerabilities, threats, and risks. Vulnerabilities are flaws or weaknesses in a security system that could be accidentally triggered or intentionally exploited and could result in a breach or a violation of security policy. Threats are the potential for a person or thing to accidentally trigger or intentionally exploit a specific vulnerability. Finally, risks are the likelihood that a given threat will trigger or exploit a particular vulnerability compared to the resulting impact. These three conditions form the foundation upon which all necessary security activities and procedures are established.

The next step is to determine appropriate security measures for the CE. This is done through a process named *risk management*. The Security Rule requires that CEs protect their ePHI by implementing and updating security measures that are sufficient to reduce risks and vulnerabilities to a level that is reasonable and appropriate for their situation. There are four conditions that must be considered in establishing their security measures relative to their situation:

1. Size, complexity, and capabilities
2. Technical hardware and software infrastructure
3. The costs of security measures
4. The likelihood and possible impact of potential risks to ePHI

The determination of what is reasonable and appropriate is made by the CE and the rationale for the decision must be documented with each specific measure. The CE must then continually review and modify their security measures to protect their ePHI in a changing environment.

The final step is to implement a *risk management policy* that incorporates the Security Rule's mandated safeguards and requirements and their associated standards and specifications. Safeguards are the specific areas the Security Rule has determined as keys to protecting ePHI. Each safeguard has standards for compliance with a set of specifications that are specific to that standard. There are three mandated safeguards.

1. Technical safeguards require the CE to develop, implement, and manage automated processes to protect data and control access to data.
2. Physical safeguards require the CE to develop, design, install, and maintain mechanisms to protect against threats, environmental hazards, and unauthorized intrusion.
3. Administrative safeguards require the CE to develop and promulgate written administrative policies and procedures that specify how security standards will be met.

In addition to the safeguards, there are two additional requirements for implementing the risk management policy.

1. CEs must meet organizational requirements that require contracts or other arrangements with BAs that will have access to their ePHI.
2. In addition, CEs must comply with the Policies and Procedures Documentation requirements:
   (a) The CE must implement reasonable and appropriate policies and procedures to comply with the Security Rule.
   (b) The CE must maintain the policies and procedures implemented in written form, including any subsequent action, activity, or assessment [6].

The Security Rule has multiple specific requirements that have been summarized in this chapter. These work with the Privacy Rule to provide the protections that HIPAA provides to PHI. This forms the foundation for ensuring that an individual's right to control their PHI is met while considering the public health needs of society. HIPAA was implemented when EHR and HIT were in their early stages of development. This law did nothing to encourage the adoption of HIT and the use of EHR systems. As this field developed and the full opportunities for improving healthcare became more apparent, a new law, HITECH, was passed to encourage the use of HIT. This led to the need for new security provisions to protect the privacy of PHI. This is the next area we will explore.

25.13 The HITECH Security Provisions

HITECH was designed to encourage healthcare providers to use EHRs and HIT by using financial incentives to motivate them. From a historical perspective, these incentives were available to three specific categories of providers and were tied to various escalating stages of "Meaningful Use." These providers had to report their use of a certified EHR system to receive the incentives. While it has changed over the years, Meaningful Use was originally defined as having three requirements.

1. Using a certified EHR in a meaningful manner, such as electronic prescribing
2. Ensuring that their system was connected to an EHR system that provided for the exchange of PHI to improve the quality of healthcare
3. Using an EHR system to submit information to DHHS on clinical measures

HITECH established the Office of National Coordinator (ONC) to determine whether meaningful use has been accomplished and to allocate the appropriate payments [16]. *HITECH required that any physician or hospital that attests to Meaningful Use must have performed a HIPAA security risk assessment and create a risk management plan as a condition to receiving payment. HITECH also stipulated that technologies and technology standards created under HITECH would not compromise HIPAA privacy and security laws. HITECH expands HIPAA privacy and security rules to hold that business associates and service providers were independently responsible for disclosing breaches* [16]. *Only the OCR enforces the privacy and security rules (Office for Civil Rights (OCR* [17]*). We will now look at breaches and enforcement.*

25.14 Enforcement of HIPAA Privacy and Security Rule Provisions

The rights of individuals to secure health information needs to be protected by the federal government for HIPAA to meet its stated objectives. There are two parts to this. First, violations of PHI privacy requirements must be defined, and methods must be in place to mitigate these violations. Second, the consequences of violating the HIPAA requirements must be addressed. These two components are subject to two additional rules called the Breach Notification Rule and the Enforcement Rule.

25.15 The Breach Notification Rule: Addressing Violations of the Security Rule

The unauthorized disclosure or use of PHI is labeled a breach. A breach is defined as an impermissible acquisition, access, use, or disclosure of PHI that compromises its security or privacy. An impermissible use or disclosure is *automatically* presumed to be a breach. The process for addressing breaches is the scope of the Breach Notification Rule. The Breach Notification rule [18] requires that a CE provides the OCR with notification following a breach of PHI. Breaches can be corrected if the CE can demonstrate low probability of data compromise, but they first must be reported. Breaches must be addressed at the time the CE the violation is discovered. There are three types of notification that are required:

1. Individual notification: Each individual whose PHI is or could be reasonably included in the breach must be notified by the CE. A breach is considered to be discovered on the first day it is known by the covered entity. Notification must be provided to each individual no later than 60 calendar days after its discovery [19].
2. Media notification: Notification must be given to the local media outlets when breach of unsecured PHI occurs involving *more than 500 residents* of a state or jurisdiction This notification must occur without unreasonable delay but no later than 60 calendar days after discovery of the breach. The purpose of this notification is to communicate the breach's occurrence to those who are affected by the breach but do not have access to mail [19].
3. Notification to the Secretary of the Department of HHS: Notification is required under all circumstances but the requirements vary based on the number of individuals who might be involved. If the breach involves 500 or more individuals, the CE must notify affected individuals and the HHS Secretary no later than 60 days after the discovery. If the breach involves less than 500 individuals, the CE must maintain a log of the breach. This can be individually reported at the time of discover or the CE can submit the log of small breaches to the Secretary of HHS during the next calendar year, no later than 60 days after the end of each calendar year [19].

Notification by a Business Associate: A BA must notify the CE of any breach of PHI within its own organization when it is discovered or known. This notification must be made no later than 60 calendar days after discovery of a breach. Subsequent laws have modified this requirement to require BAs to also report breaches directly to individuals, the media, and the HHS following the same rules that apply to the CE [19].

Law enforcement officials can require a delay of notification if the required notification, notice, or posting would impede a criminal investigation or cause damage to national security.

25.16 The Enforcement Rule: Consequences of Security Rule Violations

The enforcement of HIPAA is dictated by the Enforcement Rule, which establishes the process for correcting PHI violations and applying the appropriate consequences for the violators. The OCR is responsible for discovering breaches and enforcing the privacy and security rules. Breaches are discovered by the OCR through CE reporting

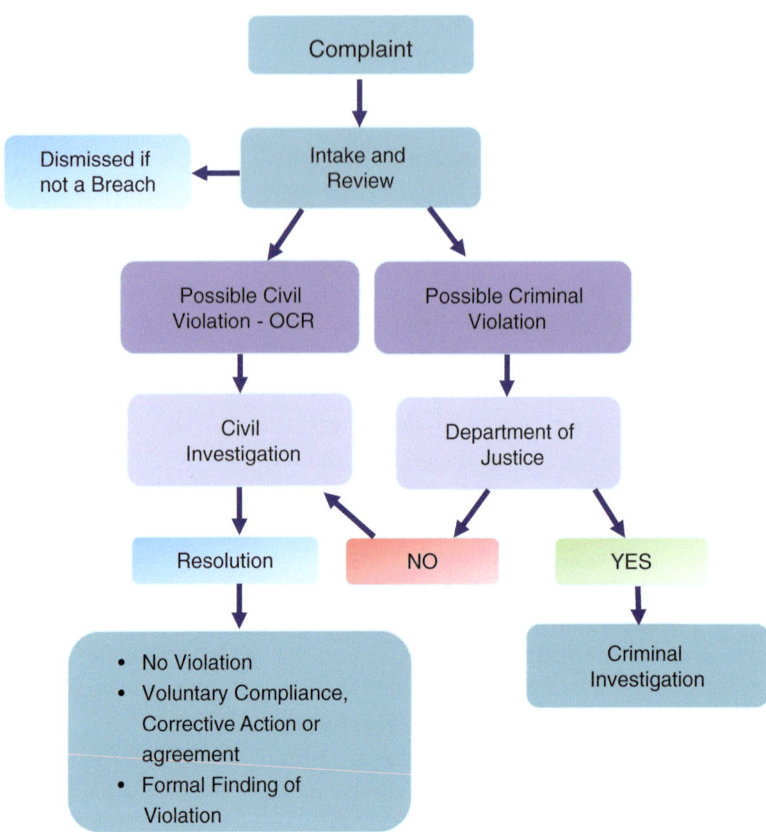

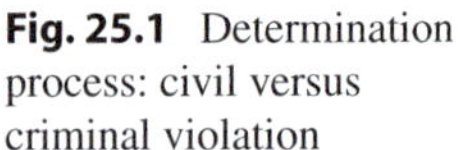
Fig. 25.1 Determination process: civil versus criminal violation

and complaints from the public. Violations fit into two categories. *Civil violations* occur when CEs do not comply with the Security Rule requirements for protecting PHI. These are the jurisdiction of the OCR. *Criminal violations* occur when PHI is misappropriated and used to illegally benefit the perpetrator. The US Department of Justice is responsible for prosecuting criminal violations. These two types of violations can result in very different consequences for the CE. The process for determining the type of violation is illustrated in the following Fig. 25.1.

25.17 Civil Violations

The Enforcement Rule establishes a process for determining whether and what type of violation has occurred. Complaints or Breaches are initially reviewed by the OCR with three outcomes. If it does not meet the conditions of a breach, the complaint is dismissed. If it meets the definition of a civil violation of the Privacy or Security Rule, the OCR begins its investigation. If it meets the definition of a criminal violation, it is referred to the Department of Justice for investigation. We will individually look at civil and criminal processes [17].

The OCR investigates the potential violation by contacting the CE to conduct its investigation. This involves a review of the CE's documentation and meetings with the relevant parties. The CE is an active participant in this investigation. The OCR then reaches three outcomes. If no violation is found, the investigation is closed and dismissed. If there is a violation and the CE voluntarily complies with the OCR's preliminary findings and requirements, corrective action, or other agreements, the CE is allowed to proceed without any penalty. If there is a violation and the CE does not agree to comply, the OCR issues a formal finding that leads to the penalty determination by the Secretary of DHHS [17].

The consequences of civil violations for noncompliance are civil monetary penalties that are imposed on the CE. Civil monetary penalties are prohibited if the violation is corrected within 30 days of the formal finding. Civil monetary penalties range from $100 to $50,000 per violation, where each patient record is considered a separate violation, depending on the severity of the violation and whether it is corrected by the CE. The amount of the penalty is determined at the discretion of the Secretary of DHHS [17].

25.18 Criminal Violations

Criminal violations are addressed in a different manner. The Department of Justice receives the matter and initiates a criminal review. These reviews have two outcomes. If no criminal violation is found to have occurred, the criminal review is dismissed and the case is returned to the OCR for a civil investigation. If a potential criminal violation is discovered, a criminal complaint is issued and the case proceeds into an investigation for possible prosecution. Criminal violations occur when Covered Entities and specified individuals "knowingly" obtain or disclose PHI, in violation of HIPAA. The complaint then goes to trial for adjudication. If found guilty, the case will move to the penalty phase [20]. The consequences of criminal violations are based on the severity of the crime. If the violation is a straightforward act of illegally disclosing or using the PHI, each convicted individual faces a fine of up to $50,000, as well as imprisonment up to 1 year. Violations committed under false pretenses allow penalties to be increased to a $100,000 fine, with up to 5 years in prison. Violations committed with the intent to sell, transfer, or use individually identifiable health information for commercial advantage, personal gain, or malicious harm permit fines of $250,000 and imprisonment up to 10 years. The extent of the criminal penalty is determined by the court that hears the case and is subject to appeal [20].

25.19 Summary of Privacy and Security in HIPAA and HITECH

This completes our chapter on the privacy and security provisions of HIPAA and HITECH. This has been a high-level overview of these laws and the associated rules and regulations. You can see that this provides protection of an individual's PHI through the establishment of the right to privacy for unauthorized disclosure and use by those who are covered by these laws. There is a lot more detail to these rules and regulations that we presented here but even this overview makes you more knowledgeable the majority of people working with heath information using health informatics. HIPAA provides great opportunities for those who are interested in applying their health informatics knowledge to improving healthcare.

This chapter provides the underlying framework for protecting PHI. The next chapter digs deeper into cybercrime related to health information, one of the biggest threats to PHI. It will then describe the cybersecurity measures that can prevent this intentional misuse of some of the most valuable information each of us possess.

Chapter Questions

1. How does the HIPAA Privacy Rule balance an individual's right to privacy with the need to support public health and high-quality care?
2. What are the main differences between regulated data, de-identified data, and limited data under the HIPAA Privacy Rule?
3. List five of the direct identifiers of PHI?
4. What are the four types of covered entities?
5. What are three types of permitted uses and disclosures under HIPAA?

Chapter Answers

1. The Privacy Rule limits how PHI can be used or disclosed while still allowing necessary information sharing for treatment, operations, and public health activities. This balance helps protect personal privacy without hindering efforts to improve population health and care quality.
2. Regulated data includes identifiable PHI and is fully protected under all HIPAA requirements, while de-identified data has all identifiers removed and is not subject to HIPAA. Limited data excludes direct identifiers and can be used for research, healthcare operations, and public health, but only with a data use agreement in place.
3. Potential answers include:

Patient Names	Medical Record Numbers
Geographic subdivisions smaller than a state: Street address, city, county, precinct, ZIP codes beyond the first three digits	Certificate/license numbers
All elements of dates (except year) for birth date, admission date, discharge date, death or exact age of a patient older than 89	Vehicle identifier and license plate numbers
Telephone numbers	Device identifiers and serial numbers
Fax numbers	Web Universal Resource Locators (URLs)
Email addresses	Internet Protocol (IP) addresses
Social security numbers	Biometric identifiers, including finger and voice prints
Health plan beneficiary numbers	Full-face photographs and any comparable images
Account numbers	Any other unique identifying numbers, characteristics, or codes

4. Covered entities include four types of organizations or people.
   (a) Health Care Providers
   (b) Health Plans
   (c) Health Insurance Companies
   (d) Healthcare Clearinghouses
5. Potential answers include:
   (a) Individual authorization
   (b) Uses and disclosures related to providing healthcare services
   (c) When the individual has the opportunity to agree or object to the disclosure or use
   (d) Disclosure incident to an otherwise permitted use or disclosure
   (e) Use or disclosure for public interest and benefit activities.

Chapter Assessment Exercise

Let's see what you have learned from this chapter. Recall that we started with you receiving medical care while on vacation, paying for it with your credit card and then receiving notification that your information was being used without your permission. You asked, "What is going on?". These questions below will allow you to apply your newfound knowledge to understand how this fits into your rights under HIPAA.

1. Discuss your rights in this scenario and if they were violated.
2. Identify the CEs in your scenario. Discuss their liability in this scenario.
3. Discuss the uses and disclosures that were made in this situation and whether they were authorized.
4. Discuss areas in which the Security Rule may not have been followed.
5. Discuss whether this was a breach and why that is so.
6. Discuss the type of notice of the breach that should have been provided if it was a breach.
7. Discuss how the OCR could learn about your incident.
8. Discuss the type(s) of violations that might have occurred and the potential consequences.

Chapter Assessment Answers

1. Your rights under HIPAA and if they were violated:
   Under HIPAA, you have the right to keep your personal health information (PHI) and payment details private and secure. The scenario describes a clear violation of these rights, as your health information was shared on social media, and unauthorized access occurred. This breach potentially indicates a failure in implementing the required security measures designed to protect electronic PHI (ePHI).
2. Identifying the Covered Entities (CEs) and discussing their liability:
   The Covered Entities in this scenario are the nurse practitioner and the pharmacy. Their liability stems from their status as providers and their failure to keep your health information safe and secure. The lack of proper encryption and access controls suggests non-compliance with HIPAA's Security Rule, which mandates the use of safeguards to monitor and protect health information.
3. Authorized uses and disclosures in this situation:
   The uses and disclosures made in this situation were not authorized under HIPAA. Sharing your health information on WhatsApp and TikTok without your consent violates your privacy rights. From a technical perspective, the unauthorized disclosures indicate a failure to enforce policies for the secure transmission of PHI, violating HIPAA's Privacy Rule.
4. Areas where the Security Rule may not have been followed:
   The Security Rule requires special digital locks (encryption) and access controls to keep health information secure. In this scenario, the clinic and pharmacy failed to implement these safeguards, allowing unauthorized access and disclosure. The lack of encryption and inadequate access controls highlights a disregard for the technical safeguards mandated by the Security Rule.
5. Determining if this was a breach and why:
   Yes, this incident qualifies as a breach under HIPAA. The unauthorized sharing of your health details online without your permission constitutes a breach of the Privacy Rule. The lack of privacy measures, such as encryption, underscores the importance of safeguarding ePHI, which was neglected in this case.
6. Type of breach notification that should have been provided:
   Following a breach, the clinic and pharmacy should have provided timely notification, within 60 days to you, explaining what happened, what information was compromised, and steps for protecting yourself. This is part of the required breach notification protocol under HIPAA's Breach Notification Rule, emphasizing transparent communication and remediation efforts.
7. How the OCR could learn about the incident:
   The Office for Civil Rights (OCR) could learn about the incident through your complaint, reports from the Covered Entities, or during an investigation or audit. The OCR plays a role in ensuring compliance with HIPAA's Privacy and Security Rules and may initiate an investigation to understand the extent of the violation.
8. Types of violations that might have occurred and potential consequences:
   Violations of HIPAA rules, such as unauthorized disclosures and failure to implement security safeguards, may result in significant financial penalties. The consequences could range from corrective actions to address security lapses to potential criminal charges for intentional violations for personal gain or malicious intent. The severity of the penalties depends on the nature and intent of the rule violations.

References

1. Health IT [Internet]. [cited 2024 Mar 1]. What is PHI (Protected/Personal Health Information)? Available from: https://www.techtarget.com/searchhealthit/definition/personal-health-information.
2. Why PHI Is Valuable to Hackers: Understanding Its Value [Internet]. 2023 [cited 2024 Mar 1]. Available from: https://www.ifaxapp.com/hipaa/phi-hackers-risks-implications/, https://www.ifaxapp.com/hipaa/phi-hackers-risks-implications/.

3. Data Sources for Health Care Quality Measures [Internet]. [cited 2024 Mar 1]. Available from: https://www.ahrq.gov/talkingquality/measures/understand/index.html.
4. Murray-Watson R. 2022 Healthcare Data Breach Report [Internet]. HIPAA Journal. 2023 [cited 2024 Mar 1]. Available from: https://www.hipaajournal.com/2022-healthcare-data-breach-report/.
5. Rights (OCR) O for C. Summary of the HIPAA Privacy Rule [Internet]. 2008 [cited 2024 Mar 1]. Available from: https://www.hhs.gov/hipaa/for-professionals/privacy/laws-regulations/index.html.
6. Rights (OCR) O for C. Summary of the HIPAA Security Rule [Internet]. 2009 [cited 2024 Mar 1]. Available from: https://www.hhs.gov/hipaa/for-professionals/security/laws-regulations/index.html.
7. Hernandez E. The differences between HIPAA and HITECH [Internet]. Compliance Home 2023 [cited 2024 Mar 1]. Available from: https://www.compliancehome.com/hipaa-hitech/.
8. Health Insurance Portability and Accountability Act of 1996 (HIPAA) | CDC [Internet]. 2022 [cited 2024 Mar 1]. Available from: https://www.cdc.gov/phlp/publications/topic/hipaa.html.
9. Rights (OCR) O for C. Covered Entities and Business Associates [Internet]. 2015 [cited 2024 Mar 1]. Available from: https://www.hhs.gov/hipaa/for-professionals/covered-entities/index.html.
10. HIPAA basics for providers: privacy, security, & breach notification rules. 2023.
11. Rights (OCR) O for C. HIPAA FAQs for Individuals [Internet]. 2015 [cited 2024 Mar 1]. Available from: https://www.hhs.gov/hipaa/for-individuals/faq/index.html.
12. What are the 18 PHI identifiers? [Internet]. [cited 2024 Mar 2]. Available from: https://www.paubox.com/blog/what-are-the-18-phi-identifiers.
13. PHI - Difference Between De-Identified and Limited Data Sets [Internet]. [cited 2024 Mar 1]. Available from: https://extranet.fredhutch.org/en/u/consortium-clinical-data-access/data.html.
14. Alder S. The HIPAA minimum necessary rule standard - updated for 2024 [internet]. HIPAA Journal 2023 [cited 2024 Mar 1]. Available from: https://www.hipaajournal.com/ahima-hipaa-minimum-necessary-standard-3481/.
15. LII / Legal Information Institute [Internet]. [cited 2024 Mar 1]. 45 CFR § 164.512 - Uses and disclosures for which an authorization or opportunity to agree or object is not required. Available from: https://www.law.cornell.edu/cfr/text/45/164.512.
16. Burde H. THE HITECH ACT: an overview. AMA J Ethics. 2011;13(3):172–5.
17. Rights (OCR) O for C. How OCR Enforces the HIPAA Privacy & Security Rules [Internet]. 2008 [cited 2024 Mar 1]. Available from: https://www.hhs.gov/hipaa/for-professionals/compliance-enforcement/examples/how-ocr-enforces-the-hipaa-privacy-and-security-rules/index.html.
18. Rights (OCR) O for C. Submitting Notice of a Breach to the Secretary [Internet]. 2009 [cited 2024 Mar 1]. Available from: https://www.hhs.gov/hipaa/for-professionals/breach-notification/breach-reporting/index.html.
19. Indiana University The Definitive Guide to Complying with the HIPAA/HITECH Privacy and Security Rules [Internet]. [cited 2024 Mar 1]. Available from: https://iu.skillport.com/skillportfe/main.action?assetid=RW$25386:_ss_book:51917#summary/BOOKS/RW$25386:_ss_book:51917.
20. Greenwood PW, Chaiken JM, Petersiua J, Prusoff U, The Criminal Investigation Process Volume III: Observations and Analysis. 1975. Available from: https://www.rand.org/pubs/reports/R1778.html.

Health Information Security and Threat Prevention

26

Saptarshi Purkayastha and Megha M. Moncy

Foundational Domains

This chapter addresses the following AMIA Foundational Domains: F4—Health Information Science and Technology, F5—Human Factors and Socio-technical Systems, F8—Professionalism.

Learning Objectives

After reading this chapter, you should be able to

1. Explain the importance of health information security in the context of modern healthcare delivery.
2. Define and apply the core principles of the CIA triad (Confidentiality, Integrity, Availability) to healthcare information systems.
3. Identify and describe common and emerging threats to health information security.
4. Understand the process of conducting a risk assessment and the importance of regular risk management.

26.1 Key Definitions

- *Authentication*: Authentication ensures that the right person gains access to a system or service. It serves as the first line of defense, confirming identities through methods such as passwords, biometrics, or tokens.
- *Authorization*: Authorization governs the actions a verified individual can take within a system. It defines access levels, ensuring users only perform tasks or access data within their permission scope.
- *Cybersecurity*: While often used interchangeably with information security, cybersecurity specifically focuses on protecting computer systems, networks, programs, and data from digital attacks, unauthorized access, or damage.
- *Data breach*: This occurs when confidential information falls into the wrong hands. It could be as simple as an employee losing a laptop or as complex as a sophisticated hacker breaking into a company's network.
- *Firewall*: A network security device that monitors and filters incoming and outgoing network traffic based on predetermined security rules. Think of it as a security guard for your network.
- *Malware*: Malware, or malicious software, encompasses a variety of software programs designed to disrupt, damage, or gain unauthorized access to computer systems. Types of malwares include viruses, worms, trojans, and spyware, each with distinct characteristics and modes of operation.
- *Phishing*: This involves deceiving individuals into disclosing sensitive information, such as login credentials or personal information, by masquerading as a trustworthy entity in elec-

S. Purkayastha (✉) · M. M. Moncy
Luddy School of Informatics, Computing, and Engineering, Indiana University Indianapolis, Indianapolis, IN, USA
e-mail: saptpurk@iu.edu

C. Eldredge et al. (eds.), *Introductory Textbook in Health Informatics*, Health Informatics,
https://doi.org/10.1007/978-3-032-16657-9_26

tronic communications. Typically conducted through email, phishing can also occur via phone calls (voice phishing) or text messages (SMS phishing).

- *Protected health information (PHI)*: As defined by HIPAA, this is any information about health status, provision of healthcare, or payment for healthcare that can be linked to an individual. This includes a wide range of identifiers, from names and addresses to device identifiers and IP addresses.
- *Risk assessment*: A systematic process of evaluating potential risks that may be involved in an activity. In cybersecurity, it is about identifying what could go wrong and how bad it could be.

26.2 Foundations of Healthcare, Risk, and Regulation

The rapid digitization of the healthcare industry in recent decades has revolutionized the way patient information is collected, stored, and shared. The widespread adoption of electronic health records (EHRs), digital diagnostic tools, telemedicine platforms, and other health information systems has greatly improved the efficiency, accessibility, and quality of patient care [1]. However, this digital transformation has also introduced significant new risks related to the security and privacy of highly sensitive health data.

Health information is among the most private and personal types of data that exists. Medical records contain a goldmine of personal information, including names, birthdates, social security numbers, and detailed health histories. If this is exposed or compromised, it can have severe consequences on the affected patients, including embarrassment, discrimination, identity theft, and even safety risks in some cases. Beyond the impact on individuals, unauthorized access to data can cause data breaches and also disrupt the operations of healthcare providers and damage public trust in the healthcare system as a whole.

Recognizing the importance of safeguarding PHI in an increasingly digital world, governments have established regulations that healthcare organizations must follow to ensure the privacy and security of the health data they handle. In the United States, the Health Insurance Portability and Accountability Act (HIPAA) sets national standards for the protection of patient information and imposes strict requirements on how PHI can be used and disclosed. Similar laws exist in other countries, such as the General Data Protection Regulation (GDPR) in the European Union.

Complying with these complex regulations and implementing effective cybersecurity measures can be challenging for healthcare organizations, especially as the threat landscape continues to evolve. However, it is an essential part of healthcare risk management in the modern age. By understanding key security concepts, common threats and vulnerabilities, and best practices for protecting health information systems, healthcare organizations can help ensure the confidentiality, integrity, and availability of the sensitive data entrusted to their care [2]. The following section of this chapter will provide an in-depth exploration of these critical topics.

26.3 Vulnerability: Understanding the Weaknesses in Health Information Systems

In the context of health information security, a vulnerability refers to a weakness or flaw in a system that can be exploited by malicious actors to gain unauthorized access, steal sensitive data, or disrupt normal operations. Vulnerabilities in healthcare information systems pose significant risks to the confidentiality, integrity, and availability of patient data. These weaknesses act as unlocked doors or open windows, allowing cybercriminals to sneak into the system and wreak havoc. Let us take a closer look at three main types of vulnerabilities:

1. *Technical vulnerabilities*: (*The Cracks in the Code*) Technical vulnerabilities are the most well-known type of weakness in information

systems. They often involve flaws in the software code or misconfigurations in hardware devices. For example, imagine an electronic health record (EHR) system with a bug that allows anyone to view patient files without proper authorization. Or think of a hospital network with a misconfigured firewall that leaves sensitive data exposed to the internet. These technical vulnerabilities are like cracks in the foundation of a building—if they are not repaired, the whole structure is at risk. Healthcare organizations can fix these weaknesses by regularly installing software patches, updating systems, and following cybersecurity best practices.

2. *Process vulnerabilities*: (*The Weak Links in the Chain Process*) These vulnerabilities are often overlooked, but they can be just as critical as technical flaws. These weaknesses arise from inadequate or poorly implemented security procedures and policies. For instance, if a healthcare organization does not have a clear process for regularly backing up data or requiring strong passwords, they are leaving the door wide open for attackers. It is like having a state-of-the-art home security system but forgetting to lock the front door. To address process vulnerabilities, healthcare organizations need to establish and enforce robust security policies, train employees on best practices, and regularly assess their procedures for gaps and weaknesses.
3. *Human vulnerabilities*: (*The Achilles' Heel of Security*) At the end of the day, humans are often the weakest link in the security chain. No matter how strong your technical defenses are, all it takes is one employee clicking on a phishing email or using a weak password to compromise the entire system. Cybercriminals know this, which is why they often target healthcare staff with social engineering attacks like phishing campaigns. These scams try to trick people into revealing sensitive information or installing malware on their devices. To combat human vulnerabilities, healthcare organizations must invest in comprehensive security awareness training for all employees, from doctors and nurses to administrative staff and IT personnel. By fostering a culture of vigilance and caution, healthcare organizations can turn their greatest vulnerability into their first line of defense against cyber threats.

26.4 Threat: Recognizing the Dangers to Health Information Systems

In the world of cybersecurity, a threat refers to any potential cause of harm or damage to an information system. When it comes to health information systems, threats can come from a variety of sources, each with its own unique characteristics and methods of attack [3]. Understanding these different types of threats is essential for developing effective strategies to protect sensitive patient data. Let us explore three main categories of threats:

1. *Natural threats*: (*The Unpredictable Forces of Nature*) Natural threats, such as hurricanes, floods, and earthquakes, may not be the first thing that comes to mind when you think of cybersecurity risks. However, these disasters can have a devastating impact on healthcare information systems. Imagine a hospital in the path of a massive hurricane. If the storm knocks out power and floods the server room, all the electronic health records and other critical data could be lost or damaged. While we cannot prevent natural disasters from occurring, healthcare organizations can mitigate their impact by implementing comprehensive disaster recovery plans. This includes strategies like maintaining secure offsite backups, using cloud-based storage solutions, and ensuring that critical systems have redundancies in place to keep them running during emergencies.
2. *Human-made threats*: (*The Malicious Actions of Cybercriminals*) Unfortunately, not all threats to health information systems come from natural causes. In many cases, the greatest risks stem from the intentional actions of malicious individuals or groups. These

human-made threats can take many forms, but they all share a common goal: to gain unauthorized access to sensitive data or disrupt normal operations. For example, a hacker might try to break into a hospital's network to steal patient records and sell them on the dark web. Or a disgruntled employee might intentionally delete important files or install malware on the system. To defend against these threats, healthcare organizations need to implement a multilayered security approach that includes tools like firewalls, intrusion detection systems, and regular security audits. They also need to have strict access controls in place to ensure that only authorized individuals can view or modify sensitive data.

3. *Technical threats*: (*The Risks of Technology Failures*) In today's digital age, healthcare organizations rely heavily on technology to store, process, and transmit patient information. However, this reliance on technology also introduces new risks. Even the most well-designed systems can experience failures or malfunctions that jeopardize data security. For instance, a software bug might cause an EHR system to accidentally expose patient records online. Or a hardware failure could result in the permanent loss of important data. To minimize these technical threats, healthcare providers need to implement rigorous testing and quality assurance procedures before deploying new systems. They also need to perform regular maintenance and updates to keep their technology running smoothly and securely. By proactively addressing potential technical issues, organizations can reduce the risk of data breaches and other security incidents.

26.5 Attack: When Threats Become Reality

In the context of cybersecurity, an attack is the actual execution of a plan by a malicious actor to exploit a vulnerability in a system. It is the moment when a threat goes from being a theoretical risk to a real-world incident. Attacks can take many different forms, but they all involve an unauthorized entity actively trying to gain access to sensitive data, disrupt normal operations, or cause some other form of harm. Let us dive into three main categories of attacks:

1. *Passive attacks*: (*The Silent Observers*) In the digital world, passive attacks involve an attacker monitoring or intercepting communications to gather information about a system or its users. For example, an attacker might eavesdrop on network traffic to learn about the types of data being transmitted or the protocols being used. While passive attacks do not directly damage the system or its data, they can still pose a significant threat. The information gathered can be used to plan future active attacks or to exploit vulnerabilities in the system. To defend against passive attacks, healthcare organizations should use strong encryption and secure communication protocols to protect sensitive data in transit.
2. *Active attacks*: (*The Direct Assault*) These attacks involve direct engagement with the target system to inflict damage or extract data. Active attacks can take many different forms, but some common examples include
   (a) Malware infections that give attackers remote access to a system
   (b) Ransomware attacks that encrypt sensitive data and demand payment for the decryption key
   (c) SQL injection attacks that exploit vulnerabilities in web applications to steal data

To defend against active attacks, healthcare organizations need to have a comprehensive security strategy that includes firewalls, intrusion detection systems, antivirus software, and regular security audits.

3. *Social engineering attacks*: (*The Art of Deception*) Not all attacks rely on technical

exploits or brute force. A brute-force attack is when hackers use trial and error to guess passwords or encryption keys, often using automated software to test countless combinations rapidly. Some of the most effective attacks use social engineering techniques to trick people into revealing sensitive information or granting access to restricted systems. Social engineering attacks come in many different flavors, but some common examples include

(a) Phishing emails that lure recipients into clicking on malicious links or attachments
(b) Pretexting scams where attackers impersonate legitimate entities to obtain personal data
(c) Baiting schemes that promise free goods or services in exchange for login credentials.

Social engineering attacks can be particularly difficult to defend against because they target the human element rather than technical vulnerabilities. To reduce the risk of these attacks, healthcare organizations should provide regular security awareness training to all employees, teaching them how to recognize and report suspicious activities. They should also implement strict access controls and authentication procedures to ensure that only authorized individuals can access sensitive systems and data.

26.6 Data Breaches in Healthcare Settings

In recent years, data breaches have become an increasingly common and severe threat to the healthcare industry. The consequences of a healthcare data breach can be devastating. For patients, the exposure of their sensitive information can lead to identity theft, financial fraud, and significant emotional distress. For healthcare organizations, data breaches can result in substantial financial losses, legal liabilities, regulatory penalties, and irreparable damage to their reputation.

26.7 Real-World Examples of Healthcare Data Breaches

Change Healthcare (2024) What could potentially be the largest healthcare data breach in history occurred at Change Healthcare in February 2024. A ransomware attack may have compromised the protected health information of up to one-third of Americans. The full extent of this breach is still being determined, but it is poised to surpass the previous record holder, demonstrating the escalating scale of cyber threats in healthcare [4].

Magellan Health (2019) In 2019, Magellan Health fell victim to a sophisticated phishing and ransomware attack. Cybercriminals initially targeted a third-party vendor with phishing emails, eventually gaining access to the systems and deploying ransomware. The breach compromised the personal health information of approximately 237,000 patients, including names, addresses, birthdates, and medical information. Magellan was required to pay $1.43 million in a class action lawsuit, illustrating the potential legal consequences of data breaches.

Texas Tech University Health Sciences Center (2021) In December 2021, Texas Tech University Health Sciences Center (TTUHSC) experienced a breach through its electronic health records vendor, Eye Care Leaders. The incident compromised over 1.2 million patient records, exposing information such as names, addresses, health insurance details, and medical record data. This case underscores the vulnerabilities that can arise from third-party vendors and the importance of supply chain security in healthcare.

Humana (2023) Humana faced a data breach in 2023 when a third-party vendor, Prospect

Medical, had its SQL database compromised. The leaked data, which included names, IDs, email addresses, and medical treatment information of over 6000 patients, was found for sale on a hacker forum.

These incidents serve as stark reminders of the ongoing and evolving challenges in healthcare cybersecurity. They underscore the critical need for robust, up-to-date security measures, continuous monitoring, and rapid incident response capabilities in the healthcare industry.

26.8 Emerging Threats

26.8.1 Ransomware

Ransomware is a type of malware that encrypts files on a victim's system, demanding payment in exchange for the decryption key. Healthcare organizations have become prime targets for ransomware attacks due to the critical nature of their data and the potential for significant disruption to medical services. Preventing ransomware attacks requires a multilayered security approach, including regular data backups, employee training on recognizing phishing emails (a common vector for ransomware), and deploying up-to-date antivirus and antimalware solutions.

26.8.2 AI-Driven Attacks

Artificial intelligence (AI) has the potential to significantly enhance cybersecurity defenses, but it also presents new opportunities for attackers. AI-driven attacks can involve the use of machine learning algorithms to identify vulnerabilities, automate the creation of malware or phishing campaigns, or conduct social engineering attacks at scale. Defending against AI-driven threats requires the adoption of advanced security technologies, including AI-based detection systems capable of identifying and responding to anomalous behaviors and threats in real-time. Additionally, organizations must stay informed about the latest developments in AI and cybersecurity to anticipate and mitigate potential threats.

26.9 The CIA Triad: Cornerstone of Health Information Security

The CIA triad is a fundamental model in information security that guides the protection of sensitive data, including PHI. It consists of three core principles: Confidentiality, Integrity, and Availability. Let us explore each of these in the context of healthcare (Fig. 26.1).

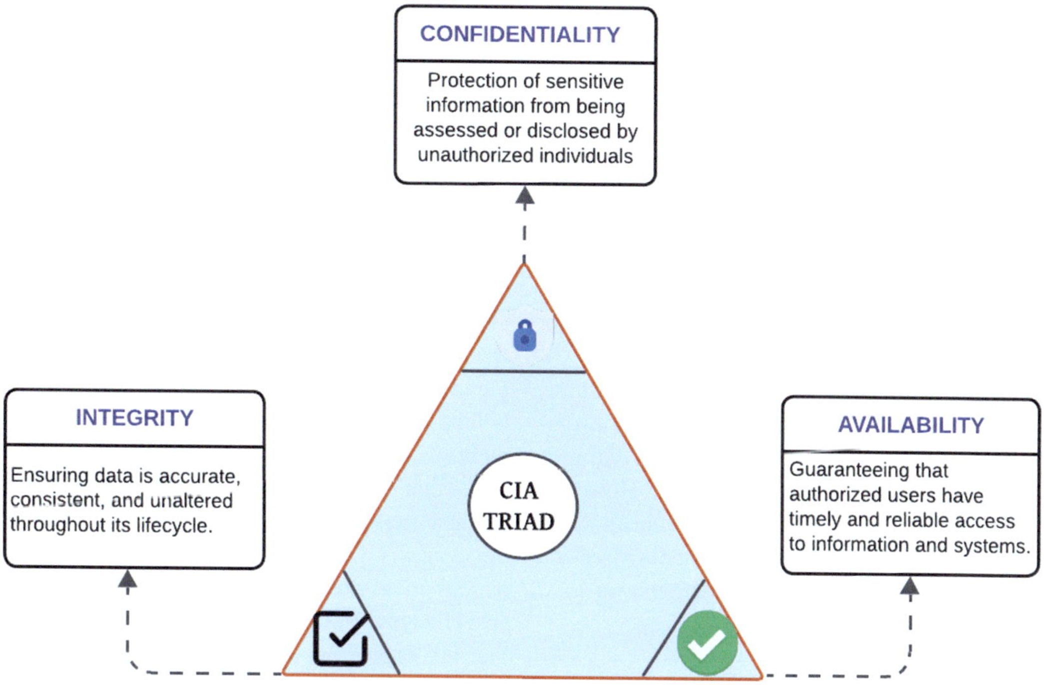

Fig. 26.1 The three pillars of the CIA model: Confidentiality, Integrity, and Availability

26.10 Confidentiality: Safeguarding Patient Privacy

Confidentiality ensures that data is kept private and is only accessible to authorized individuals or systems. In healthcare, this principle is paramount due to the sensitive nature of patient information. It protects patient privacy, maintains trust in the healthcare system, and complies with legal and ethical standards such as HIPAA in the United States [5].

In practice, confidentiality is maintained through measures like encryption of electronic health records (EHRs), role-based access control, and secure messaging systems for communication between healthcare providers. However, balancing accessibility for care providers with strict access controls remains a significant challenge.

26.11 Integrity: Ensuring Accuracy and Trustworthiness

Integrity refers to maintaining the accuracy, consistency, and trustworthiness of data throughout its entire lifecycle. In healthcare, where data integrity can literally be a matter of life and death, this principle ensures that medical decisions are based on accurate, unaltered information.

Healthcare organizations implement integrity through digital signatures to verify the authenticity of medical orders, audit trails that track changes to patient records, and robust backup systems. The challenge lies in protecting data integrity during system upgrades or data migrations and detecting sophisticated attacks that might alter data subtly.

26.12 Availability: Ensuring Timely Access to Critical Information

Availability ensures that information is accessible to authorized users when and where it is needed. In healthcare, timely access to information can be crucial for patient care, enabling informed decision-making in critical situations and supporting continuity of care across different healthcare settings.

To maintain availability, healthcare systems often employ redundant systems, fail-over mechanisms, and cloud-based EHR systems that provide access from multiple locations. However, balancing high availability with security measures and protecting against denial-of-service attacks present ongoing challenges.

26.13 Balancing the CIA Triad in Healthcare

The true challenge lies in balancing all three components of the CIA triad simultaneously. Stringent confidentiality measures might impact the availability of data in emergencies, while ensuring high availability could introduce vulnerabilities compromising data integrity or confidentiality. Healthcare organizations must carefully navigate these trade-offs, considering regulatory requirements, specific needs of different departments, technological capabilities, and resource constraints. By understanding and applying the CIA triad, healthcare organizations can develop comprehensive information security strategies that protect patient data while supporting efficient and effective care delivery.

26.14 Risk Management and Threat Analysis

Risk management and threat analysis are critical components of an organization's security strategy, especially in the healthcare sector where the stakes involve not just financial loss but also patient safety and privacy. Understanding the types of risks—strategic, operational, and compliance—is essential for developing effective mitigation strategies [6].

26.14.1 Strategic Risks

Strategic risks are those that affect the overall goals, direction, and long-term viability of an organization. In the context of healthcare, strategic risks could include changes in healthcare policies, shifts in patient demographics, advancements in medical technology, or emerging health crises that could alter the demand for services or the way those services are delivered. For example, a new regulation that significantly changes patient privacy requirements could require extensive changes to IT systems and processes, affecting an organization's ability to compete or maintain profitability.

To manage strategic risks, healthcare organizations must engage in continuous environmental scanning and scenario planning to anticipate changes that could impact their strategic objectives. Developing flexible strategic plans that can adapt to changing circumstances and investing in technologies that offer scalability, and adaptability can help mitigate these risks.

26.14.2 Operational Risks

Operational risks are associated with the day-to-day functioning of the organization and can affect its ability to execute its mission effectively. These risks can arise from internal processes, people, systems, or external events. In healthcare, operational risks might include data breaches, IT system failures, medical equipment malfunctions, or human errors that lead to patient safety incidents.

Managing operational risks involves implementing robust internal controls, including policies and procedures, training programs, and technology solutions designed to minimize errors and disruptions. Regular audits and monitoring can identify potential operational vulnerabilities, while incident response plans and business continuity planning ensure the organization can respond effectively to incidents and minimize their impact.

26.14.3 Compliance Risks

Compliance risks are related to the need to comply with laws, regulations, and standards governing the healthcare industry. These can include privacy regulations such as HIPAA in the United States, data protection laws like the GDPR in the European Union, and various other healthcare-specific regulations regarding patient care, billing, and reporting. Noncompliance can result in legal penalties, financial losses, and damage to reputation.

To mitigate compliance risks, healthcare organizations must maintain a comprehensive compliance program that includes regular training for employees, periodic risk assessments to identify areas of potential noncompliance, and ongoing monitoring and auditing of compliance efforts. Engaging legal and regulatory experts to stay informed of changes in the regulatory landscape is also crucial for ensuring that policies and practices remain in compliance.

26.14.4 Conducting a Risk Assessment

Risk assessment is a systematic process to identify, analyze, and evaluate the risks associated with vulnerabilities and threats to an organization's assets. In the healthcare sector, this means pinpointing potential risks to patient data, healthcare IT systems, and operational capabilities [7]. The steps to conduct a comprehensive risk assessment include

- *Identify the assets*: Begin by cataloging all assets that could be affected by cybersecurity threats, including hardware, software, data, and even personnel and physical space.
- *Identify threats and vulnerabilities*: Determine what potential threats could exploit and what vulnerabilities exist within the system. Threats can range from malware and phishing attacks to natural disasters and human error, while vulnerabilities might include outdated software, weak passwords, or lack of employee training.
- *Assess current security measures*: Evaluate the effectiveness of existing security measures and controls in place to protect against identified threats and vulnerabilities. This can help to uncover areas where security could be strengthened.
- *Determine the likelihood and impact*: For each identified threat and vulnerability, assess the likelihood of it occurring and the potential impact it could have on the organization. This step involves considering factors such as the value of the affected assets and the organization's current security posture.
- *Document and plan*: Document the findings of the risk assessment and develop a plan to address the identified risks. This plan should include specific security measures to mitigate high-priority risks, responsibilities for implementing these measures, and timelines for completion.

26.15 Navigating the Future of Health Information Security

As we look to the future, the fields of AI and blockchain offer exciting possibilities for enhancing the security of health information. AI's advanced threat detection capabilities and blockchain's potential for secure, patient-centered data management could significantly strengthen defenses against cyber threats. However, these technologies also bring new challenges and ethical considerations that must be addressed.

Healthcare organizations must remain agile, ready to adopt and adapt these technologies while navigating their complexities. By doing so, they can ensure the protection of sensitive health data in an increasingly digital world, maintaining patient trust and upholding the highest standards of care. The evolution of health information security is a journey that requires continuous innovation, vigilance, and a commitment to ethical principles. As we embrace the possibilities of AI and blockchain, the healthcare sector has the opportunity to set new benchmarks for security, privacy, and patient empowerment in the digital age.

Knowledge Check Questions

1. What makes healthcare data a prime target for cybercriminals?
2. Describe the difference between authentication and authorization.
3. Define the CIA triad and explain how each component applies to health information security.
4. What role does compliance risk management play in healthcare cybersecurity?
5. Identify a health information system and evaluate how it addresses each aspect of the CIA triad.

Answers

1. Healthcare data is a prime target because it contains sensitive personal information, including medical history, financial data, and personal identification. This information can be exploited for identity theft, fraud, or blackmail. Additionally, healthcare organizations often store large amounts of valuable data with varying levels of security, making them vulnerable to cyberattacks.
2. Authentication is the process of verifying the identity of a user or system, typically through credentials like usernames and passwords, biometric data, or security tokens.

   Authorization refers to granting or denying access to specific resources or actions based on the user's permissions or role, which are determined after authentication.
3. Confidentiality ensures that patient data is only accessible by authorized individuals or systems, protecting privacy.

   Integrity ensures that health data remains accurate and unaltered, which is crucial for making informed medical decisions.

   Availability ensures that patient data is accessible when needed, allowing healthcare providers to deliver timely and effective care.

   In healthcare, the CIA triad protects sensitive patient information while ensuring proper access and usage for medical decision-making.
4. Compliance risk management ensures healthcare organizations adhere to laws and regulations like HIPAA, protecting patient privacy and avoiding legal or financial penalties. It involves developing policies and procedures, training staff, conducting regular audits, and maintaining up-to-date knowledge of changing regulations to ensure adherence.
5. An example is *electronic health records (EHRs):*
   - Confidentiality is maintained through encryption, role-based access control, and secure communication channels.
   - Integrity is ensured by using audit trails and digital signatures to track changes and verify authenticity.
   - Availability is addressed through redundant systems, backup mechanisms, and cloud-based solutions that ensure continuous access to patient records.

References

1. Khatamjonovich FM. Security threats in information systems classification. Miasto Przyszłości. 2024;53:1128–9.
2. Loumbas EZ, Peters M. Data security implications in digital health: a cautionary tale. In: Nursing and infor-

matics for the 21st century-embracing a digital world. 3rd ed, Book 4. Productivity Press; 2022. p. 109–28.
3. Seh AH, Zarour M, Alenezi M, Sarkar AK, Agrawal A, Kumar R, Ahmad Khan R. Healthcare data breaches: insights and implications. Healthcare. 2020;8(2):133. MDPI.
4. The Most Damaging Healthcare Data Breaches (List & Analysis) [Internet]. soteri.io. Available from: https://soteri.io/blog/healthcare-data-breaches-and-analysis.
5. Cochran KA. The CIA triad: safeguarding data in the digital realm. In: Cybersecurity essentials: practical tools for today's digital defenders. Berkeley: Apress; 2024. p. 17–32.
6. Force JT. Risk management framework for information systems and organizations: [Internet]. National Institute of Standards and Technology; 2018 Dec. Available from: http://dx.doi.org/10.6028/nist.sp.800-37r2.
7. Shaikh FA, Siponen M. Information security risk assessments following cybersecurity breaches: the mediating role of top management attention to cybersecurity. Comput Secur. 2023;124:102974.

Project Management

27

Katie A. McCarthy

Foundational Domains
This chapter addresses the following AMIA Foundational Domains: F7—Social, Behavioral, and Information Science and Technology Applied to Health, F9—Interprofessional Collaborative Practice, and F10—Leadership.

Learning Objectives
After reading this chapter, you should be able to

1. Define project, project management, project manager, project management office, and project portfolio.
2. Identify and describe the phases of the project.
3. Explain the impact of budget, scope, and resources on successful project completion.
4. Describe the importance of stakeholders, milestones, and deliverables within projects.
5. Compare and contrast project management with change management and vendor management.

27.1 Introduction

To illustrate the concepts within this chapter, we will use a hypothetical case study that focuses on Sheila, who is the Director of Clinical Informatics for a large healthcare system that includes 10 hospitals and several hundred clinics. One of the hospitals is an academic medical center aligned with the region's largest research university. During a recent senior leadership meeting, she is informed that the organization needs to begin tracking social determinants of health within the electronic health record (EHR) system, and she is assigned to lead this project. Per the senior leadership team, the project must be completed by the first of the year, 9 months from now.

Sheila assembles a team and assigns Clarissa, a senior clinical informaticist, as the team lead. Sheila and Clarissa meet regularly to discuss the status of the work. During the first month, Clarissa reports that work is progressing well, the team is collaborating effectively, and they are on track to complete the work by the first of the year.

Early in the second month, though, Clarissa shares that the team disagrees about the definition of "social determinants of health" and progress has slowed. In addition, Sheila hears from the Chief Nursing Officer (CNO) that nurses within the organization have heard about additional documentation they will need to complete, and they are concerned about the time involved. In addition, the Chief Technology Officer (CTO) has asked for a meeting with Sheila to discuss significant concerns about the ability to store additional data within the EHR system.

Sheila knows that this project is important to the healthcare system, as well as its providers and

K. A. McCarthy (✉)
Sullivan School of Business, Engineering, and Technology, Carroll University, Waukesha, WI, USA
e-mail: kamccart@carrollu.edu

C. Eldredge et al. (eds.), *Introductory Textbook in Health Informatics*, Health Informatics,
https://doi.org/10.1007/978-3-032-16657-9_27

patients, so she quickly needs to determine what to do next. She reaches out to another senior leader, who recommends assigning a project manager to the project.

27.2 What Is a Project?

Sheila learns that the healthcare system has a department that helps manage projects. She meets with the director of the Project Management Office (PMO), who starts by asking Sheila about the work that needs to be completed to determine if that work meets the definition of a "project."

A project is a temporary set of activities that have a clear start, a clear end, and produce an outcome [1, 2]. Examples of informatics-related projects include

- A software upgrade to an existing EHR system that needs to be completed within the next 24 months.
- Optimization of nursing workflow within an intensive care unit (ICU) to reduce the time needed to complete all the necessary documentation within the EHR system.
- Creation of new clinical decision support to identify patients at high risk for heart disease to prompt clinicians to monitor cholesterol levels and blood pressure.

In comparison, operational processes are repetitive, functional activities that support an organization in achieving its mission and vision. Examples of informatics-related operational processes include

- Ongoing response to and resolution of EHR system issues that are reported by clinicians throughout a healthcare system.
- Monthly review and analysis of reports of patient safety issues and medical errors to find and address systemic patterns.
- Regular updates to laboratory test reference ranges within the laboratory information system (LIS).

Based on these definitions and Sheila's description of the work, the director determines that the work is a project because it has a defined start (2 months ago), a defined end (by the first of the year), and an identified outcome (documentation of social determinants of health within the EHR).

27.2.1 What Is a Project Management Office (PMO)?

As a next step, the director explains more about the project support that the PMO department can provide.

Although every PMO is different, this PMO has standard policies and processes for capturing project requests within the healthcare system, prioritizing them based on organizational strategic imperatives, and assigning project managers to assist with the prioritized projects [2, 3].

The PMO has software to track projects that are requested by leaders throughout the healthcare system. Project requests can include renovations of existing facilities, implementation of new software, installation of new equipment, and development of new training for clinicians or staff. These projects are then placed in a "project portfolio." In this portfolio, the projects are categorized based on the organizational strategies they support. For example, the healthcare system has a strategic imperative to focus on patient wellness, so Sheila's project request may be categorized under this strategy.

Once projects are organized within the portfolio, the PMO works with organizational leaders to prioritize the projects within each strategic imperative and across the entire portfolio. Prioritization is based on impact to achieving the strategy, the cost of each project, and the personnel needed to complete the project work.

Sheila's project was not requested through this process, so no documentation exists within the tracking software; as a result, the project request has not been formally approved nor assigned to a project manager.

27.2.2 Who Is a Project Manager (PM)?

A project manager (PM) leads the team tasked with achieving the project outcome [2]. They are responsible for a variety of tasks, including allocating work, defining project roles, tracking tasks and responsibilities, addressing and escalating issues, and communicating project status [3]. The PMO director and Sheila agree that having PM support is critical to getting the project back on track.

The PMO director provides two options. First, the director could assign one of their project managers who has training and experience leading projects and can work quickly to get the project request approved and on track. The downside is that they will need to rely on the team to help identify tasks and issues. A second option is to provide a PM mentor for one of the existing team members. Existing team members are already familiar with the project and the issues that are occurring but may not have the time to learn project management. The PM mentor can provide "just in time" training on key project management tasks and responsibilities.

Sheila asks that a project manager be assigned to the project (the first option), and the PMO director assigns Ahmad as the PM.

27.2.3 What Is Project Management?

Sheila meets with Ahmad and provides him with an overview of the project and the issues that have been reported. She asks about the approach he will use to ensure the project meets the established timeline.

Ahmad explains that project management is a form of management. Its goal, like other forms of management, is to provide direction for a group of people who are working to achieve a goal. So, PMs need to know how to manage budgets, people, and processes [1, 2]. The difference between project management and the type of management Sheila performs is that project management focuses on the achievement of a project goal instead of managing operational work [2].

As part of the project management process, Ahmad will lead the team through a set of processes that help initiate, plan, execute, monitor and control, and close a project. Some of these steps may have already been completed, and Ahmad will first assess the project team's progress and then fill in any gaps that may exist.

27.3 How Is a Project Initiated and Approved?

Initiating processes define a new project or a new phase of an existing project. As part of these processes, authorization is received to start the project (or phase) [2].

Without an approved project request, Ahmad's first initiating task is to work with senior leadership, Sheila, and the existing project team to understand the project background and justification. He learns that the project is an extension of a pilot project that was performed in one of the healthcare system's primary care clinics. In this clinic, clinicians and staff identified a significant increase in anxiety levels for patients between 10 and 16 years of age based on mental health questionnaires completed during annual wellness visits. After collecting and analyzing data, they identified three factors correlated with this increase: use of social media, nutrition, and time spent outdoors. With two local middle schools, they implemented a community garden, cooking classes, and a social media challenge based on these factors. These interventions were successful, and the healthcare system would like to expand these interventions to additional clinics and schools. (For more information about this pilot project, refer to the data science chapter in this textbook.)

In speaking with the existing team, Ahmad learns that social determinants of health is a large area of informatics-related research and can include a variety of factors such as economic stability, access and quality of education, access to quality healthcare, geographic factors, and social and community factors [4]. Ahmad quickly determines that a more detailed scope and plan of work will be needed as soon as the project request is approved.

To obtain approval, he creates a project request and submits it through the PMO tracking software. The request is aligned with the patient wellness strategic imperative and is assigned a high priority because of its potential positive impact on patients.

27.4 How Is a Project Planned?

With the project request approved, Ahmad works with the project team to identify questions that need to be answered, including

- What is meant by "social determinants of health"? What exactly would the organization like to track?
- Can the existing EHR system support tracking of social determinants of health? If so, what options exist? If not, will the system need to be modified by the vendor?
- What is the role for each project team member? Have the roles been clearly defined?
- What budget (if any) was allocated for this project?
- Who are considered the stakeholders for this project?
- What outcome determines if/when the project is "done"?

To answer these questions, Ahmad will work through project planning processes, which are used to establish the scope of the project, refine the project's goals and objectives, and determine the project management approach that will be used [2].

27.4.1 Identifying the Project Goal and Objectives

Because this project is an extension of another project, Ahmad schedules a meeting with representatives from this pilot team (Chen, Malia, and Sarah) and the current social determinants team.

In the meeting, Ahmad begins by asking Chen, Malia, and Sarah to describe the work completed as part of the pilot project. They explain that they used data from paper mental health questionnaires and the number of referrals to mental health services to determine the patient population with the highest anxiety levels.

During the pilot, they experienced several challenges. First, they needed to manually enter data from the paper questionnaires into a database. Second, because of illegible handwriting and other issues, some answers could not be entered into the database. Finally, the database they used was not connected to the EHR, which meant the data could only be used by the pilot team. At the end of the pilot, the team recommended implementing the questionnaire within the EHR system and a standard report so that the results could be viewed by clinicians and staff within the clinics. The current project is a result of this recommendation.

In addition, the pilot team explains that changing the paper questionnaires to an electronic questionnaire in the EHR will change the workflow for clinicians and patients. A *workflow* is a set of steps or activities that need to be completed to finish a task and/or achieve a goal [5]. Right now, the existing workflow includes steps to hand out the paper questionnaire to patients and their caregivers and then steps to scan the completed questionnaires into the EHR. These steps within the workflow will need to be changed if the questionnaires are completed electronically within the EHR.

Ahmad explains that the next step is to develop a project goal and objectives for the current project.

Based on the information from the pilot team and input from the project team, the goal for the current project is to implement mental health questionnaires and a standard report of the questionnaire results within the EHR system.

To achieve this goal, the project will have the following objectives:

- Create and implement a mental health questionnaire within the EHR system.
- Create and implement a standard report of the results of the answers from these questionnaires.
- Identify and implement modifications to workflow to include mental health screening using the EHR questionnaire during annual wellness visits and use of the standard report.

The team verifies that each of these objectives are *specific*, *measurable*, *achievable*, *relevant*, and *time-bound* (known as SMART objectives) [6]. For example, the implementation of a mental health questionnaire is a clear and specific task and can be measured by identifying when the questionnaire is available for patients to complete within the EHR. Completing this objective is achievable because the questionnaire is already available in paper form (so the questions are already known) and the EHR has functionality to provide questionnaires. This objective is also relevant to the current project because the questionnaire is needed to achieve the goal of the project. Finally, the objective is time-bound because it must be implemented by the end of the project.

27.4.2 Defining the Project Scope

Next, Ahmad works with the pilot team and the project team to develop a project scope. Scope is the work that must be performed to meet the requirements of the project [2]. Ahmad explains that scope must be achievable within the limitations and constraints of the project. Often, these limitations and constraints are related to time or resources (budget, personal, supplies, facilities, etc.).

For example, from a timing perspective, this project must be completed by the first of the year. From a funding perspective, the current project was not part of the initial portfolio prioritization and funding process, so funding will be limited and still needs to be requested and approved. From a team perspective, members of the existing project team will be the individuals assigned to complete the project. Therefore, the team will include a project manager (Ahmad), a senior clinical informaticist (Clarissa), a database administrator (Michael), a systems analyst (Santiago), and a reporting specialist (Ruth). Chen, Malia, and Sarah will be available to answer questions but will not be assigned to the project.

Although a new EHR questionnaire and report can be available to anyone throughout the healthcare system once they are implemented, work is needed to ensure that the questionnaire and report are integrated appropriately into clinical workflows. Therefore, the team determines that they will need to limit the current project to a maximum of three clinics. In addition, the questionnaires will be provided to patients 10–16 years of age (similar to the pilot project).

Finally, Ahmad explains that the team should also identify the work that is not included in the scope of the current project (known as *exclusions*). The scope will not include any clinical areas other than the three selected for this project. In addition, the scope will not include analyzing the data captured using the EHR mental health questionnaires or implementing any interventions. Finally, clinic workflows for assessing mental health of patients younger than 10 years of age and older than 16 years of age will not be included within this project.

Ahmad documents the project goal, objectives, and scope and reviews the document with the team. They agree that it represents their discussion and understanding of the project.

27.4.3 Identifying the Project Requirements

In the next project team meeting, Ahmad explains that another step in planning a project is identifying requirements. A *requirement* is a characteristic, function, or capability that meets a business need and should be achieved at the end of the project [2]. The requirements provide further details to specify what needs to be achieved based on the project goal, objectives, and scope.

The team brainstorms a series of requirements for the project, and Ahmad documents a list of the requirements and assigns each one a unique identifier (so the team can easily refer to them during the project). Examples of these requirements are shown in Table 27.1.

27.4.4 Defining Project Team Roles and Responsibilities

Next, Ahmad works with the team to further define their roles and responsibilities within the project.

Sheila will be the *project champion* and sponsor. In her role, she will share project information and status with leaders within the healthcare system. In addition, she will help address any resistance or barriers that the project team experiences.

As project manager, Ahmad will be responsible for maintaining project documentation according to PMO processes, including the project charter, plan, budget, and issues list. He will schedule regular meetings with Sheila, the project team, and project stakeholders.

Clarissa will work with clinic representatives to understand the mental health assessment within each clinic. She will also work with them to document the current workflows and then identify changes that are needed to integrate the new questionnaire and standard report. She will develop communication and training plans to ensure clinicians, staff, and leaders are ready for the changes.

Table 27.1 Example project requirements

ID	Requirement
QUES-001	Mental health questionnaire is available as a survey within the EHR system
QUES-002	Mental health questionnaire is provided within the patient portal for patients (or their guardians) to complete
QUES-003	Mental health questionnaire is available as a paper form for individuals without access to the patient portal
ERPT-001	Standard report is available within the EHR system to obtain data from the mental health questionnaires
ERPT-002	Standard report for the mental health questionnaires includes options to filter information by area (clinic, unit, etc.); patient age or age range; and date range
WKFW-001	Clinic workflow is modified to include entry of paper mental health questionnaires into the EHR if the questionnaire could not be completed electronically

Clarissa, Santiago, and Ruth will work with the EHR vendor to create the mental health questionnaire and standard report. They will test these changes and, when approved, will implement the changes into the EHR.

Throughout the project, Michael will be monitoring the EHR database and providing metrics to his Information Technology (IT) team and the project team to ensure the database structure and storage is sufficient to meet the needs of the project. In addition, he will work with Clarissa and the Security team to ensure appropriate security access is set up for the questionnaire and report following the guidelines from the Compliance Department.

27.4.5 Identifying Stakeholders

As part of these roles and responsibilities, each team member will work with project stakeholders. Ahmad explains that *stakeholders* are individuals, group, or organizations that may be affected by a decision, activity, or outcome of the project [2].

Some of the stakeholders include the clinicians, staff, and leaders within the three selected clinics for this project. Ahmad works with Sheila and other leaders within the healthcare system to select these clinics. They select two primary care clinics and one pediatric clinic based on their current mental health assessment workflows and work with patients 10–16 years of age. Each clinic leader assigns a representative (Abbie, Ben, and Xin) to work with the project team.

Teams within the organization will also be stakeholders. For example, the Clinical Informatics team will need to be aware of the EHR changes so that they can be tested in future upgrades of the system. The Reporting team will need to be aware of the new standard report in case they are asked to run the report for a clinic. The Data Science team will need to be aware of the EHR changes and report, as they may be asked to help clinics analyze the data. The Compliance team will provide guidelines for appropriate access to the new EHR questionnaire and report. The IT Database team will need to be aware of the database changes. And the IT Security team will need to set up the security recommended by the Compliance Department.

Ahmad also needs to consider stakeholders who want regular updates about the project progress. For example, the Chief Nursing Officer (CNO) and Chief Technology Officer (CTO) have both expressed concerns about the project, so they may be potential stakeholders. And senior leaders within the organization have asked for regular updates, so they will need to be included on the list of stakeholders.

27.4.6 Estimating the Project Budget

Next, Ahmad works with the team to create an initial budget estimate for the project.

First, Ahmad meets with Chen, Malia, and Sarah to understand the costs involved with the pilot project, which were mostly for the interventions performed at the two middle schools. Because implementing interventions is excluded from the scope of the current project, these costs do not need to be included within the initial budget estimate.

Ahmad also works with leadership to determine what costs should be included for project team members. Leadership states that all the team members will currently work on this project as part of their regular job duties, so no additional staffing costs need to be included. They do recommend, though, that Ahmad add a small contingency budget to cover the costs of consultants should a project team member leave the project.

Next, Clarissa and Santiago reach out to the EHR vendor to obtain an estimate to implement the mental health questionnaire and standard report before the first of the year. The vendor provides a documented estimate, which Clarissa and Santiago provide to Ahmad.

Based on their input from the project team and the estimates Ahmad has received, he creates a budget estimate for the project and adds a small contingency budget (to handle any unexpected expenses/costs that arise).

27.4.7 Identifying Project Deliverables

Next, Ahmad works with the team to identify all the deliverables for the project. A deliverable is something that needs to be completed for the goal and requirements of the project to be met [2].

For example, Clarissa will work with Chen, Malia, Abbie, Ben, and Xin to understand the current workflows within each clinic and modify these workflows. Deliverables from this work include

- A current state workflow diagram
- A future state (modified) workflow diagram
- A plan for training clinic staff, leaders, and clinicians
- A list of individuals who need training and security access to the EHR changes
- A schedule for implementing the changes in each clinic

Clarissa, Santiago, and Ruth will be working with the EHR vendor on the mental health questionnaire and standard report. Based on this work, their deliverables will be

- The questionnaire and standard report
- A testing plan
- A list of changes needed based on testing
- The final versions of the questionnaire and report

Michael, Clarissa, and the IT Security team will work with the Compliance and IT Security teams to set up the appropriate security for clinicians, staff, and leaders. Their deliverables will include a description of the security setup that is needed and a listing of individuals and the security they have been assigned.

As Michael monitors the EHR database, his deliverable will be a monthly metrics report to IT leaders and the IT Database team.

Ahmad continues working with each team member to identify the project deliverables. Together, they determine the sequence for completing these deliverables as well as the deadline for their completion. This information is documented for the team to review and share with their teams and stakeholders.

27.4.8 Creating the Project Management Plan

Based on his work with the project team, Ahmad creates the *project management plan* (also known as a project plan). A project plan lists the tasks, timelines, and responsibilities for completing the work of the project. Ahmad will use this plan to manage the project from start to finish [7].

As part of this planning, Ahmad identifies milestones for the project. A *milestone* is a significant point in the project, typically when a significant task or deliverable is complete [2]. For example, completion of the future state (modified) workflow is significant as it determines the training that will be needed for clinic staff, leaders, and clinicians as well as the security changes that will need to be implemented. Therefore, completion of the future state workflow deliverable is one of the milestones for the project.

Next, Ahmad determines the critical path for the project to determine if the first of the year deadline can be met (6 months from now). The *critical path* is the sequence of activities that have the longest duration and, therefore, determine the shortest possible duration of the project [2].

In making this determination, he works with the team to understand the large activities of the project and how long it will take. They also identify which activities can occur concurrently (at the same time) and which need to happen sequentially. Based on this information, he creates a chart showing the activities that can "overlap," as shown in Fig. 27.1.

Based on this information, the team can make the first of the year deadline if the deadline for the EHR changes is met, as these changes are needed to finalize the workflow modifications, training development, and security changes. Once these are complete, then the 4 weeks of training for clinic leadership, staff, and clinicians can begin. Therefore, the timeline for the EHR changes plus the 4 weeks of training create the critical path for this project (as indicated by the darker rows in Fig. 27.1).

Following PMO processes, Ahmad documents the project plan, milestones, and critical path using Microsoft® Project™, which is *project management software* to help organize projects. While other software exists for this purpose such as Monday.com, Jira, Asana, and ClickUp, the PMO has selected Microsoft® Project™ as its software of choice for projects led by PMs, and Microsoft® Excel™ as the software for teams led by a team member with a PM mentor.

27.4.9 Obtaining Management Support

Ahmad uses all the information he has gathered to create a *project charter* document, which includes the requirements, scope, stakeholder list, estimated budget, and project organization (including team roles and responsibilities). In addition, he finalizes the project plan after reviewing it with the project team and key stakeholders. He will use this plan to monitor the progress of the project and provide status information to Sheila and other stakeholders.

As a next step, he meets with Sheila, who approves the project charter and plan. Then, Sheila presents the project to organizational leaders, including the CNO and CTO. She emphasizes that, for the project to be successful, the clinics and project team will need support from organizational management. In addition, the scope will need to be limited to the three identified clinics to meet the first of the year deadline.

The leaders agree to the project charter and plan. They request monthly progress updates so that they can provide the necessary support. The CNO and CTO state that their concerns have been addressed and pledge their support for the project.

Task	Month					
	1	2	3	4	5	6
Workflow changes						
Training development						
EHR changes						
Security						
Training delivery						

Fig. 27.1 Timeline for key project activities

27.5 How Are Projects Managed?

With the project planning complete, Ahmad begins the *execute* and *monitor and control phases* of project management.

In the execution phase, the team members begin working on the activities within the project [7]. They will be completing tasks, creating deliverables, and doing the work to reach each milestone in the project.

In the monitor and control phase, Ahmad will monitor the project work and ensure that deadlines are being met. He will ensure the project remains within budget. If any variances occur from the project plan or the budget, he will document the issue and work with the team and Sheila to resolve the variances.

27.5.1 Managing Communication

To support the execution phase, Ahmad begins scheduling the ongoing meetings needed for the project.

- He starts with the project status meeting that will occur weekly. In this meeting, team members will provide an update on the work they have completed, the issues they have encountered, and the work they have planned for the upcoming week.
- Next, he schedules a meeting with Sheila every other week to provide progress updates and discuss issues and roadblocks that the team experiences.
- Finally, he schedules a monthly meeting with stakeholders to provide an overall status of the project and answer any questions they have.

For each meeting, Ahmad prepares an agenda that lists the items to be discussed. In addition, he documents meetings minutes during each meeting for the team to reference.

27.5.2 Managing Vendors and Contracts

As a next step in the execution phase, Ahmad reaches out to the EHR vendor. A *vendor* is a supplier that can provide a service or product for the project [7]. In this case, the EHR vendor will be providing the mental health questionnaire and standard report for the project.

Because of this relationship, Ahmad will need to manage the vendor throughout the project. *Vendor management* is an approach for selecting appropriate vendors, ensuring the right vendor contracts are in place, controlling costs and managing other vendor metrics, and mitigating risks when using vendors [8]. Because the project is using the existing EHR vendor, most of the vendor management is completed by the Clinical Informatics and IT teams.

Ahmad focuses on ensuring the appropriate contract is approved for this project. A contract is a legally binding agreement to require a supplier (in this case, the EHR vendor) to provide a product, service, or result to the buyer for payment [2]. Ahmad reviews the contract, which includes the expected budget and timeline. He obtains the appropriate leadership signatures and forwards the signed contract to the vendor.

27.5.3 Managing Issues and Action Items

Ahmad starts the monitor and control phase by setting up issue tracking and escalation for the project. An *issue* is a situation that could impact the achievement of the project goal or requirements [2]. To track these issues, Ahmad sets up a list in which he enters a description of the issue, the person who reported it, the current status of the issue, the next steps to resolve the issue, and its eventual resolution.

For example, during the second project team status meeting, Michael states that the IT Database team is planning an upgrade to the EHR. The IT Database team would like to begin testing the upgrade at the same time as the project team will be finalizing the EHR changes, which may cause conflicts. Ahmad documents this issue on the issues list, and then the team identifies the action items (next steps) to take to resolve this issue. They decide that Michael will work with the IT Database team to see if the upgrade can be rescheduled for after the EHR changes for this project are complete. This action item is documented as a next step on the issues list.

In addition, Ahmad works with Sheila to identify an escalation plan for the project. An *escalation plan* is a step-by-step process identifying who should be contacted when an issue cannot be resolved between teams and/or the issue is significant and requires immediate attention. For example, Michael reports back that the IT Database team did not agree to reschedule the EHR database upgrade. Therefore, following the escalation plan, Ahmad contacts Sheila and asks her to reach out to the IT Database team leader and the CTO to make them aware of the conflict. Sheila works with the appropriate leaders to resolve the issue. The resolution is documented in the issues list, and the status of the issue is changed to resolved.

Finally, Ahmad creates a change request log for the project. A *change request* is a formal, documented proposal for changing the project scope or a project document, deliverable, or requirement [2]. If issues cannot be resolved (even if escalated), then a change may need to be made to the existing project. For example, if the EHR database issue could not be resolved, then Ahmad may have needed to enter a change request to modify the scope or timeline of the project to adjust for this upgrade.

Throughout the project, Ahmad reviews the issues list with the project team during their regular meeting and documents updates and resolutions. As needed, he escalates issues to Sheila and other leaders.

27.5.4 Managing Change

As the project progresses, Ahmad ensures the stakeholders receive regular updates. This communication is critical for change management. *Change management* is a comprehensive, structured approach for supporting individuals, groups, and organizations in transitioning from what is currently happening to what will be happening in the future [2].

Because of this regular and transparent communication, the stakeholders ask questions and raise concerns so that they can be addressed before the changes are implemented. For example, one of the clinic managers raised a concern that two clinicians would be on leave during the planned implementation, which could cause problems with scheduling training. Clarissa works with the clinic manager to adjust the training schedule for these two clinicians.

27.5.5 Organizing and Managing Project Work

As the PM, Ahmad continues organizing and managing the work of the project as the team continues working on their tasks. The PMO has a structure for maintaining project documentation, so Ahmad ensures all the documents for the project are stored in the correct location. By organizing these documents, Ahmad ensures they are available for the project team and stakeholders, as well as future project teams who may want to refer to them.

27.6 How Do We Know When a Project Is Done?

As the project nears completion, Ahmad begins the *close phase* of project management.

First, he ensures that all the project tasks are completed including transferring maintenance of the EHR questionnaire and report to the appropriate teams. For example, Clarissa works with the Clinical Informatics team to update the testing plans for future EHR upgrades so that the questionnaire and report are verified as part of that work. In addition, Ahmad meets with Sheila and leadership from the three clinics to review the project, its deliverables, and maintenance plan. Sheila and the leaders approve this work, signifying the closure of the project.

During the final meeting for the project, the project team and stakeholders meet to reflect on the lessons they learned while working on the project. *Lessons learned* are the knowledge and skills gained during the project, which can be applied to future projects to avoid issues and improve project performance [2]. For example, the team has recommended a process for implementing the EHR mental health questionnaire and report for additional clinics. Ahmad documents these lessons in the project closeout report and stores this document following PMO policies.

At the end of the meeting, Ahmad surprises the project team with lunch and handwritten thank you notes to celebrate the work they completed.

27.7 Summary

As project manager, Ahmad provided direction to the project team as they worked to implement a mental health questionnaire within the EHR system and a standard report to view the results.

With the support of healthcare system leadership, they worked through the initiate, plan, execute, monitor and control, and close phases of the project including key activities like identifying a project goal, objectives, and scope; creating a project plan; communicating with stakeholders; and resolving issues.

Ahmad continually monitored progress and ensured the team completed the project within budget. By the end of the project, the team completed all their work, and the work was approved by Sheila (the project sponsor) and the clinic leadership. The team reflected on their work to identify lessons learned and celebrated their accomplishments.

27.8 Resources

See Table 27.2 for a list of project management resources.

Table 27.2 Project management resources

Resource	Website (link)
Information about project management careers	Project manager on Indeed (https://www.indeed.com/career/project-manager)
Professional organization for project management	Project Management Institute (PMI) (https://www.pmi.org/)
Project management software	Asana (https://asana.com/uses/project-management) ClickUp (https://clickup.com/) Jira (https://www.atlassian.com/software/jira) Microsoft® Project™ (https://www.microsoft.com/en-us/microsoft-365/project/project-management-software) Monday.com (https://monday.com/)

Knowledge Check Questions

1. *Define project, project management, project manager, and project portfolio.*
2. *List the phases of project management.*
3. *Describe the activities involved in each phase of project management.*
4. *Explain how budget, scope, and resources impact the success of a project.*
5. *Compare and contrast project management, change management, and vendor management. How are they the same and how are they different?*

Answers

1. A project is a temporary set of activities that have a clear start, a clear end, and produces an outcome.
   Project management is a form of management that provides direction for a group of people who are working to achieve a project goal.
   A project manager leads the team that is tasked with achieving a project outcome.
   A project portfolio is a listing of projects that have been requested within an organization to support achievement of the organization's mission, vision, and strategies.
2. The phases of project management are as follows:
   - Initiating
   - Planning
   - Executing
   - Monitoring and controlling
   - Closing
3.

Phase	Activities
Initiating	Define the project or a new phase of an existing project Create project request and submit for approval Receive authorization to start the project (or phase)
Planning	Identify project goals and objectives Define project scope Identify project requirements Define project team roles and responsibilities Identify stakeholders Estimate the project budget Identify project deliverables Create the project management plan Obtain management support
Executing	Complete tasks in the project plan Create deliverables Complete milestones identified in the project plan
Monitoring and controlling	Monitor the project work and ensure deadlines are met Review the project budget and address variances Manage communication, vendors and contracts, and issues and action items Organize and manage project documentation
Closing	Transfer maintenance of project work to operational teams Reflect on and document lessons learn Celebrate

4. The scope of the project identifies the work that must be performed to complete project requirements. To complete this work, adequate resources are needed such as personnel, budget, and time. For example, if the project scope requires updating a database, then the project team will need someone with the appropriate skills and knowledge to do these updates. If the project scope requires the purchase of new equipment, then the budget must include money for this purchase. If the project scope requires the creation of three new screens within an EHR, time must be allotted in the project plan to ensure there is sufficient time to complete these tasks (assuming personnel have the skills and knowledge to complete this work, and the budget includes any money needed to support this work). Finally, the team must only complete work that is within this project scope, as this work is what drives the resources and budget needed—completing work outside of scope can negatively impact resources and budget.

5. Project management is a form of management that provides direction to a group of people who are working to achieve a goal.
   Change management is a comprehensive, structured approach for supporting individuals, groups, and organizations in transitioning from what is currently happening to what will be happening in the future.
   Vendor management is an approach for selecting appropriate vendors; ensuring the right vendor contracts are in place; controlling costs and managing other vendor metrics; and mitigating risks when using vendors.
   For each of these areas, specific tasks and items are monitored and controlled to contribute to the success of a project. Project management monitors and controls the project progress. Change management monitors and controls the changes that are planned as well as associated communication. Vendor management controls the vendor selection and approval process and monitors the vendors to ensure they are meeting the intended goals.
   These areas are different in several ways. First, each monitors and controls something different. Second, project management occurs within the context of a project, while change management and vendor management can occur within a project and as ongoing efforts within an organization. Third, each area is typically led by individuals with different skill sets. Project management is typically handled by someone trained in project management. Change management can be handled by a project manager or another leader trained in change management. Vendor management may involve legal personnel to review contracts.

Glossary of Terms

Term	Definition
Budget	An estimate of the expenses and costs involved with completing the tasks and activities within a project.
Change management	A comprehensive, structured approach for supporting individuals, groups, and organizations in transitioning from what is currently happening to what will be happening in the future.
Deliverable	A task, activity, document, etc., that needs to be completed for the goal and requirements of the project to be met.
Exclusion	Work that is not included within the scope pf a project.
Milestone	A significant point or even in the project, typically when a significant task or deliverable is complete.
Project	A project is a temporary set of activities that have a clear start, a clear end, and produce an outcome.
Project management	A form of management that provides direction for a group of people who are working to achieve a goal. Project management focuses on the application of knowledge, skills, tools, and techniques to activities that support achievement of a project goal.
Project management office (PMO)	A management structure to support projects within an organization. Within this structure, standard policies and processes exist for capturing project requests within the organization; prioritizing them based on organizational strategic imperatives; and assigning project managers to assist with the prioritized projects.

Term	Definition
Project manager (PM)	A project manager leads the team tasked with achieving the project outcome. They are responsible for a variety of tasks, including allocating work; defining project roles; tracking tasks and responsibilities; addressing and escalating issues; and communicating project status.
Project portfolio	A listing of projects that have been requested within an organization to support achievement of the organization's mission, vision, and strategies. An organization may have a single project portfolio, multiple portfolios, or a larger portfolio that contains "sub" portfolios.
Requirement	A characteristic, function, or capability that meets a business need and should be available at the end of the project.
Resources	Individuals or items needed to complete a project. Examples of resources include people, money, supplies, or facilities.
Scope	Work that must be performed to complete a project that meets the requirements.
SMART objective	A project objective that is specific, measurable, achievable, relevant, and time-bound.
Stakeholders	An individual, group, or organization who may be affected by the project and its activities.
Vendor management	An approach for selecting appropriate vendors; ensuring the right vendor contracts are in place; controlling costs and managing other vendor metrics; and mitigating risks when using vendors.
Workflow	A set of steps or activities that need to be completed to finish a task and/or achieve a goal.

References

1. Hallows J. Information systems project management: how to deliver function and value in information technology projects. American Management Association (AMA); 1998.
2. Project Management Institute (PMI). A guide to the project management body of knowledge (PMBOK) guide. 7th ed. Project Management Institute (PMI); 2021.
3. Balgrosky JA. Understanding health information systems for the health professions. Jones & Bartlett Learning; 2020.
4. Office of Disease Prevention and Health Promotion. Social determinants of health. Healthy People 2030. https://health.gov/healthypeople/priority-areas/social-determinants-health. Accessed 23 May 2023.
5. Hashemi-Pour C. Workflow. November 2023. https://www.techtarget.com/searchcio/definition/workflow.
6. Eby K. 28 SMART goals for SMART project managers: a complete guide with examples. 2023. https://www.smartsheet.com/content/project-management-smart-goals.
7. Coplan S, Masuda. Project management for healthcare information technology. The McGraw-Hill Companies, Inc.; 2011.
8. Gartner. Vendor Management. https://www.gartner.com/en/information-technology/glossary/vendor-management.

Governance Considerations in Health Informatics

28

Sue S. Feldman

Foundational Domains

This chapter addresses the following AMIA Foundational Domains: F7—Social, Behavioral, and Information Science and Technology Applied to Health, F8—Professionalism, F9—Interprofessional Collaborative Practice.

Learning Objectives

After reading this chapter, you should be able to

1. Describe governance archetypes.
2. Explain the value of visualizing governance on one page.
3. Articulate the fundamentals of governance.

Definitions

- Governance—The system of rules, practices, and processes by which an organization is directed and controlled.
- Compliance—The act of adhering to laws, regulations, standards, and ethical practices that apply to the organization.
- Risk—The possibility of events or actions that may negatively impact an organization's ability to achieve its objectives, safeguard its assets, or maintain compliance with legal, ethical, or regulatory standards.
- Accountability—The obligation of individuals or organizations to account for their actions and decisions and accept responsibility, and disclose results in a transparent manner.
- Ethics—The principles and values that guide behavior and decision-making within an organization. Ethical governance ensures that actions are not only legally compliant but also align with moral and societal standards.
- Strategy—The long-term plan an organization follows to achieve its goals and objectives. Governance includes establishing and monitoring strategy to ensure alignment with stakeholder interests and organizational mission.

28.1 Introduction

Governance is basically the rules of the road for effective practices within an organization. It is the decision rights and accountability framework for encouraging desirable behaviors [1]. Information technology (IT) governance, in general, and health IT governance, more specifically, should always be aligned with broader organizational goals and values. Because of these linkages to the broader organizational goals, IT governance cannot be planned, executed, or measured in isolation, but rather as a shared process.

S. S. Feldman (✉)
Graduate Programs in Health Informatics,
University of Alabama at Birmingham,
Birmingham, AL, USA
e-mail: sfeldman@uab.edu

C. Eldredge et al. (eds.), *Introductory Textbook in Health Informatics*, Health Informatics,
https://doi.org/10.1007/978-3-032-16657-9_28

IT governance as a shared process includes understanding

- Costs
- Asset utilization
- Growth
- Business agility

All too often, IT governance is seen as an IT issue. When we take the time to understand the shared processes that exist just under the surface of IT governance, we see that it is really an initiative that cuts across the entire organization and impacts more than just processes, but also decision-making. For example, the cost of governance is not just about the tools and technologies, but also about the human resources needed across the organization, decision-making time (which will likely be slower), and risk assessment. Likewise, asset utilization is not just about *how* the tools and technologies are used, but also consider accountability and transparency of those tools and technologies and the decisions they enable. Some may think that having governance in place may restrict growth in that there are constraints to innovation. However, if governance is enacted properly, there is tighter alignment with the overall strategic plan of the organization, allowing for faster growth. Once people recognize IT as a strategic role in driving business success, organizations will no longer view IT, and the associated governance, as just a support function. Instead, IT will be viewed as a critical enabler of innovation, efficiency, and competitive advantage. Lastly, IT governance must be enacted in an environment of change to foster business agility. Shared decision-making in IT governance allows businesses to harness the perspectives of multiple stakeholders, aligning IT initiatives with broader organizational goals. Consider the use of artificial intelligence (AI) in organizations. Although AI has been around and used in healthcare for decades, the recent elevation of it to a mainstream application has many organizations integrating AI tools and processes into their core strategies. IT governance frameworks are being adapted to focus not only on compliance, but also on innovation and strategic growth to facilitate rapid adoption of AI.

Governance is essential. However, governance is not a "one and done" initiative. In fact, when organizations or initiatives are newly formed, oftentimes, the governance is very loose [2]. This is purposeful and stimulates innovation. However, as the initiative or the organization matures, the governance needs to tighten so that there are appropriate guardrails in place. However, one must be cautious not to tighten governance so much that innovation is impeded. As such, governance quality is a continuous process, and leaders must never become complacent with the level of performance afforded by governance. Leaders must be willing to shift governance policies and procedures as needed to support the strategic direction of an agile organization. Staying steadfast on policies and procedures that are outdated, risk making the organization obsolete—*because of* governance. In general, governance structures can ultimately determine the degree of success or failure of an organization. But on the way to that success or failure are a lot of contributing activities—each that carry risk. Regardless of whether there is a loosely structured or tightly structured governance, there must be a coherent set of principles with a shared understanding of those principles by those doing the governing.

Simply adopting technical policies and procedures is not enough—the system must be aligned and there must be system-level accountability. This responsibility extends to all levels moving from simple task to a systems-thinking level [3]. Systems-thinking is a holistic approach to governance that focuses on the way that a system's individual parts interrelate and how systems work over time and within the context of larger systems [4]. While this has been thought of in terms of more global systems, it can easily be applied to the healthcare domain [5–7]. While the temptation might be to think that taking a systems-thinking approach, that is, considering the entire system, will make governance unnecessarily complicated, that is not always the case.

28.2 Simplifying Governance

Governance can and should be uncomplicated and not complex. As such, there are methods to simplify governance. However, before doing so, it is essential to understand IT governance decision domains and archetypes.

28.2.1 Decision Domains

Decision domains refer to the five governance areas in which decisions are made. When participating in decisions, one must consider the questions contained in these domains. These domains are described in Table 28.1 with the associated example questions for consideration.

28.2.2 Governance Archetypes

Governance archetypes [1] have to do with the decision-making types—basically, the flow of decisions. There are six governance archetypes. The governance archetypes, with a description and example of each, are provided in Table 28.2.

28.2.3 Tools to Simplify Governance

As mentioned, governance does not need to be unnecessarily complicated or complex. In fact, it can be distilled to structure, process, and outcomes where structure is who has input and who makes the decision, process is ensuring that decisions align to the business strategies and organizational objectives, and outcomes give attention to the key performance indicators [1, 8]. Below are some tools that can help break apart governance in a simple manner such that it is easier to understand relative to the business strategies, organizational objectives, and decision-making influence.

Table 28.1 Decision domains

Decision domain	Description	Example questions to consider
IT principles	Understanding the role and uses of the IT	What is the role of this IT product to support the strategic mission of the organization? How will the product be used across business lines?
IT infrastructure	Understanding the strategic direction for coordinated or shared service	How does the infrastructure support the strategic mission across the organization? What needs and uses across all business services are being considered in the infrastructure?
IT architecture	Policies, procedures, principles, and rules setting the direction of accepted uses and purchases of IT	How does the architecture support privacy and security? What are the down-stream considerations of this purchase relative to our existing needs and infrastructure?
Business application needs	Ensuring that the business needs underpin IT requirements, expenditures, and uses	How does the IT support the business needs of the organization? How does the IT align with the strategic direction of the organization?
IT prioritization and investment	Planning for IT costs in terms of the total cost of operation	What is the value of the IT investment? How does the investment align with the strategic direction of the organization?

Adapted from Ref. [1]

28.2.3.1 Balanced Scorecards

Balanced scorecards (BSCs) were first introduced in the late 1980s and early 1990s as a mechanism to translate strategy into results and provide visualizations as to the degree of performance of a unit, business line, etc. [9]. By the mid-1990s, the use of BSCs was mainstream, but

Table 28.2 Governance archetypes

Archetype	Description	Decision-making examples by role
Leadership monarchy	A group of individual senior manager	C-suite level individual or group decisions (may or may not include IT, but not exclusively IT leadership)
IT monarch	Groups of or individual IT senior managers	C-suite level (inclusive of IT) individual or group decisions
Feudal	Unit leaders, key process owners, or their delegates	Director and process owner together
Federal	Shared by senior management and business unit leaders	C-suite, director, and process owners
Duopoly	Senior management and one other group	C-suite and director, for example
Anarchy	Every unit or even users act independently	One group or one person making a decision unilaterally

Adapted from Ref. [1]

primarily in business and not in IT. It was not until a decade later that the use of BSCs was being used in IT as a mechanism to align, support, and enable IT and business governance and performance [10]. Since this time, there are many variations of BSCs in use, all of which contain similar guiding principles. These guiding principles depend on the orientation of the organization and the internal forces that drive those relationships. Regardless, the BSC should consider the following three perspectives [9–11]:

- Perspective 1: a fusion of business and IT in a manner to support IT governance processes, policies, and procedures
- Perspective 2: a measurement of business and IT strategies such that the IT supports the organization's key performance indicators
- Perspective 3: attention to user orientation, operational excellence, business contribution, and future roadmap/initiatives

28.2.3.2 Governance on One Page

The value of seeing something all on one page lies in providing clarity, coherence, and efficiency for improved comprehension, reliability, and decision-making. This can be done in a list form, charts, tables, or other visualizations [12–14]. The clarity, coherence, and efficiency can be further unpacked as such:

- Holistic view for better understanding—seeing all content at once allows grasping the entire context and the relationships between those contexts without needing to scroll or flip through pages
- Quick reference and comparisons—time savings as the need to navigate multiple sections is eliminated
- Cognitive ease—especially with complex information or information from multiple sources, seeing everything in one place reduces cognitive load because the need to hold information in one's memory is eliminated
- Better decision-making—seeing everything at once supports more informed and immediate decision-making
- Visual flow—it aids in maintaining a natural flow of reading or analyzing data without interruptions, which can make understanding easier and more intuitive

Table 28.3 can be used to plot governance on one page. This table is an essential component of every governance plan and is populated with roles and not people [1].

28.2.3.3 Barriers and Best Practices

Even the best strategic planning and organizational strategies can be met with barriers [15]. Learning from best practices can help increase awareness and identification of those barriers. Governance requires a culture of psychological safety to talk about failures and risks. For example, sometimes those responsible for systematic measurement against key performance indicators

Table 28.3 Governance on one page

	IT principles		IT infrastructure		IT architecture		Business applications		IT prioritization and investment	
	Input	Decision	Input	Decision	Input	Decision	Input	Decision	Input	Decision
Business monarchy										
IT monarchy										
Feudal										
Federal										
Duopoly										
Anarchy										

Used with permission from Ref. [1]

may run up against data that are not adequate or accurate enough to produce what is being asked of them. Instead of seeing this as a failure, a culture of opportunity creates an environment where an example like this is turned into learning and progress. Regardless, governance cannot happen in a culture where there is no accountability [15].

Learning from best practices can help mitigate risk of failure [16]. Some best practices include [15, 16].

- Leadership must create a culture of psychological safety.
- A systems-thinking approach must prevail.
- Ensure infrastructure for data use supports business goals and strategic direction.
- Integrating data collection and IT.
- Use data to drive quality and value.
- Creating an environment for creating and collecting useful and usable data.
- Outcomes tracking against key performance indicators from the beginning.

28.3 Ethical and Legal Considerations

Ethical and legal considerations are also a part of every governance plan. Quite simply, this includes privacy and security regulations, professional codes of conduct, and ethical implications of technology use in healthcare.

28.3.1 Privacy and Security

The largest and most well-known privacy and security governance controls (in the United States) are around the Health Insurance Portability and Accountability Act (HIPAA), which has less to do with insurance and more to do with information. The HIPAA privacy rule offers protections of personally identifiable information (PII) and protected health information (PHI). PII is any information that can be used to identify a person, such as name, address, Social Security number, and email address. It limits the use and disclosure of PII without consent. PHI is a subset of PII and is specific to health-related information that can be used to identify a person. In other words, PHI is the medical definition of PII and takes PII a step further. Such examples include PII elements plus biometrics, medical record numbers, and device attributes. There are long lists of both PII and PHI examples that can be found online.

The Confidentiality of Substance Use Disorder Patient Records, commonly referred to as 42CFR part 2, is another extremely important governance control that provides further privacy protection of sensitive data on top of PII and PHI protections. Examples of sensitive data include substance use disorder treatment, certain diagnoses, and certain prescriptions.

Governance rules provide protections over patient data and information such that there are privacy protections around disclosure and use of data and security protections around encryption. Typically, patients will sign a release of information (ROI) that will allow data associated with payment, treatment, and operations to flow from one system to another. Sensitive data or data used for something other than payment, treatment, and operations (e.g., for Social Security Disability Determination) can still be transmitted, but instead of an ROI, patients sign an authorization. The difference between an ROI and an authorization is that an ROI is a blanket release and an authorization is a specific release for only certain records, to only a certain organization, and for only a certain period of time.

The Health Information Technology for Economic and Clinical Health Act (HITECH) expanded the scope of HIPAA's privacy and security protections in the context of electronic health records (EHRs). This expansion provided governance for breach notifications and the enforcement of penalties (enforcement is governed by the US Office of Civil Rights) around those breaches.

Other governance controls around privacy and security include the 21st Century Cures Act that promotes patient access to their data and requires healthcare providers to support interoperability standards to facilitate the flow of patient data between systems.

There are several key governance concepts related to privacy and security that should appear in every governance plan. These concepts should also include policies and procedures for enacting and enforcing appropriate controls. They are

- Data minimization—ensuring that only necessary data are collected and processed
- Access control—limiting access to PHI to authorized personnel only
- Encryption—using encryption to secure health data both in transit and at rest
- Audit trails—implementing logging and monitoring to track access to health information
- Data breach response—establishing a clear procedure for responding to security incidents, including timely breach notification

Governance refers to the processes, systems, and structures through which decisions are made, authority is exercised, and actions are taken to manage and regulate a group of people or an organization. It encompasses various aspects of leadership, management, and administration aimed at achieving goals, ensuring accountability, and promoting the well-being of the entity being governed. Privacy and security mandates administrative, physical, and technical safeguards to ensure the confidentiality, integrity, and availability of PHI.

28.4 Chapter Summary

This chapter discusses the fundamentals of a simplified governance. It provides tools for strategic planning and measuring and visualizing governance. It laid out the governance archetypes and how to appropriately represent governance on one page to increase understanding and relatability. Lastly, this chapter discussed the ethical and legal considerations around governance. The information provided in this chapter are also the components of a governance plan, and therefore, could provide a foundation actionable governance practices.

Knowledge Check Questions

1. A federal archetype:
   (a) Has the unit leader solely responsible
   (b) Is where there is shared responsibility between senior management and unit leaders
   (c) Includes the director and process owner together
   (d) Includes the C-suite, director, and process owners together
2. The value of visualizing governance on one page is to provide a
   (a) Holistic view for better understanding of relationships
   (b) Fusion of business and IT

    (c) Measure of key performance indicators relative to the governance structure
    (d) Roadmap for future governance-related initiatives
3. In order for governance to occur in an organization, the organization must have
    (a) A culture of psychological safety
    (b) Accountability
    (c) Someone in leadership who is willing to let accountability slide, as long as things are running smoothly
    (d) Clean separations between data collection and IT to allow for separate and independent governance over each

Answers

1. (b) and (d)
2. (a)
3. (a) and (b)

References

1. Weill P, Ross JW. IT governance on one page. Available at SSRN 664612. 2004.
2. Feldman SS, Horan TA, Drew D. Understanding the value proposition of health information exchange: the case of uncompensated care cost recovery. Health Syst. 2012.
3. Nelson EC, Batalden PB, Huber TP, Mohr JJ, Godfrey MM, Headrick LA, et al. Microsystems in health care: Part 1. Learning from high-performing front-line clinical units. Joint Comm J Qual Improv. 2002;28(9):472–93.
4. Wikipedia. Systems Thinking 2024 [cited 2024 October 15]. Available from: https://en.wikipedia.org/wiki/Systems_thinking.
5. Ison R, Straw E. The hidden power of systems thinking: governance in a climate emergency. Routledge; 2020.
6. Jaradat RM, Keating CB, Elakramine F, El Amrani S, Oumaima L. Systems thinking for complex system governance. In: Complex system governance: theory and practice. Springer; 2022. p. 411–53.
7. Voulvoulis N, Giakoumis T, Hunt C, Kioupi V, Petrou N, Souliotis I, et al. Systems thinking as a paradigm shift for sustainability transformation. Glob Environ Change. 2022;75:102544.
8. Donabedian A. The quality of care. How can it be assessed? JAMA. 1988:260.
9. Kaplan RS. The balanced scorecard as a strategic management system. Harv Bus Rev. 1992;1992:61–6.
10. Van Grembergen W, Saull R. Information technology governance through the balanced scorecard. In: Information technology evaluation methods and management. IGI Global; 2001. p. 199–211.
11. Van Grembergen W, De Haes S. Measuring and improving IT governance through the balanced scorecard. Inf Syst Control J. 2005;2(1):35–42.
12. Torcasio S, Sweller J. The use of illustrations when learning to read: a cognitive load theory approach. Appl Cognit Psychol. 2010;24(5):659–72.
13. Rayner K. The 35th Sir Frederick Bartlett Lecture: eye movements and attention in reading, scene perception, and visual search. Q J Exp Psychol. 2009;62(8):1457–506.
14. Lurie NH, Mason CH. Visual representation: implications for decision making. J Market. 2007;71(1):160–77.
15. Storey J, Buchanan D. Healthcare governance and organizational barriers to learning from mistakes. J Health Organ Manag. 2008;22(6):642–51.
16. Nelson EC, Batalden PB, Homa K, Godfrey MM, Campbell C, Headrick LA, et al. Microsystems in health care: Part 2. Creating a rich information environment. Joint Comm J Qual Saf. 2003;29(1):5–15.

29 Data Management

Katie A. McCarthy

Foundational Domains

This chapter addresses the following AMIA Foundational Domains: F2—Information Science and Technology, F4—Health Information Science and Technology.

Learning Objectives

After reading this chapter, you should be able to

1. Define data, big data, and data management.
2. Identify and describe the key areas within data management.
3. Describe the role of data governance in data management.
4. Explain and provide examples of each stage within the data lifecycle.

29.1 Introduction

To illustrate the concepts within this chapter, we will use a hypothetical case study that focuses on Michael, who is a database administrator who works for a large healthcare system that includes 10 hospitals and several hundred clinics. One of the hospitals is an academic medical center aligned with the region's largest research university.

K. A. McCarthy (✉)
Sullivan School of Business, Engineering, and Technology, Carroll University, Waukesha, WI, USA
e-mail: kamccart@carrollu.edu

In his role, he works with clinicians, researchers, administrators, and leaders to understand their data needs and maintain the organization's databases so that individuals have the information they need to care for patients, lead the organization, and do cutting-edge research. For example, one of his colleagues, Sarah, recently reached out about a project she's working on to capture social determinants of health within the organization's electronic health record (EHR). They have a meeting coming up to discuss the specifics and how Michael may be able to help with this effort.

In addition to his full-time position, Michael teaches an undergraduate course in data management one night a week. He loves sharing "real-world" examples, and he's wondering if Sarah's project could be an interesting example for class.

29.2 What Is Data?

On the first night of class, Michael starts by defining "data." *Data* are facts or observations about the world [1, 2]. For example, a website might report that today's high temperature was 96.7 °F for Houston, TX. For organizations, though, the term "data" is often used more generally to include information such as names and addresses, treatment plans for patients, and national identification numbers for providers and insurers [1]. Therefore, Michael states that the class will use this broader definition of data.

C. Eldredge et al. (eds.), *Introductory Textbook in Health Informatics*, Health Informatics,
https://doi.org/10.1007/978-3-032-16657-9_29

In addition, data is an *asset* for an organization. Assets are economic resources that hold or produce value for an organization and can be owned or controlled by that organization [1]. Because data is an asset and has significant value to the organization, it requires management just like any other asset—which is why data management is important.

29.2.1 What Is Big Data?

Next, a student raises their hand and asks, "Is data the same thing as big data?" Micheal answers that, yes—big data is a form of data. In general, big data has several characteristics that make it unique. Initially, three characteristics were identified, which are known as the "three V's of big data."

- *Volume*, which means the amount of data being captured, stored, and managed. For example, big data may be greater than 100 terabytes or in the range of petabytes or exabytes [1, 3].
- *Velocity*, which means how quickly the data is being generated, accumulated, and stored. For example, the number of Google searches per day has increased from 32.8 million in 2000, to 5.6 billion in 2018; therefore, data related to these searches is accumulating more and more quickly as time progresses [1, 3].
- *Variety*, which is the variety of ways that these data are structured. One example is structured data, which is data that follows a formal, defined structure and can be stored in database tables. Traditionally, this type of data is what we think of when we think about data within databases. Semi-structured data may have some format, but that format is not as "strict" as structured data. For example, documents that are formatted using XML may use "tags" to identify some of the data, but the document is not as structured as a database table. Finally, unstructured data does not have any formal, defined structure. Text files, emails, images, videos, etc., could be examples of this type of data. Big data often consists of structured, semi-structured, and unstructured data that all must be stored and accessed [3].

Over time, the list of V's has expanded and may continue to grow. For example, veracity is often included in the V's as it is the trustworthiness of data, including its quality, integrity, credibility, and accuracy.

From a data management perspective, big data is still data that needs to be managed as an asset for an organization. The storage and maintenance of these data may be different, though, because of its characteristics.

29.2.2 Challenges

When working with data, several challenges are common.

First, data requires explanation, meaning someone must interpret the data to identify what it means, how it should be used, and how to evaluate its quality [4]. For example, 96.0 could be a patient's temperature, a student's grade on an exam, or someone's age, so more information is needed to know exactly how to interpret the data.

Second, data is shared and used by different people for a variety of purposes—so who owns the data and makes decisions about how the data should be handled? [4] For instance, a patient shares that they are working with a nutritionist to lose weight. The doctor documents this information in the patient's record within the EHR. In addition, the insurance company is paying the nutritionist and the doctor on behalf of the patient. Who "owns" the information about the nutrition plan the patient is using? The patient who is following the plan? The nutritionist who created the plan? The insurance company that is paying the nutritionist?

Finally, many people may be involved in the creation, storage, and modification of data, so how do we know when the data are incorrect? And how do we determine who should be allowed to modify or correct the data? [4] For example, a doctor prescribes a heart medication for their patient. During the patient's next visit, they state that they cannot afford the medication and ask the doctor for a different prescription. The doctor documents in their EHR progress note that the patient refuses to take their heart medication. The patient sees this information in their after-visit summary and wants the note changed because they are not refusing the medication—they cannot afford it. Is the note correct? If not, who should be allowed to change the note?

29.3 What Is Data Management?

Challenges like these happen every day within organizations. Therefore, after spending the first week of the course discussing data, big data, and its challenges, Michael decides to spend the second week defining and describing data management, which helps address these challenges.

Data management includes the plans, policies, programs, and practices needed to deliver, control, protect, and enhance the value of data assets within organizations [1]. Data management is all the activities that occur to manage the data and information that are valuable to an organization. For example, data management could include procedures for how data are collected, or policies related to who will be allowed to access sensitive data.

29.3.1 Key Areas Within Data Management

Next, to better understand the scope of data management, Michael explains the key areas that exist within the field (shown in Table 29.1) [1].

29.3.2 Role of Data Governance in Data Management

Within these areas, data governance has a unique role, as it guides all other areas of data management and ensures that data is managed according to established policies and best practices and focuses on how decisions are made about data [1].

Table 29.1 Areas within data management

Area	Description
Data governance	Provides direction and oversight by establishing policies, processes, and procedures to make decisions related to the data assets within an organization
Data architecture	Based on organizational strategies, identifies the data needed and designs a plan for managing these data assets
Data modeling and design	Creates a formal representation (known as a "data model") of the data within an organization
Data storage and operations	Designs, implements, and supports the storage of data within an organization
Data security	Maintains the privacy and confidentiality of data throughout its lifecycle
Data integration and interoperability	Moves data between different systems and storage locations (such as moving data between two databases)
Document and content management	Plans, implements, and controls activities related to unstructured data within an organization, especially documents required for legal and regulatory compliance
Reference and master data	Maintains the accuracy, timeliness, and relevancy of the most critical, business essential information within an organization
Data warehousing and business intelligence	Enables analysis and reporting of data to support decision making within an organization
Metadata	Creates and maintains the definitions, models, data flows, and other information needed to understand the data within an organization
Data quality	Measures, assesses, and improves the fitness (or quality) of data used within an organization

Therefore, data governance creates an inherent "separation of duties" between those who enforce these policies and best practices (individuals working within data governance) and those complying with these policies and best practices (individuals working within other data management areas). For more information about the role of data governance and its importance, refer to the data governance chapter in this textbook.

Table 29.2 Roles within data management

Role	Responsibilities	Training and education
Data architect	Creates an organization's data strategy, which is the plan or "blueprint" to organize, retrieve, interpret, store, maintain, and share data to meet the requirements of the organization [5, 6] Usually leads the data management team [5]	Significant technical expertise in data architecture, modeling, integration, design, management, security, and governance [5]
Data engineer	Builds the technological foundation to implement the organization's data strategy [7] Ensures that data are received, transformed, and stored so that they are accessible to individuals such as data scientists, data analysts, informaticists, and other data users [7] Builds and optimizes databases, data tools, and data pipelines [7]	Works with database systems (such as SQL and NoSQL) [5] Experience migrating, integrating, processing, and cleaning data; using programming languages (such as Python) [5] Works with cloud computing and distributed systems [5]
Database administrator (DBA)	Responsible for managing and ensuring reliable access to an organization's databases [8, 9] Ensures data is safe and accessible by configuring database systems and tracking their performance Resolves problems and implements backup and recovery plans [10]	Strong understanding of data management systems, data structures, and programming languages

For example, Michael maintains a database that contains accounting data for the healthcare system. According to data governance within the organization, this data is "owned" by the chief financial officer (CFO). Therefore, when Michael wants to make changes to this database, data governance requires him to contact the CFO to obtain approval. And data governance provides a process for documenting this approval before Michael makes the changes.

Michael is responsible for complying with the data governance policies and best practices required by the healthcare system. Individuals within the data governance team work with Michael to ensure he is following the correct data governance policies, processes, and procedures while working with the organization's data.

29.3.3 Common Roles Within Data Management

During the next class, Michael describes common roles within data management, including data architects, data engineers, and database administrators. More information about these roles is shown in Table 29.2.

29.4 What Is the Data Lifecycle?

As the course continues, Michael meets with Sarah to learn more about the social determinants of health project to determine if it could be a good "real-world" example to use in class. In this project, the team will be building a mental health questionnaire within the EHR to capture anxiety levels of patients from 10 to 16 years of age. In addition, the EHR vendor will be creating a standard report that can be used to obtain the results from these questionnaires.

Although Sarah has worked with Michael before, she asks about the support he and his team can provide during the project. Michael explains that his team works with data throughout its lifecycle. The *data lifecycle* describes how data are created and used and, when the data are no longer needed, how they are destroyed securely and appropriately [11].

Based on his discussion with Sarah, Michael agrees to be part of the social determinants project team to gather more information about the data and its lifecycle, including the data to be captured and its sources, who needs access to the data, where the data should be stored, the quality of the data, and how the data need to be maintained.

29.4.1 What Data Do We Have?

Ahmad, the project manager for the social determinants of health project, schedules a meeting for the project team to discuss the data that will be captured as part of the project.

Ahmad explains that the current project is an extension of a pilot project that was performed in one of the healthcare system's primary care clinics. (To learn more about this pilot project, refer to the project management chapter in this textbook.) In this clinic, clinicians and staff identified a significant increase in anxiety levels for patients between 10 and 16 years of age. After collecting and analyzing data, they identified three factors correlated with this increase: use of social media, nutrition, and time spent outdoors. With two local middle schools, they implemented a community garden, cooking classes, and a social media challenge based on these factors. These interventions were successful, and the healthcare system would like to expand these interventions to additional clinics and schools.

During this pilot project, the team gathered data from paper mental health questionnaires and stored this information within a database. Michael realizes that he and Ericka set up this database together, so he has a good understanding of the data it contains. Clarissa, a senior informaticist on the current project team, explains that this same data will be captured for the current project. Instead of using paper forms, the questionnaires will be built within the EHR system so that the data can be captured electronically.

Next, Michael asks how these data will be used. Ahmad explains that the EHR vendor will create a standard report, which leaders and clinicians can use to review and analyze results. From this analysis, clinics can replicate the interventions of the pilot primary care clinic and partner schools or develop new interventions based on their analysis.

Based on this information, Michael knows this project would be a great example within his course. The project team agrees, and they receive appropriate approvals from leadership to share the project information with Michael's class. The project team also agrees to participate in some of Michael's classes so that they can work directly with the students. During the next class, Michael and the team explain the project to the students, including the purpose of the project, the role of each team member, and the data to be captured.

29.4.2 What Data Do We Need?

Next, Michael and the project team share a copy of the paper mental health questionnaire with the students. After reviewing this information, a student asks, "Shouldn't we also capture data such as whether a patient has experienced abuse or bullying? This information is not included within the current questionnaire but could affect someone's mental health."

The team explains that several factors need to be considered when answering this question.

First, does the project scope include adding this information? Right now, the scope is to implement the existing questions on the mental health questionnaire. The answers to these questions are the "needed" data for this project. Any other information is outside of the project scope and may be considered "desired" data. Unless additional resources (time, people, money, etc.) and approvals are obtained, the project team cannot add "desired" data to the scope of the project.

Next, is this information especially sensitive such as information that may require intervention by law enforcement or other agencies? If so, does the project team have the appropriate resources and knowledge to work with this data appropriately? In this example, suspected abuse of minors does need to be reported, and the current team does not include experts in this process. Therefore, unless a change to the project scope is approved and experts are added to the team, this data should not be added.

Finally, does this additional data support the purpose of the project? In this case, information about potential abuse and bullying is correlated within mental health and, therefore, could be an important addition to the questionnaire. Because clinicians and researchers are needed to identify the appropriate questions to obtain this information, Chen and Malia agree to take this suggestion to clinician leadership for consideration in a future project.

29.4.3 What Is Metadata?

The next step in identifying the data that will be captured and used is documenting "data about the data," also known as metadata. This information is captured and documented so that everyone in the project team (and, eventually, the organization) understands what the data does (and does not) represent and how it should (and should not) be used [4].

For example, the mental health questionnaires capture the level of anxiety using a scale of 1–5 (with 1 being low anxiety and 5 being high anxiety). In addition, Clarissa states that the pilot team used answers to several nutrition-related questions to calculate an "overall quality of nutrition" value. This information is metadata about the needed data for the project.

One of the students asks, "How do you keep track of the metadata?" Michael explains that a data dictionary is a document that lists the data that needs to be captured and its metadata. The metadata can include definitions of terms, business rules, appropriate values, the source of the data, and any other information that may be helpful for correctly interpreting and using the data. Michael, the project team, and students begin documenting the data and its metadata within a data dictionary (a portion of which is shown in Table 29.3).

Table 29.3 Example data dictionary

Data	Definition	Data source	Metadata
Anxiety	Level of anxiety reported by patient (or guardian)	EHR mental health questionnaire (question 3)	Uses a 1–5 scale (1 being low anxiety, 5 being high anxiety) Level is self-reported and not based on an objective measure
Nutrition	Identifies an overall quality of nutrition reported by the patient (or their guardian)	EHR mental health questionnaire (questions 4, 5, and 6)	Calculation based on answers to questions 4, 5, and 6: (Answer 4 × Answer 6)/Answer 5 Higher values indicate better quality of nutrition Calculation developed by clinicians in pilot clinic (Chen and Malia) with assistance from Ivan, Diane, and Sarah

29.4.4 Who Needs Access to the Data?

During the next class, Michael explains the importance of protecting this data within the EHR. The data security area of data management focuses on the security policies and procedures that ensure data and information assets are protected in alignment with laws and regulations; contractual agreements; and business requirements and expectations [1].

As a first step within data security, the project team needs to work with organizational leadership to identify who "owns" the mental health questionnaire data. This data owner is responsible for ensuring appropriate individuals have authorization (approval) to access this data; their identify can be verified (authentication); and a record is maintained indicating who accessed, modified, or deleted information (auditing) [1]. (For more information about data security, refer to the health information security chapter in this textbook.)

Currently, the paper mental health questionnaires are collected by clinics and then sent to the Health Information Management (HIM) department for scanning into the EHR (as an image) and then storing the paper copy. Organizational leadership determines that the HIM department will own the paper questionnaires and the EHR data, as they are a centralized department that can work with clinicians, staff, and leaders throughout the health system. As data owners, the HIM department will work with organizational leadership to determine who needs access to this information and ensure appropriate security controls are in place.

29.4.5 How Will the Data Be Stored?

Michael explains that the next step in the data lifecycle is determining how the data will be stored and maintained. For this project, the answers from the mental health questionnaire will be stored in the EHR system and its associated database. Michael explains, though, that this is only the first step in making this decision.

Within the healthcare system, the data strategy includes databases, data warehouses, and data lakes.

- A database is a collection of data or information, typically focusing on a single topic or system. Database management systems (DBMSs) are used to create and maintain databases, including adding, modifying, and deleting data. For these transactions to be efficient, databases have a defined structure and rules to support the quality and integrity of the data [12–14].
- Data warehouses are highly structured repositories that contain data from a variety of disparate sources (such as multiple databases). To maintain the structure, data are extracted (copied) from their original source, transformed into the structure of the data warehouse, and then loaded into the data warehouse (known as the ETL or extract transform load process) [12–15]. Often, this process is completed using a data pipeline, which is a method for extracting, transforming, and loading data [16].
- Data lakes are repositories that contain data from a variety of disparate sources. Data are stored in their raw form from their original sources; therefore, data lakes can store information in a variety of formats within the same repository [12–14]. To create and maintain a data lake, an extract load and transform (ELT) process may be used in which data are extracted from their original source and loaded into the data lake. Then, when someone uses these data, they perform any necessary data transformations [15]. Data pipelines can be created for some or all of these extraction, loading, and transformation steps [16].

A student asks, "Why does the organization need all three?" Michael explains that the health system has data within a variety of systems, including their EHR, their finance and accounting system, and their materials management system. By combining these data into a single repository, the organization can analyze situations holistically. For example, the organization could determine the cost of a surgery based on recent data about the personnel involved, the length of the surgery, the cost of facilities and supplies, etc.

Another student asks, "Why use both a data warehouse and a data lake?" Michael explains that the type of data storage needed depends on the work that will be done with the data. For example, simple reporting and analysis can usually be supported by data warehouses. For more complex analysis, data scientists and programmers may want to transform data based on a specific technique they are using. In this case, a data lake would be more appropriate [12].

Next, Michael explains that the organization uses an environment strategy to ensure the databases, data warehouses, and data lakes are appropriately maintained and managed. An environment strategy includes plans and procedures for effectively managing changes to related technology systems and data. Michael explains that the EHR system has an environment strategy (as shown in Fig. 29.1).

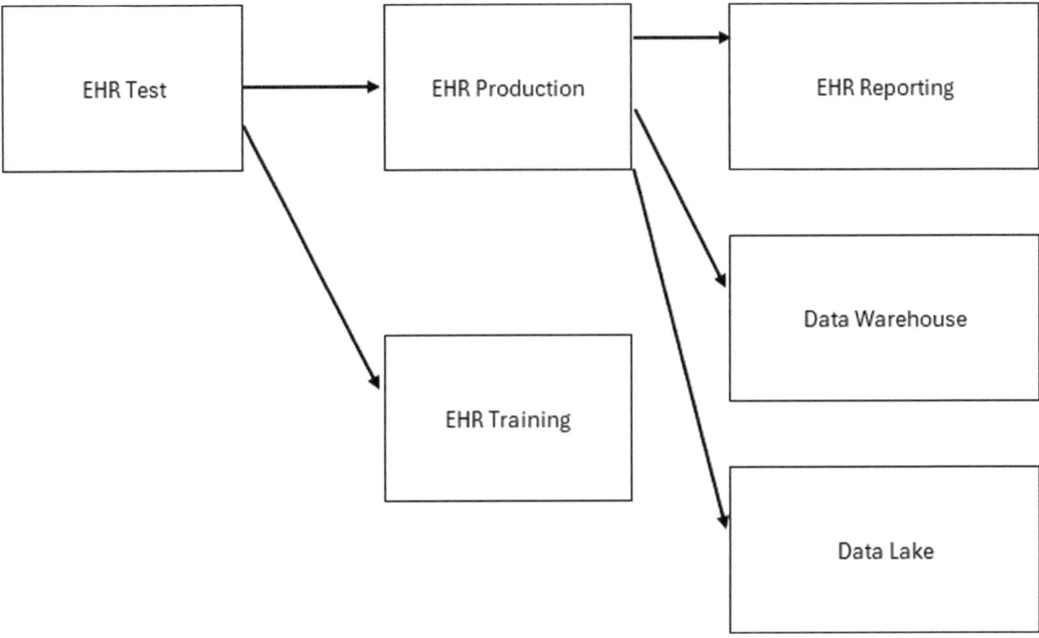

Fig. 29.1 Example environment strategy

For example, the healthcare organization has six "environments" for the EHR system. Each environment has a copy of the EHR software and has its own database. Whenever a change is proposed for the EHR, the Informatics team builds and tests the change in the EHR Test environment. If the change is approved, the change is made in the EHR Training environment so that individuals can be trained on the changes. Then the change is made in the EHR Production environment, which is the environment that clinicians, staff, and leaders use on a daily basis. On a regular basis, information from the EHR Production environment is copied to the EHR Reporting environment and the organization's data warehouse and data lake so that reporting and analysis can be performed. A backup copy of the EHR Production database is also created on a regular basis as part of the disaster recovery plan for the EHR system (which is explained later in this chapter).

29.4.6 What Data Structure Will Be Used?

At the start of the next class, a student asks, "How do you decide how the data will be stored?" Michael explains that this decision is based on several factors, including

- What type(s) of data and information need to be stored?
- Who will need access to this information (a small group of people or many)?
- What is the purpose of gathering the data?
- How will the organization be using the data?

Based on this information, the project team first determines if a database, data warehouse, or data lake is appropriate. For this project, all three will be needed. The EHR database will store the original data, and then this data will be added to the data warehouse and data lake.

If a database is appropriate, then the next step is to determine the type of database. Michael explains that five basic database types are used within the organization: relational, nonrelational, hierarchical, network, and object-oriented.

29.4.6.1 What Is a Relational Database?

A relational database organizes and stores data in tables consisting of columns and rows (as shown in Fig. 29.2). Within this type of database, each table has a *primary key*, which is a value that uniquely identifies each record (row) [17]. Other tables within the database have a column (or combination of columns) that reference this primary key in the original table. This column or combination of columns is known as the *foreign key*.

For example, in the Provider table, the primary key for Sarah Smith is 156170. In the Provider Clinic table, the Provider column is the foreign key because it uses Sarah Smith's primary key from the Provider table.

Relational databases represent relationships (or links) between information by using the primary key as a foreign key within another table [17]. Sarah Smith (primary key 156170) works in the Pulmonary Care clinic (primary key 459). Within the Provider Clinic table, a record (primary key 89) represents this relationship by including the provider ID and location ID as foreign keys. The health system has a Specialty Clinics Center (primary key 13) in which the Pulmonary Care clinic is located; therefore, in the Location table, the Pulmonary Care clinic is related to the Specialty Clinics Center using foreign key 13.

Relational databases have a structure that is easy to understand and is built to avoid duplication of data. Because of this standardization, information can be easily queried (searched for and obtained) using well-known languages such as *Structured Query Language* (SQL). This structure, though, can also be costly to create and maintain. In addition, as additional data needs are identified and implemented, the database and its relationships can become complex. When this occurs, database performance can decrease, meaning obtaining data may be slower [18].

29.4.6.2 What Is a Nonrelational Database?

Nonrelational databases store information such as documents and network graphs [19, 20]. Also known as NoSQL databases, nonrelational databases tend to be more flexible than other database types because they can store different formats of data within a single database [21]. As a result, they can manage large quantities of complex and diverse data [20].

Without a defined structure, though, the data lack standardization, making it difficult to ensure the information is consistent and maintained appropriately. Relationships cannot be easily defined between data. In addition, standard lan-

Provider Table

ID	First Name	Last Name	Provider ID
156170	Sarah	Smith	456981
156171	Ahmad	Khan	950780
156172	Hilda	Roman	450690

Provider Clinic Table

ID	Provider	Clinic
89	156170	459
90	156170	458
91	156171	460

Location Table

ID	Location Title	Building
458	South Specialty Clinics	12
459	Pulmonary Care	13
460	Cardiology Specialists	13

Building Table

ID	Building
12	Main Campus
13	Specialty Clinics Center

Fig. 29.2 Example of relational database tables

guages like SQL cannot be used to obtain data [21]. As a result, reporting can be challenging, and individuals may need significant training to use these databases effectively.

29.4.6.3 What Is a Hierarchical Database?

In *hierarchical databases*, information is stored in a tree-like structure in which a "parent" concept can have one or more "child" concepts related to that patient concept. A "child" can have one and only one "parent." Hierarchical databases tend to "classify" information into categories or levels as shown in Fig. 29.3.

In this example, the "root" of the "tree" is a clinic (the Pulmonary Care clinic) within a health system. Within this clinic, multiple providers (Sarah Smith and Ahmad Khan) see patients. Jose Martinez and Maddie Jefferson have seen Sarah Smith within the Pulmonary Care clinic. He Chen and Brigette Marcon have seen Ahmad Khan within the clinic.

The hierarchical organization of the data can make searching for data simple and fast, as many programming languages have built-in support for tree structures. In addition, if a "parent" concept needs to be added, modified, or deleted, the implications of these changes can be easily identified as the "child" concepts can be quickly identified. This structure, though, can be inflexible as only one "parent" is allowed for a "child," which can result in duplication of data. For example, if Sarah Smith and Ahmad Khan both see Maddie Jefferson, then Maddie Jefferson's information would need to be duplicated to be listed under both providers. Also, if many levels exist within the hierarchical structure, searching for and obtaining data can be time consuming [22].

29.4.6.4 What Is a Network Database?

Network databases are similar to hierarchical databases with one significant difference—they allow a "child" concept to have more than one parent "concept" as shown in Fig. 29.4 [19].

One advantage of this structure is that relationships do not need to be strictly "parent" and "child"; instead, relationships can exist in multiple directions and not just "top down." This flexibility is critical for highly interconnected data,

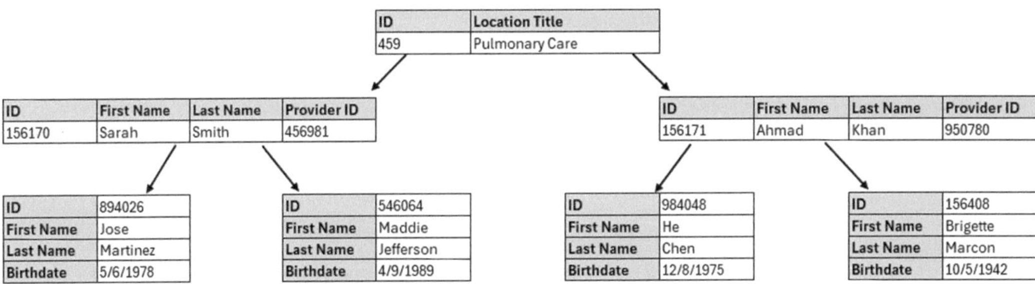

Fig. 29.3 Example of a hierarchical database

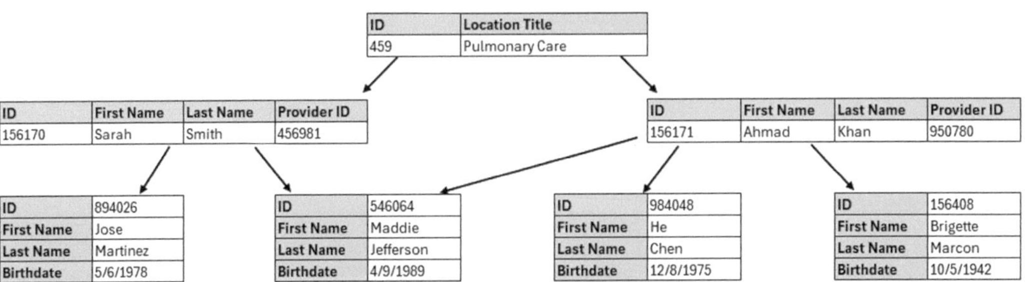

Fig. 29.4 Example of a network database

which is common in healthcare (i.e., patients may be seen in multiple clinics, by a variety of providers, etc.). In network databases, these interconnected relationship can be easily represented without the need to duplicate data [23]. In addition, new relationships can be added, which allows the database to scale and grow.

With this growth, though, comes challenges. These databases can become complex and difficult to maintain because of these interconnected relationships. In addition, standardizing the database may be difficult because of changing relationships, so duplication of data may occur and obtaining data may be time consuming and require significant database knowledge [23].

29.4.6.5 What Is an Object-Oriented Database?

Object-oriented databases are based on objects, which are real-world concepts that have certain attributes and behaviors [24, 25]. These objects and their relationships are represented within the database, as shown in Fig. 29.5.

In this example, three objects exist: Location, Unit, and Person. Each object has certain attributes to further define the object. For example, a Location (such as a hospital or clinic building) has an ID, a title, and an address. Each object can also have methods or ways that the object can interact with other objects. For example, a Person object can manage a unit; work in a unit; train in a unit (such as a nurse educator); or learn in a unit (such as a student nurse).

The depth of data that objects contain as well as clear relationships among objects is a key advantage of this data structure. In addition, software can be written using object-oriented programming languages, which means the software and its associated database can use similar structures. Within this structure, though, the complexity of the objects and their relationships can decrease the efficiency of the database. In addition, individuals working with these databases may require significant programming knowledge [24, 25].

29.4.6.6 What Software Is Needed to Support Databases?

After explaining the basic types of databases, Michael explains that two types of software exist to support these databases: database management systems (DBMSs) and query languages.

Database management systems (DBMSs) are software used to create and manage the database, including creating the data structure; ensuring appropriate protections and security are setup; and additions, modifications, and deletions of data are handled correctly and logged for future reference [26]. For example, Microsoft SQL Database, IBM, Db2, Oracle Database, and Sybase are all examples of DBMS for relational databases [26]. MongoDB and Db2 are examples for object-oriented databases [26].

Second, a *query language* may be needed. Obtaining data from a database (also known as querying the database) often requires a specific

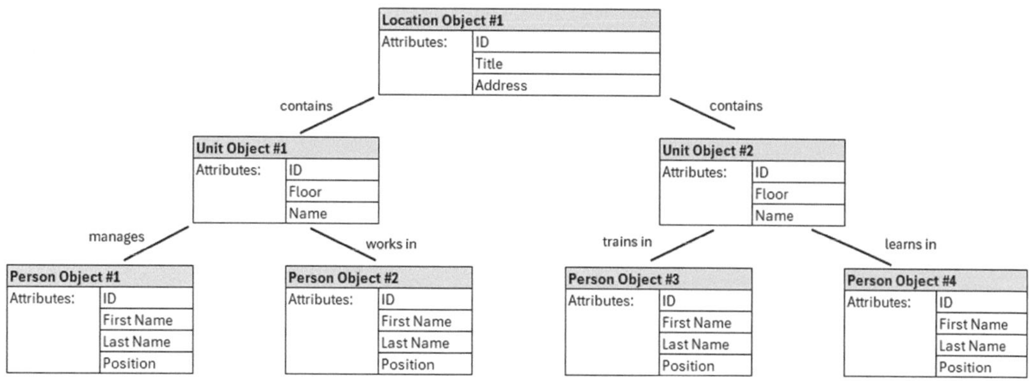

Fig. 29.5 Example of an object-oriented database

language based on the type of database. For example, relational databases often use SQL to obtain data from the tables within the database [27]. Other database types may have specific query languages based on the DBMS used. For example, MongoDB Query Language (MQL) works with the MongoDB DBMS [27].

29.4.7 How Do We Know if the Data Are Correct?

As the course continues, Michael explains another area within data management—*data quality*. Data quality measures, assesses, and improves the fitness (or quality) of data used within an organization [1]. Data quality involves several dimensions, which are described in Table 29.4 [4].

When the project team meets with the class, they discuss how they will ensure data quality within the project. Primarily, the project team will work with the EHR vendor to implement business rules for the questions. For example, based on the metadata for anxiety level, only numbers 1–5 will be able to be entered in response to that question. The team also develops a process to complete daily review of the standard report of questionnaire results for the first six months after the EHR mental health questionnaire is implemented. If they identify any issues during this review, the team will review the data to determine the source of the problem and resolve the issue.

Table 29.4 Dimensions of data quality

Dimension	Description	Example
Completeness	The degree to which required data is entered or obtained based on the business rules within an organization	A clinic has a business rule that requires the first name and last name for a patient be entered into the EHR before the patient can schedule an appointment. If both of these values are entered prior to scheduling an appointment, the data has a high degree of completeness based on this business rule
Uniqueness	The degree to which data can have duplicated values	A hospital has a business rule that each physician must have a unique provider identifier. If no provider identifier numbers are duplicated, then the data has a high degree of uniqueness based on this business rule
Validity	The degree to which data conforms to established business rules for acceptable content, which may include format, data type, and valid values	A pharmacy has a business rule that a patient's birthdate must be entered in MM/DD/YYYY format, with MM being a two-digit month, DD being a two-digit date, and YYYY being a four-digit year. If a birthdate is unknown, it should be entered as 01/01/1801. If a patient's birthdate is unknown and their birthdate is entered as 2/2/2020, then this data would have low validity based on the pharmacy's business rule
Reasonableness	The degree to which data are reasonable and logical based on real-world scenarios and comparison with other data within the organization	A database administrator is reviewing entries within the analytics reporting system for the heights (in inches) of adult human patients. The database administrator finds a patient height value of 310 inches (or the equivalent of more than 25 feet tall). This data would have low reasonableness based on logical values within the real world (where no humans are more than 25 feet tall)
Integrity	The degree to which data are consistent across multiple databases capturing the same or similar information	A hospital has a system that tracks payments within their cafeteria. These payments are then uploaded into the hospital's accounting system. If both the cafeteria system and the hospital's accounting system have the same amount of payments for April 1, then the data have a high degree of integrity

(continued)

Table 29.4 (continued)

Dimension	Description	Example
Timeliness	The degree to which data are available when needed by the organization	On the first of each month, a clinic runs a report to find patients who have been newly diagnosed with diabetes so they can follow up with these patients and provide additional support. Therefore, the reporting system must have an upload of patients, their diagnoses, and the dates of diagnoses before the first of the month (usually, the week before the next month). If the needed uploaded is performed late (after the first of the month), it would have a low degree of timeliness based on the needs of the clinic
Coverage	The degree to which data supports all the business operations within an organization	A nursing school needs to track information for their students including their grades, overall grade point average (GPA), preferred clinical sites, and immunization status. The database the school is currently using only tracks grades and GPA; therefore, this data has a low degree of coverage based on the needs of the nursing school
Accuracy	The degree to which data corresponds to correct real-world values	A patient sets up a well-person visit with their primary care doctor. On the day of the visit, the scale in the clinic is broken, so the patient's weight cannot be measured. When the provider sees the patient, the patient reports that he weighs 215 lbs., even though he weighed 230 lbs. on his home scale that morning. This data would have a low degree of accuracy based on the real-world value

29.4.8 How Do I Maintain the Data?

Nearing the end of the course, Michael covers another aspect of the data lifecycle, which is maintaining the data. In this project, the project team needs to consider the existing data as well as the data once the questionnaire is implemented within the EHR.

Currently, during annual wellness visits, patients (or their guardians) complete a standard paper questionnaire about the patient's mental health. During the pilot project, information from these completed questionnaires was manually abstracted and entered into a database. For the current project, this questionnaire will be created within the EHR, and the data will be stored within the EHR database.

A student asks, "What happens to the existing database when the questionnaire is implemented within the EHR? Does this data get converted into the EHR?" Michael explains to the class that this question is important. Once this project is complete, answers to the mental health questionnaires could be found in one of three places: a completed paper form, an entry into the pilot project database, and within the EHR. So, if a clinician wants to find this information, how do they know where to look? And how can they determine which information is "current"?

Michael explains that the project team works with the HIM department (the data owner) to identify the "*system of record*" for mental health questionnaire data. A system of record is the system where the best version of the information is created/captured and maintained [1]. For this project, the HIM department determined that the paper questionnaires will be the "system of record" for any information captured prior to the completion of this project. Once this project is complete, the EHR database will be the system of record.

Because these data are assets for the organization and critical information for clinicians and their patients, Michael explains the importance of business continuity, disaster recovery, and backups in maintaining the data.

Organizations can be impacted by a variety of situations, including electrical outages, natural disasters, and civil unrest. When disasters or adverse events occur, healthcare organizations must continue to function to serve their communities; therefore, they must have plans and procedures to ensure critical functions are operational. These plans, known as *business continuity plans*, include procedures for maintaining critical services such as ensuring appropriate staffing; having access to water, electricity, and sanitation; obtaining supplies for sanitation and emergency care; and accessing critical data [28].

As part of the business continuity plan, IT, informatics, and data management teams have a *disaster recovery plan*, which outlines the steps needed to restore access to data, systems, and other technology resources should these be impacted by the event. The disaster recovery plan would outline the steps needed to restore this access as quickly as possible [29].

For data and databases, the disaster recovery plan may include standby databases and backups. A standby database is a separate database that is maintained as a "copy" of the main database [30]. Should the main database be unavailable, the organization can switch to the standby database. A backup is a copy of the data stored within the database, and this backup is maintained in a separate storage location from the original data and database [30]. Should a database be negatively impacted, the backup can be used to either re-create the database or restore the data within the database to a known state.

29.5 Summary

As described in this hypothetical case study, Michael is a database administrator who is responsible for managing and ensuring reliable access to an organization's databases. As part of the social determinants of health project, he ensures that the data from the mental health questionnaires are appropriately managed throughout the data lifecycle, including the data to be captured and its sources; who needs access to the data; where the data should be stored; the quality of the data; and how the data need to be maintained.

Throughout the project, Michael shares his expertise and experience with students in his undergraduate course. Most importantly, they learn that data is an asset for an organization and, like any other asset, it requires careful and intentional management, including plans for unexpected situations such as natural disasters and cybersecurity attacks.

29.6 Resources

See Table 29.5 for a list of data management resources.

Table 29.5 Data management resources

Resource	Website (link)
Professional organization for data management professionals and information	DAMA International (https://www.dama.org/cpages/home)
Information about careers in data management	Database administrator on Indeed (https://www.indeed.com/career/database-administrator) Data engineer on Indeed (https://www.indeed.com/career/data-engineer) Key roles for a data management team (https://www.techtarget.com/searchdatamanagement/tip/What-key-roles-should-a-data-management-team-include) U.S. Bureau of Labor Statistics: Database Administrators and Architects (https://www.bls.gov/ooh/computer-and-information-technology/database-administrators.htm)

Glossary of Terms

Term	Definition
Accuracy	A dimension of data quality. The degree to which data corresponds to correct real-world values.
Asset	Economic resources that hold or produce value for an organization and can be owned or controlled by that organization.
Backup	A copy of data that is stored separately from the original data; part of a disaster recovery plan.
Big data	Datasets or data collections that are extremely large and fast growing, and may contain a variety of structured, semi-structured, and unstructured data.
Business continuity	Procedures for maintaining critical services such as ensuring appropriate staffing; having access to water, electricity, and sanitation; obtaining supplies for sanitation and emergency care; and accessing critical data during an unplanned event (such as a natural disaster or cybersecurity attack).
Completeness	A dimension of data quality. The degree to which required data is entered or obtained based on the business rules within an organization.
Coverage	A dimension of data quality. The degree to which data supports all the business operations within an organization.
Data	Facts or observations about the world such as names and addresses, treatment plans for patients, and national identification numbers for providers and insurers.
Data architect	Individual who creates an organization's data strategy
Data architecture	A key area within data management that, based on organizational strategies, identifies the data needed and designs a plan for managing these data assets.
Data engineer	Individual who builds the technological foundation to implement the organization's data strategy.
Data governance	A key area within data management that provides direction and oversight by establishing policies, processes, and procedures to make decisions related to the data assets within an organization.

Term	Definition
Data integration and interoperability	A key area within data management that moves data between different systems and storage locations (such as moving data between two databases).
Data lake	A repository of data from disparate sources that can support a variety of data formats and structures. Within a data lake, data are stored in their original, raw form (no transformation).
Data management	The plans, policies, programs, and practices needed to deliver, control, protect, and enhance the value of data assets within organizations.
Data pipeline	A method used to obtain data from a variety of sources, transform the data, and then load the data into the appropriate storage location (such as a database, data lake, or data warehouse).
Data quality	A key area within data management that measures, assesses, and improves the fitness (or quality) of data used within an organization.
Data security	A key area within data management that maintains the privacy and confidentiality of data throughout its lifecycle.
Data storage and operations	A key area within data management that designs, implements, and supports the storage of data within an organization.
Data strategy	The plan or "blueprint" to organize, retrieve, interpret, store, maintain, and share data to meet the requirements of the organization.
Data warehouse	A repository of data from disparate sources. The repository has a well-defined structure, and data are transformed into this structure prior to being loaded into the data warehouse.
Data warehousing and business intelligence	A key area within data management that enables analysis and reporting of data to support decision making within an organization.
Database	Collection of data and information. Typical database types include relational, non-relational, hierarchical, network, and object-oriented.
Database administrator (DBA)	Individual who manages and ensures reliable access to an organization's databases.

(continued)

Term	Definition
Disaster recovery	Plans and procedures that outline the steps needed to restore access to data, systems, and other technology resources should these be impacted by disasters or adverse events.
Document and content management	A key area within data management that plans, implements, and controls activities related to unstructured data within an organization, especially documents required for legal and regulatory compliance.
Environment strategy	A strategy (including plans and procedures) for effectively managing changes to related technology systems and data.
Integrity	A dimension of data quality. The degree to which data are consistent across multiple databases capturing the same or similar information.
Metadata	A key area within data management that creates and maintains the definitions, models, data flows, and other information needed to understand the data within an organization.
Reasonableness	A dimension of data quality. The degree to which data are reasonable and logical based on real-world scenarios and comparison with other data within the organization.
Reference and master data	A key area within data management that maintains the accuracy, timeliness, and relevancy of the most critical, business essential information within an organization.
Timeliness	A dimension of data quality. The degree to which data are available when needed by the organization.
Uniqueness	A dimension of data quality. The degree to which data can have duplicated values.
Validity	A dimension of data quality. The degree to which data conforms to established business rules for acceptable content, which may include format, data type, and valid values.

Knowledge Check Questions

1. *Take 10 min and write a list of the data you use in your daily life. Select one data item from your list that you think is the most important in your life. Why is this data important to you? What value do you derive from this data?*
2. *For the data item you selected, explain the lifecycle of that data using the stages described in this chapter.*
3. *Why is data management important within an organization?*
4. *Identify and describe the areas within data management.*
5. *Explain why big data is different from other types of data.*

Answers

1. (Answers will vary depending on the results of student brainstorming for 10 min. An example of the "select one" answer is provided below.)
   Financial data (such as the balance in my checking account) is the most important data in my life, as it determines if I am making enough money to pay my bills, buy groceries, etc. Without knowing if I have sufficient funds, I cannot make informed decisions in other aspects of my life. For example, if I want to avoid debt and know that I have $100 for groceries this month, then I know I need to plan carefully to know I can purchase sufficient food for the month while staying in that budget. The main value of this information is being able to make informed decisions in my life that align with my goals and values.
2. (Answers will vary depending on the answer to the first question. This example answer is based on the example answer to the previous question.)
   Financial data are created each time I deposit or withdraw money from my accounts. In addition, my bank may create data by charging fees, adding rewards, or doing other tasks that impact my account balance. I use my financial data on a regular basis (such as planning my weekly grocery budget or deciding if I can purchase a new sweater). To use this data, I first need to know all my account numbers and their associated usernames and passwords. I also need to know how to access the information (such as through a bank website). Depending on the type of information, it may be stored in a database (listing credits and debits) or in documents

(such as tax forms that need to be completed each year). To ensure the data are correct, I can compare my receipts to what appears within my account and also look for unusual activity (such as fees that I did not expect). I can maintain information on my own (such as having my own spreadsheet) in addition to the bank keeping their records. For all of this information, I need to maintain it in a secure manner (such as encrypted files that are password protected) and not share my usernames and passwords. If I decide to close an account, then information about that account may need to be deleted after an appropriate amount of time (e.g., I may want to keep the information for the length of time needed to support my tax return).

3. Data management includes the plans, policies, programs, and practices needed to deliver, control, protect, and enhance the value of data assets within organizations. It involves all the activities that occur to manage the data and information that are valuable to an organization. Without these activities, data may be compromised and result in decision-making that is based on incorrect information. For example, one aspect of data management is data security. If a hacker is able to access important data and modify it without the organization knowing, leadership may make incorrect decisions based on the comprised data, which could negatively impact organizational profits and strategies.
4. The areas within data management include:
   - Data governance: Provides direction and oversight by establishing policies, processes, and procedures to make decisions related to the data assets within an organization.
   - Data architecture: Based on organizational strategies, identifies the data needed and designs a plan for managing these data assets.
   - Data modeling and design: Creates a formal representation (known as a "data model") of the data within an organization.
   - Data storage and operations: Designs, implements, and supports the storage of data within an organization.
   - Data security: Maintains the privacy and confidentiality of data throughout its lifecycle.
   - Data integration and interoperability: Moves data between different systems and storage locations (such as moving data between two databases).
   - Document and content management: Plans, implements, and controls activities related to unstructured data within an organization, especially documents required for legal and regulatory compliance.
   - Reference and master data: Maintains the accuracy, timeliness, and relevancy of the most critical, business essential information within an organization.
   - Data warehousing and business intelligence: Enables analysis and reporting of data to support decision-making within an organization.
   - Metadata: Creates and maintains the definitions, models, data flows, and other information needed to understand the data within an organization.
   - Data quality: Measures, assesses, and improves the fitness (or quality) of data used within an organization.
5. Big data has three characteristics that differentiate it from other types of data. First, the volume of data captured for big data is large (greater than 100 terabytes). Second, big data is generated very quickly (such as significant increases in the number of Google searches year to year). Finally, big data is stored in a variety of ways including databases, documents, and videos (structured, semi-structured, and unstructured).

References

1. DAMA International. DAMA – DMBOK: data management body of knowledge. 2nd ed. Technics Publicatons; 2017.
2. Bernstam EV, Johnson TR, Cohen T. Healthcare data, information, and knowledge. In: Health informatics: practical guide. 7th ed. Informatics Education; 2018.
3. Gutta S. Data Science: THe 5V's of Big Data. Medium. April 5, 2020. https://medium.com/analytics-vidhya/the-5-vs-of-big-data-2758bfcc51d

4. Plotkin D. Data stewardship: an actionable guide to effective data management and data governance. 2nd ed. Academic; 2020.
5. Kutay J. Data Architect vs. Data engineer: an overview of two in-demand roles. https://www.striim.com/blog/data-architect-vs-data-engineer-an-overview-of-two-in-demand-roles/
6. Indeed Editorial Team. Data Architect vs. Data Engineer: What's the Difference? February 3, 2023. https://www.indeed.com/career-advice/finding-a-job/data-architect-vs-data-engineer
7. Dataquest. Data Engineer, Data Analyst, Data Scientist – What's the Difference. April 12, 2021. Accessed February 5, 2024. https://www.dataquest.io/blog/data-analyst-data-scientist-data-engineer/?utm_source=google&utm_medium=&matchtype=&device=c&utm_campaign=ai_launch_sale&campaignid=20758249356&adgroupid=&adid=&utm_content=&gad_source=5&gclid=EAIaIQobChMIysq78aGUhAMVRmVHAR2h3g7AEAAYBCAAEgIMU_D_BwE
8. Foot C. What key roles should a data management team include? December 15, 2022. https://www.techtarget.com/searchdatamanagement/tip/What-key-roles-should-a-data-management-team-include
9. Indeed. What Does a Database Administrator Do? https://www.indeed.com/career/database-administrator
10. Gulati A. Database administrator vs. data engineer: skills, salary, responsibilities. September 6, 2023. https://www.knowledgehut.com/blog/data-science/database-engineer-vs-database-administrator
11. Steenbeek I. The data management toolkit: a step-by-step implementation guide for the pioneers of data management. Data Crossroads; 2019.
12. Kidd C. Data storage explained: data lake vs. warehouse vs. database. October 28, 2020. https://www.bmc.com/blogs/data-lake-vs-data-warehouse-vs-database-whats-the-difference/
13. MongoDB. Databases vs. data warehouses vs. data lakes. https://www.mongodb.com/resources/basics/databases/data-lake-vs-data-warehouse-vs-database
14. Confluent. Databases vs. data lakes vs. data warehouses: comparing data sources. https://www.confluent.io/learn/databases-data-lakes-and-data-warehouses-compared/
15. AWS. What is ETL (Extract Transform Load)? https://aws.amazon.com/what-is/etl/
16. Stryker C. What is a data pipeline? IBM. https://www.ibm.com/think/topics/data-pipeline
17. Google Cloud. What is a relational database? https://cloud.google.com/learn/what-is-a-relational-database
18. DatabaseTown. Relational database benefits & limitations (Advantages & disadvantages). https://databasetown.com/relational-database-benefits-and-limitations/
19. Data Science Wizards. 5 basic types of databases. November 2, 2022. https://medium.com/@datasciencewizards/5-basic-types-of-databases-9f8d10c73ebf
20. MongoDB. What is a non-relational database? https://www.mongodb.com/resources/basics/databases/non-relational
21. Foote KD. NoSQL databases: advantages and disadvantages. November 17, 2022. https://www.dataversity.net/nosql-databases-advantages-and-disadvantages/
22. HeavyAI. Hierarchical database. https://www.heavy.ai/technical-glossary/hierarchical-database
23. Spasojevic A. What is a network database? March 21, 2024. https://phoenixnap.com/glossary/network-database
24. Dancuk M. What is an object-oriented database. April 15, 2021. https://phoenixnap.com/kb/object-oriented-database
25. MongoDB. What is an object-oriented database? https://www.mongodb.com/resources/basics/databases/what-is-an-object-oriented-database
26. KingswaySoft. The 10 most popular database management systems in 2023. October 18, 2023. https://www.kingswaysoft.com/resources/industry-analysis/top-database-management-systems
27. Chia A. Query languages: a simple introduction. https://www.splunk.com/en_us/blog/learn/query-languages.html
28. Cisco. What is business continuity? https://www.cisco.com/c/en/us/solutions/hybrid-work/what-is-business-continuity.html#~planning-activities
29. Google Cloud. What is a disaster recovery plan? https://cloud.google.com/learn/what-is-disaster-recovery
30. DBVisit. Disaster recovery versus backups. https://dbvisit.com/disaster-recovery-vs-backups

30 Artificial Intelligence

Robert E. Hoyt

Foundational Domains
This chapter addresses the following AMIA Foundational Domains: F2—Information Science, F4—Health Information Science and Technology, F7—Social, Behavioral, and Information Science and Technology Applied to Health.

Learning Objectives
After reading this chapter, you should be able to

1. Discuss how artificial intelligence (AI) is applied to the field of medicine.
2. Compare machine learning and artificial intelligence.
3. Enumerate different applications of large language models (LLMs).
4. Discuss the impact of image analysis in medicine.
5. List the challenges facing AI today.

30.1 Background of Artificial Intelligence and Machine Learning

The history of artificial intelligence (AI) can be traced back to the mid-twentieth century. The term "artificial intelligence" was coined by John McCarthy in 1956 at a conference at Dartmouth College. Early AI research focused on "expert systems," such as Mycin in the 1970s and 1980s. These systems were based on predefined rules, such as if-then statements and were used primarily for medical diagnosis [1].

In the 1980s and 1990s, there was a shift toward statistical methods, such as logistic regression, and machine learning, with the development of algorithms capable of learning from data. Neural networks emerged, and with additional computational layers, deep learning evolved. In the 2010s, deep learning gained significant traction and led to breakthroughs in natural language processing and computer vision. In 2016, Google's DeepMind project AlphaGo defeated the Go champion Lee Sedol. In 2018, Google DeepMind launched AlphaFold, which predicted the 3-D structure of proteins. Generative AI appeared in approximately 2021, with the ability to generate images, text, audio, and video. ChatGPT 3.5 was launched in November 2022 and GPT-5.1 in 2025. Large language models (LLMs) are revolutionary and will be discussed in other sections [2, 3].

Artificial intelligence (AI) is a field where computer systems can perform tasks that traditionally required human intelligence. In the context of health informatics, AI holds great promise for improving patient care, clinical workflows, and medical research. AI applications in healthcare range from predictive analyt-

R. E. Hoyt (✉)
Department of Internal Medicine, Virginia Commonwealth University, Richmond, VA, USA
e-mail: robert.hoyt@vcuhealth.org

C. Eldredge et al. (eds.), *Introductory Textbook in Health Informatics*, Health Informatics,
https://doi.org/10.1007/978-3-032-16657-9_30

ics and personalized (precision) medicine to medical image analysis and drug discovery. AI-powered predictive models can forecast disease, identify high-risk patients, and optimize resource allocation.

Narrow artificial intelligence refers to AI used for specific tasks, such as interpreting a chest x-ray. *Artificial general intelligence* (AGI) refers to more advanced AI that can perform multiple tasks and can think like a human. General AI would have the capacity to reason, solve problems, and comprehend complex ideas in various domains. AGI would be capable of adapting to new situations and learning from experience. AGI has not been achieved at this time, but AI continues to evolve at a rapid pace [4].

Machine learning (ML), a subset of AI, utilizes ML algorithms to learn from data, identify patterns, and make predictions without being explicitly programmed. In healthcare, ML is used for tasks such as disease diagnosis, patient risk stratification, and treatment outcome prediction. By analyzing large volumes of patient data, ML models can assist healthcare professionals in making more accurate and timely clinical decisions [4]. For example, machine learning (predictive modeling) can be used to predict the risk of readmission to a hospital.

Figure 30.1 displays a Venn diagram of AI, machine learning, deep learning, and generative AI. Figure 30.2 displays how artificial intelligence fits into the data–information–knowledge–wisdom (DIKW) pyramid and how AI can augment human intelligence. AI could serve to expand differential diagnoses and cite the newest developments published in the medical literature, thus improving quality and safety [3, 5].

Artificial intelligence (AI) is a rapidly evolving field that can handle a variety of tasks such as learning from data, text and image generation and analysis, problem-solving, text summarization, and brainstorming. AI has the potential to revolutionize various industries, including healthcare, by automating processes, providing insights from large datasets, and assisting in decision-making.

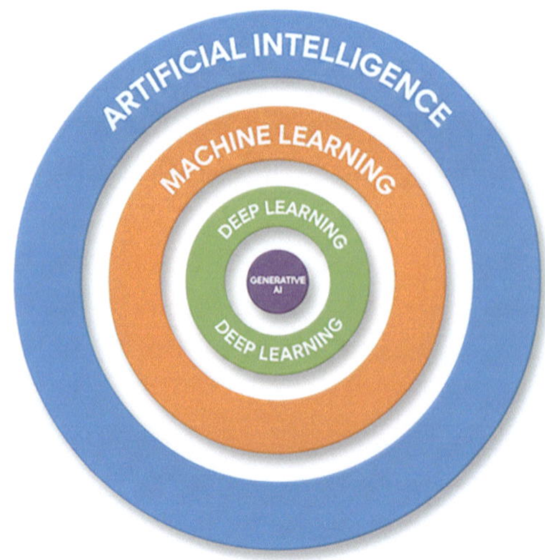

Fig. 30.1 Venn diagram of AI, machine learning, deep learning, and generative AI

Artificial intelligence is necessary in the medical field for multiple reasons. Medical knowledge is said to double every 73 days, and the amount of total worldwide data is estimated to be 181 zettabytes by 2025 (a zettabyte is equal to 1 billion terabytes) [3]. When you consider how much medical data there is to analyze, its complexity and diversity, and the rate it appears, it becomes clear that AI is the only way to come to grips with this data avalanche.

In summary, AI and ML have the potential to transform medicine, offering opportunities to enhance patient outcomes, streamline healthcare operations, and drive innovation in medical research. Understanding the principles and applications of AI in healthcare is essential for preparing future healthcare informatics professionals to leverage these technologies effectively and ethically.

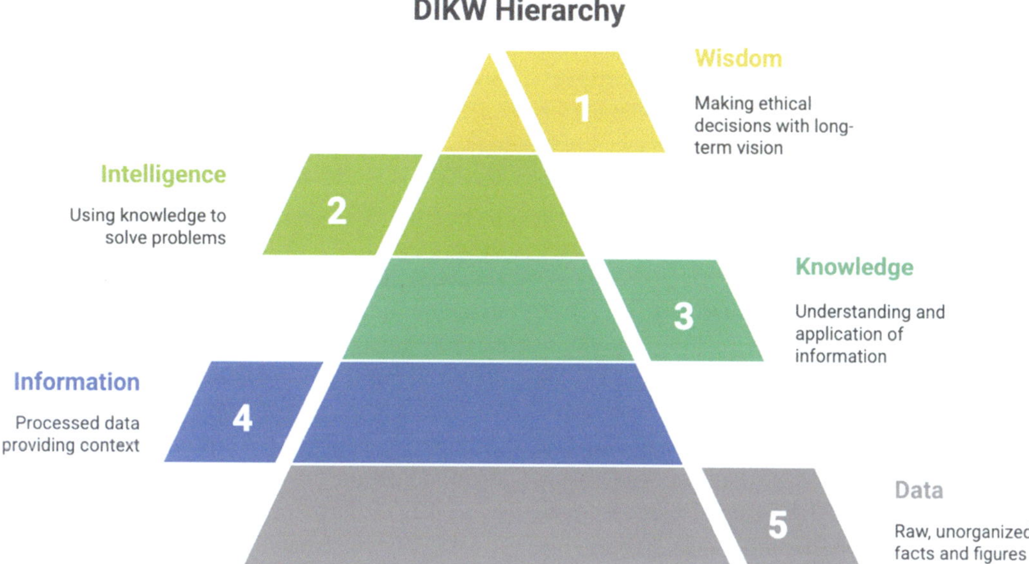

Fig. 30.2 DIKW pyramid augmented by AI [3]. (The image was created using Napkin AI, 2025)

30.2 Machine Learning

Machine learning is mostly used to create prediction models, so they are the backbone of predictive analytics. Machine learning follows a standard workflow or pipeline. Data is collected from a variety of sources, such as an enterprise data warehouse or a data lake. The data is cleaned to take care of acronyms and unclear text, such as M for males, or different date formats. Missing data is handled by a variety of methods, such as imputation. Data are then explored with descriptive statistics and data visualization, such as histograms and heatmaps. There is feature engineering where variables can be added, deleted, or combined. These steps are in preparation for the modeling phase where different families of algorithms are selected and run.

There are two major types of machine learning: supervised and unsupervised learning.

30.2.1 Supervised Learning

Supervised learning refers to a situation where you know what you want to predict, and you have data to accomplish this. For example, you are trying to predict who will develop pancreatic cancer. You have a dataset of 1000 patients who developed a variety of cancers plus data on the usual risk factors. Of the 1000 patients, 100 have pancreatic cancer. One column is labeled outcome, and if they developed pancreatic cancer, it is labeled 1, if not 0. The supervised learning outcome is frequently binary such as benign or malignant, readmitted or not readmitted, but predicting more than two outcomes is possible. When the outcome involves categorical data (zero vs. one, benign vs. malignant), this is a classification model. This is the most common type of predictive analytics. When the outcome is numerical (heart rate, cost of hospitalization, length of stay, etc.), this is a regression model [5].

Most commonly, the dataset is split (e.g., 75%/25%) into train and test data. Multiple algorithms are used to train on just the training data but tested on the test data. Older statistical algorithms could be used, such as logistic regression, linear regression, and Naive Bayes. Newer machine learning algorithms include random forest, xgboost, gradient boosting, SVM, and neural networks [5].

Classification model performance is based on sensitivity, specificity, positive and negative predictive values, the area under the curve (AUC), and many other metrics. Most ML algorithms can also perform regression except logistic regression and Naive Bayes. Regression model performance is based on R squared, root mean square error (RMSE), mean square error (MSE), and other metrics [5].

30.2.2 Unsupervised Learning

Frequently, you have a dataset that does not include an outcome. In other words, it is simply a dataset collected over time with many variables and you want to look for hidden patterns or groups (clusters). The unsupervised learning algorithms find clusters in the data that you can later explore. An example of this would be exploring genomic and phenotypic data to look for new relationships or clusters. Another example would be using unsupervised learning early in the COVID-19 pandemic to try to uncover hidden patterns in the data. This approach has great potential but is less commonly performed or published [6].

30.3 Artificial Intelligence

30.3.1 Artificial Neural Networks

Neural networks are a major component of machine learning and artificial intelligence. They mirror the structure and function of the human brain with interconnected neurons organized in layers. Each neuron receives input signals, processes them, and generates an output signal, which serves as input to other neurons. This interconnected structure allows neural networks to learn complex patterns and relationships from data, making them well-suited for tasks such as image and speech recognition, medical diagnosis, and predictive modeling.

The basic building block of a neural network is the perceptron, which takes multiple input values, applies weights to them, sums them up, and passes the result through an activation function to produce an output. The perceptron was introduced by Frank Rosenblatt in 1958. Multiple perceptrons are organized into layers, including an input layer, one or more hidden layers, and an output layer. The hidden layers enable the network to learn increasingly complex representations of the input data, while the output layer produces the final result of the network's computation. Modern neural networks often have 50–100 hidden layers [7]. Figure 30.3 demonstrates a simple perceptron.

1. Input layer: The input layer consists of one or more input neurons, which receive input such as data or image pixels.
2. Weights: Each input neuron is associated with a weight, which represents the strength of the connection between the input neuron and the output neuron.
3. Weighted sum: The incoming weights are summed and passed forward.
4. Activation function: The activation function determines the output of the perceptron based on the weighted sum of the inputs. This permits linear and nonlinear models. There are several types of activation functions.
5. Output: The output of the perceptron is often a binary value, such as 0 or 1, for example, predicting diabetes (1) or no diabetes (0).
6. Training algorithm: During training, the weights of the perceptron are adjusted to minimize the error between the predicted output and the true output.

Training a neural network involves adjusting the weights of the connections between neurons to minimize the difference between the network's predictions and the actual outcomes. This is typically achieved through a process called backpropagation, where the network's performance is evaluated, and the weights are updated accordingly. Through this iterative process, the network learns to make accurate predictions and generalize from the training data to new, unseen data [7].

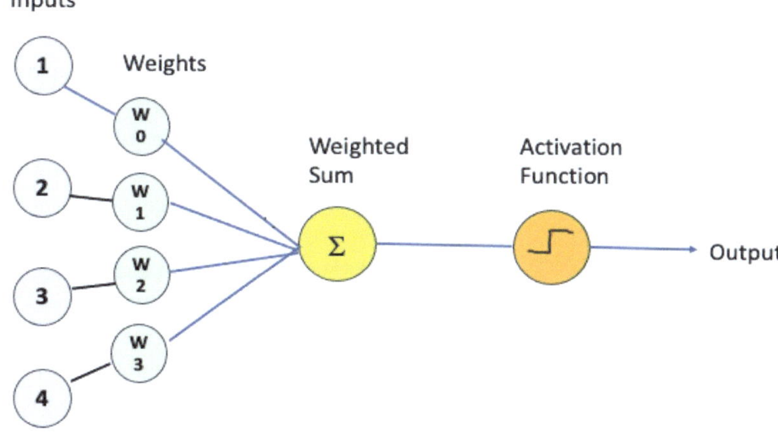

Fig. 30.3 Simple perceptron

30.3.2 Computer Vision (Image Analytics)

Computers cannot interpret images or words. They must "embed" or "vectorize" them as numbers. A convolutional neural network (CNN) "deconstructs" the image into a simpler numerical framework. In the case of images, the pixels are assigned numbers based on a grayscale, and color images can also be analyzed. A black pixel would have a value of zero and a pure white pixel would have a value as much as 255, with all other shades of gray in between. CNNs are designed to automatically learn features from input data. CNNs are made up of several layers, including convolutional layers, pooling layers, and fully connected layers. The convolutional layer applies filters to extract features, the pooling layer further reduces the image to improve computation, and the fully connected layer makes the final prediction. CNNs train on very large image databases such as ImageNet, so they understand patterns such as colors, and edges [8]. Training on an image database and then using that information on a new image it has not seen before is an example of "transfer learning." CNNs are widely used for image and video recognition, image classification, medical image analysis, and computer vision.

There are multiple use cases for CNNs in the medical field:

- Radiology image interpretation: Many studies have demonstrated that AI has high accuracy interpreting a variety of x-rays and other radiologic images [9].
- Retinal image interpretation: IDX-Dr is a software AI platform that screens retinal images. The primary goal is to screen for diabetic retinopathy by non-ophthalmologists [10].
- Dermatology image interpretation. AI is very capable of interpreting both images of skin lesions and skin pathology images [11].
- ECG interpretation: AI can successfully interpret routine 12-lead ECGs [12].

Much of what has been mentioned so far has dealt with AI identifying image patterns that are readily identifiable by humans. AI can also identify patterns humans cannot see, such as

- Determining race from a chest x-ray [13]
- Determining cardiovascular risk factors from a retinal scan [14]
- Determining age and gender from a routine 12-lead ECG [15]

It is important to keep in mind that most experts do not expect AI to replace medical specialists. Rather, they see AI augmenting medical knowledge and expertise.

30.3.3 Natural Language Processing (NLP)

There are many reasons why researchers have tried to analyze human text (natural language) using computers. This would expedite text interpretation and make language translation (e.g., English to Spanish) much easier. Early on, documents were classified using statistical methods and later machine learning was used for this task. Most recently, tremendous gains have been made using artificial intelligence. Since 2017, almost all AI-related NLP has used the AI transformer architecture. Transformers predict the next word or phrase in a sentence based on extensive training and generated probabilities.

Natural language processing (NLP) can be broken down into natural language understanding (NLU) and natural language generation (NLG). NLU involves the comprehension of human language by computers. It focuses on transforming unstructured language data into a structured representation that is easier for the computer to manipulate. NLU is essential for applications such as chatbots, voice assistants, and sentiment analysis.

NLG, on the other hand, is the use of artificial intelligence to produce written or spoken narratives from data. NLG is related to human-to-machine and machine-to-human interaction, including computational linguistics, NLP, and NLU. NLG software can mine large quantities of numerical data, identify patterns, and share that information in a way that is easy for humans to understand. It is used in applications such as chatbots and voice assistants, converting financial reports and other types of business data into easily understood content for employees and customers [3].

As with interpreting images, words must be represented as numbers in a vector or matrix for a computer to understand the words using AI. Linear algebra is required to calculate the relationships between words in a sentence or paragraph.

The applications of NLP are extensive and evolving:

- Virtual assistants like Siri and Alexa can have meaningful conversations. Patient chatbots can answer patients' questions.
- Machine translation can translate speech to text and text to speech. It also permits language translation, for example, English to German.
- Social media platforms can automatically detect and flag harmful content.
- Medical diagnoses can be aided by NLP systems that analyze patient records and identify potential health risks.

30.3.4 Large Language Models (LLMs)

In November 2022, OpenAI launched ChatGPT 3.5, and in April 2023 GPT-4 was made available [16]. Since then, there has been an avalanche of LLMs produced. Their size varies from millions to a few billion parameters (weights) to 1.76 trillion parameters for GPT-4. The models have been trained on a massive corpus from the Internet, textbooks, and other resources. In addition, there are ten or more biomedical LLMs that are trained on medical resources such as PubMed, but most are not publicly available at this point. There are also small language models (SLMs) that are useful for many tasks, as they are faster and cheaper to train and execute, compared to LLMs. Some salient points about LLMs to consider:

- GPT-4 and several other newer LLMs can interpret images such as plots and graphs [16].
- Perplexity AI provides references with its answers [17].
- Many LLMs permit the uploading of datasets for interpretation. For example, Advanced Data Analysis is a ChatGPT plugin that provides natural language description and analysis of datasets, in addition to Python code [16].
- LLMs can provide code assistance, such as debugging.
- Many LLMs permit the uploading of PDFs for summarization and analysis of content.

Creating high-yield prompts as LLM input is important to get the best answers, and this is known as prompt engineering. This has become an art and a science, and multiple prompting tips exist. It is always wise to have a comprehensive prompt that includes the context of who is requesting information, under what circumstances and providing examples. In addition, "chain-of-thought" prompting provides multiple steps or steps for the LLM to complete.

LLM performance can be improved with additional data as well as a technique known as retrieval augmented generation (RAG). RAG consists of uploading additional content (e.g., PDFs) to the LLM to improve accuracy and reduce hallucinations. For example, you might upload a PDF on a complex topic (e.g., a clinical practice guideline on cystic fibrosis) that is converted to a vector database. With a new prompt, the LLM will access its extensive knowledge base and the RAG resources to produce a more comprehensive answer.

New language models are announced weekly, so it is impossible to list more than a few models, and interesting trends are reported here. It is just a matter of time before we have widespread foundational models that can perform a variety of tasks. In medicine, we anticipate the use of "multimodal models" that can interpret text, images, and genomic information from the electronic health record. Based on this new aggregation of data, we can anticipate advances in precision and public health.

LLMs can evaluate images, text, and video, so a future goal is to have any input converted to any output. For example, input video and output text or vice versa.

30.3.5 Generative Adversarial Networks (GANs)

GANs are a type of AI that can simulate new images, tabular data, videos, and audio output. They consist of two neural networks: a generator and a discriminator. The generator creates new data instances that resemble the training data, such as images, while the discriminator's role is to distinguish between the real data and the data created by the generator. The two networks are trained together in a competitive setting, where the generator aims to produce data that is indistinguishable from real data, and the discriminator aims to correctly identify the generated data. This process results in the generator improving its ability to create realistic data, while the discriminator improves its ability to differentiate between real and generated data. GANs have wide-ranging applications, including generating realistic images, videos, and voice outputs, as well as compressing datasets and improving the accuracy of machine learning models. They are a powerful and innovative tool in the field of artificial intelligence, with the potential to create highly realistic and useful synthetic data [3].

30.4 Artificial Intelligence Challenges

30.4.1 Ethical Challenges

- *Bias and discrimination*: AI algorithms learn from the data they are trained on, and unfortunately, this data often reflects the biases and prejudices of our society. This can lead to discriminatory outcomes, such as biased hiring practices or unfair loan approvals [18, 19].
- *Transparency and explainability*: Many AI systems, like deep learning models, operate as "black boxes." Their decision-making processes are opaque, making it difficult to understand how they arrive at certain conclusions. This lack of transparency can reduce trust and accountability [20].
- *Privacy and surveillance*: The vast amounts of data collected by AI systems raise serious privacy concerns. Balancing the benefits of AI with the right to privacy is a delicate dance. Several types of AI system hacking have already been encountered.
- *Job displacement and automation*: AI's ability to automate tasks raises concerns about job displacement. While AI can create new jobs, the transition can be challenging for displaced

workers and may exacerbate existing inequalities [21].

- *Superintelligence*: Some experts warn of the potential threat posed by advanced AI, particularly if it surpasses human intelligence and develops its own goals and motivations. While this scenario may seem like science fiction, it is crucial to have open and informed discussions about the safeguards and limitations we need to implement as we develop increasingly sophisticated AI. The goal is to have AI augment human intelligence and not replace it. There is also concern that AI might induce intellectual complacency.
- Navigating the ethical landscape of AI requires a multipronged approach:
  - Robust ethical frameworks: establishing clear guidelines and principles for the development and deployment of AI, ensuring fairness, transparency, and accountability.
  - Diversity and inclusion in the AI field: encouraging diverse perspectives in the development and governance of AI to mitigate inherent biases and ensure it serves the needs of all communities.
  - Public education and awareness: fostering open dialogue and understanding about AI's capabilities and limitations, empowering individuals to make informed choices about its use in their lives.
  - Governmental guardrails are needed as AI evolves.

Incorrect information All LLMs have the tendency to "hallucinate," which means they can generate believable, but incorrect information. This can include false references as well. This is why information generated from LLMs should be verified.

Cost The user cost of an LLM is low, but the cost to train and maintain the LLM infrastructure is very high. Many features are free while in the beta-testing phase, but eventually they may be expensive. Open-source LLMs and smaller LLMs offer less expensive alternatives.

Carbon Footprint To train an LLM like GPT-4 requires tremendous energy consumption. It is estimated that it required 50–60 million kWh to train GPT-4, but much less to maintain it [22].

Lack of Expertise In the field of medicine, there are not enough knowledgeable people to understand and implement AI in multiple areas. This is complicated by the fact that AI has advanced exponentially in the past several years. Most medical schools do not include AI in their curricula so how are healthcare workers going to keep up?

30.5 Future Trends

We expect generative AI to continue to improve rapidly and be utilized for clinical and nonclinical solutions in healthcare. Multiple other innovations are being tested as well. Here are two AI-related innovations worth following.

Digital Twins Digital twins (DT) in medicine refer to the virtual replicas of patients that leverage real-time data to enhance personalized healthcare and precision medicine. Originating from the manufacturing sector, the concept has expanded into healthcare, where it has the promise of dynamic modeling of individual health states and tailored treatment strategies. By integrating a variety of data sources, such as physiological measurements, medical imaging, and genetic information, digital twins provide healthcare professionals with comprehensive insights into patient health.

Numerous challenges exist however: Regulatory hurdles, concerns regarding data security and privacy, and the complexity of integrating disparate data sources pose significant obstacles to widespread implementation. Ethical considerations, including potential disparities in access to these advanced technologies, further complicate the landscape, prompting discussions about equity in healthcare delivery. In addition, integration with the electronic health record and the lack of reimbursement could slow progress [23].

Federated Learning Federated learning represents a transformative approach in medical research and healthcare delivery, offering solutions to longstanding challenges in data privacy and collaboration.

The primary advantage of federated learning in medicine is its ability to train machine learning models across decentralized datasets while maintaining patient privacy. Healthcare institutions can collaborate on model development without sharing raw patient data, ensuring compliance with regulations like HIPAA and GDPR. Instead of exchanging data, federated learning exchanges model weights, thus preserving privacy.

A central server/entity first shares the base model weights with the local hospitals. Local hospitals train on their data (images), and they share model weights with the central entity. The central entity can then aggregate these weights, and they are then shared back to the local hospitals. No protected health information is shared.

Chang et al. demonstrated how federated learning enabled multiple hospitals to jointly develop diagnostic models for COVID-19 from chest x rays while keeping patient data local. In rare disease research, federated learning has proven particularly valuable. Traditional centralized approaches struggle with limited data, but federated learning allows researchers to share models, not data, across multiple institutions [24].

Knowledge Check Questions

1. Who coined the term artificial intelligence?
   (a) Frank Rosenblatt
   (b) Alan Turing
   (c) John McCarthy
   (d) Nikola Tesla
2. Which of the following is a regression model?
   (a) Predicting a glucose level
   (b) Predicting the presence or absence of diabetes
   (c) Predicting admission to the ICU
   (d) Predicting death from COVID
3. Which statement about machine learning is *false*?
   (a) Machine learning is used for predictive analytics
   (b) Large language models are the backbone
   (c) Machine learning uses algorithms
   (d) Machine learning can do supervised or unsupervised learning
4. Which of the following might be considered a sign of artificial general intelligence?
   (a) Interpreting a chest x ray
   (b) Writing an essay
   (c) Generating an image
   (d) Thinking abstractly
5. Which methodology might be useful to discover genetic patterns in data?
   (a) Unsupervised learning
   (b) Supervised learning
   (c) Convolutional neural networks
   (d) Natural language processing

Answers

1. (c)
2. (a)
3. (b)
4. (d)
5. (a)

References

1. Schneider J. Foundation models in brief: a historical, socio-technical focus [Internet]. arXiv [cs.AI]. 2022. Available from: http://arxiv.org/abs/2212.08967
2. Kucharavy A, Schillaci Z, Maréchal L, Würsch M, Dolamic L, Sabonnadiere R, et al. Fundamentals of generative large language models and perspectives in cyber-defense [Internet]. arXiv [cs.CL]. 2023; Available from: http://arxiv.org/abs/2303.12132
3. Chang AC. Intelligence-based medicine: artificial intelligence and human cognition in clinical medicine and healthcare. Academic; 2020.
4. Helm JM, Swiergosz AM, Haeberle HS, Karnuta JM, Schaffer JL, Krebs VE, et al. Machine learning and artificial intelligence: definitions, applications,

and future directions. Curr Rev Musculoskelet Med. 2020;13(1):69–76.
5. Patrishkoff D, Hoyt R. No-code data science. Mastering advanced analytics, machine learning and artificial intelligence. Lulu.com. 2023
6. Karim MR, Beyan O, Zappa A, Costa IG, Rebholz-Schuhmann D, Cochez M, et al. Deep learning-based clustering approaches for bioinformatics. Brief Bioinform. 2021;22(1):393–415.
7. Perceptrons [Internet]. [cited 2023 Dec 12]. Available from: https://www.w3schools.com/ai/ai_perceptrons.asp
8. ImageNet [Internet]. [cited 2023 Dec 14]. Available from: https://www.image-net.org/
9. Daugaard Jørgensen M, Antulov R, Hess S, Lysdahlgaard S. Convolutional neural network performance compared to radiologists in detecting intracranial hemorrhage from brain computed tomography: a systematic review and meta-analysis. Eur J Radiol. 2022;146(110073):110073.
10. Savoy M. IDx-DR for diabetic retinopathy screening. Am Fam Physician. 2020;101(5):307–8.
11. De A, Sarda A, Gupta S, Das S. Use of artificial intelligence in dermatology. Indian J Dermatol. 2020;65(5):352–7.
12. Martínez-Sellés M, Marina-Breysse M. Current and future use of artificial intelligence in electrocardiography. J Cardiovasc Dev Dis [Internet]. 2023;10(4) https://doi.org/10.3390/jcdd10040175.
13. National Institute of Biomedical Imaging and Bioengineering [Internet]. [cited 2023 Dec 14]. Study finds that artificial intelligence can determine race from medical images. Available from: https://www.nibib.nih.gov/news-events/newsroom/study-finds-artificial-intelligence-can-determine-race-medical-images
14. Poplin R, Varadarajan AV, Blumer K, Liu Y, McConnell MV, Corrado GS, et al. Prediction of cardiovascular risk factors from retinal fundus photographs via deep learning. Nat Biomed Eng. 2018;2(3):158–64.
15. Attia ZI, Friedman PA, Noseworthy PA, Lopez-Jimenez F, Ladewig DJ, Satam G, et al. Age and sex estimation using artificial intelligence from standard 12-lead ECGs. Circ Arrhythm Electrophysiol. 2019;12(9):e007284.
16. OpenAI. Available from: https://openai.com/
17. Perplexity AI. Available from: https://www.perplexity.ai/
18. Jobin I, Ienca M, Vayena E. The ethical impact of artificial intelligence: a systematic review. BMC Med. 2019;17(1):1–14.
19. Floridi L, Cowls J. What is data ethics? In: Buolamwini J, editor. Data ethics. Academic; 2019. p. 1–20.
20. Mittelstadt BD, Russell C, Danks D, Chouldechova A. Principles for explaining explanations in artificial intelligence. Commun ACM. 2019;62(3):56–65.
21. Marr B. The 15 Biggest risks of artificial intelligence. Forbes Magazine [Internet]. 2023 Jun 2 [cited 2023 Dec 14]; Available from: https://www.forbes.com/sites/bernardmarr/2023/06/02/the-15-biggest-risks-of-artificial-intelligence/
22. Ludvigsen KGA. Towards Data Science. 2023 [cited 2023 Dec 14]. The carbon footprint of GPT-4. Available from: https://towardsdatascience.com/the-carbon-footprint-of-gpt-4-d6c676eb21ae
23. Papachristou K, Katsakiori PF, Papadimitroulas P, Strigari L, Kagadis GC. Digital Twins' advancements and applications in healthcare, towards precision medicine. J Pers Med. 2024;14(11):1101.
24. Chang K, et al. Distributed deep learning networks among institutions for medical imaging. J Med AI. 2020;15(3):228–40.

Index

C. Eldredge et al. (eds.), *Introductory Textbook in Health Informatics*, Health Informatics, https://doi.org/10.1007/978-3-032-16657-9

Q

R

S

T

MIX
Papier aus verantwortungsvollen Quellen
Paper from responsible sources
FSC® C105338

If you have any concerns about our products,
you can contact us on
ProductSafety@springernature.com

In case Publisher is established outside the EU,
the EU authorized representative is:
Springer Nature Customer Service Center GmbH
Europaplatz 3, 69115 Heidelberg, Germany

Printed by Libri Plureos GmbH
in Hamburg, Germany